Integrated Textbook
of Geriatric Mental Health

INTEGRATED TEXTBOOK

of Geriatric Mental Health

DONNA COHEN, PH.D.   CARL EISDORFER, M.D., PH.D.

The Johns Hopkins University Press · Baltimore

© 2011 The Johns Hopkins University Press
All rights reserved. Published 2011
Printed in the United States of America on acid-free paper
9 8 7 6 5 4 3 2 1

The Johns Hopkins University Press
2715 North Charles Street
Baltimore, Maryland 21218-4363
www.press.jhu.edu

Library of Congress Cataloging-in-Publication Data
Cohen, Donna, 1947–
  Integrated textbook of geriatric mental health /
Donna Cohen and Carl Eisdorfer.
      p. ; cm.
  Includes bibliographical references and index.
  ISBN-13: 978-1-4214-0097-6 (hardcover : alk. paper)
  ISBN-13: 978-1-4214-0098-3 (pbk. : alk. paper)
  ISBN-10: 1-4214-0097-9 (hardcover : alk. paper)
  ISBN-10: 1-4214-0098-7 (pbk. : alk. paper)
  1. Geriatric psychiatry—Textbooks. 2. Older people—
Mental health—Textbooks. I. Eisdorfer, Carl. II. Title.
  [DNLM: 1. Aged. 2. Mental Disorders—psychology.
3. Dementia. 4. Mental Health Services. WT 150]
  RC451.4.A5C623 2011
  618.97'689—dc22   2010049747

A catalog record for this book is available from the
British Library.

*Special discounts are available for bulk purchases of this
book. For more information, please contact Special Sales at
410-516-6936 or specialsales@press.jhu.edu.*

The Johns Hopkins University Press uses environmentally
friendly book materials, including recycled text paper that
is composed of at least 30 percent post-consumer waste,
whenever possible.

CONTENTS

PREFACE

This is a textbook with an attitude. We have written about the foundations of geriatric mental health care with a salient point of view about what constitutes effective care for older persons. The text is intended both for clinicians in training and for those in practice who want to prepare for the challenges of geriatric mental health care in the twenty-first century.

It is a daunting task to create a textbook for students at so many levels: medical students; graduate students in psychology, nursing, and social work; and residents and fellows in psychiatry, neurology, and medicine as well as for mental health professionals in practice and primary care physicians. While initially it seemed impossible to organize and write a book to serve the educational needs of such a diverse clinical audience, we approached the challenge of structuring this textbook based on five principles:

1. Training and competency standards exist for a geriatric mental health curriculum that can serve to guide the scope of the textbook (Leif et al. 2005; Knight et al. 2009).

2. Core competencies have been developed for subspecialty training and certification in geriatric psychiatry (Leif et al. 2005), and they have been approved by the American Board of Psychiatry and Neurology.

3. References and website links in the chapters will allow readers to access technical information and clinical evidence appropriate to their level of expertise and professional needs.

4. Because clinical care and training are shifting to evidence-based strategies, a useful textbook must integrate overarching principles of care, relevant knowledge, essential skills, and accurate information sources for new research data to enlighten clinical decision-making for optimal patient care.

5. Because the creation of knowledge is ongoing and printed texts with their bibliographies are in danger of rapid obsolescence, the judicious selection of informative websites will allow readers to access the latest information and interpret it within the principles and guidelines throughout this volume.

Our framework is designed to make the most relevant information accessible to a broad audience of professionals in training and in practice despite different educational backgrounds and licensure requirements.

Effective health care involves decisions encompassing clinical, ethical, moral, family, and social dimensions, including the provision of care within a mental health delivery system constrained by cost containment. This textbook is intended to do more than provide information and resources to enhance clinical care. It also emphasizes the professional responsibilities of clinicians to know clinical consensus guidelines and evidence-based practices where they exist, stay informed about the latest research findings, think critically about the application of research discoveries to practice, understand the subjective experience of illness, actively partner with older patients and family caregivers, and integrate psychosocial and preventive approaches to clinical care.

The Challenge of Geriatric Mental Health Care

Mental health problems probably affect at least 25 percent of the older population in the United States, and as the population ages the number of adults age 65 or older who have serious psychiatric illnesses will more than double: from 7 million to at least 15 million by 2020. Yet despite the high prevalence of problems, many go unrecognized and therefore untreated. This is largely because the primary health care system is the de facto mental health care system, and most clinicians in non-mental health settings do not have adequate training—or interest, for that matter—in geriatric mental health care.

For the foreseeable future, the need for trained geriatric mental health professionals in the United States and throughout the world will continue to be largely unmet. Although more trained specialists are needed to respond to the epidemic of mental disorders in the aged, the magnitude of the problem requires more than increasing the numbers of trained specialists. Ongoing training and continuing education across the broader clinical spectrum are essential to upgrade the knowledge and skills of all health care practitioners across the spectrum of care settings. Furthermore, health care policy reform is important to remove barriers to accessing mental health care.

Mental health care involves more than the diagnosis and treatment of specific disorders. Mental health plays a powerful role in the motivations and capacities of older people to age successfully and productively with increasing longevity. This is true for the active well-aged, referred to as the "young-old," who are age 65–74; the "old-old," those age 75–84, who are more challenged by health and lifestyle changes; and the "oldest-old," persons age 85 or older, who are the fastest growing segment of the population and at the highest risk for chronic illness, disability, and dependency.

Geriatric mental health care involves an understanding and integration of information from many scientific content areas. The challenge of this textbook is to achieve an integration of information that not only presents the interdisciplinary knowledge necessary for effective care but also presents it in a way that helps both specialists in mental health care and primary care professionals to examine their standard of care and take responsibility to improve practice patterns and empirically monitor patient outcomes.

A broad spectrum of technical knowledge is a requisite for high-quality clinical care,

enabling clinicians to diagnose and treat older persons in the context of the patient's individual needs and resources. Experienced clinicians recognize that the context of care is frequently a major factor in the effectiveness of clinical decision-making. Family relationships, partnerships with specific health care organizations, legal and financial issues, the array of community and social agencies, and cultural belief systems may all play determining roles. The integration of the patient within this complex matrix of biopsychosocial and environmental-organizational variables is ignored at the peril of the practitioner and the expense of the patient and family.

The patient is not defined by a disease. The patient's condition is far more than the DSM-IV-TR diagnosis, and the determination of appropriate care interventions transcends the treatment manual. To paraphrase the famed physician William Osler: it is more important to know the patient than to know the disease. Understanding an individual's functionality, which emphasizes strengths as well as problems, is in the last analysis the target of our interventions. Patients are people first, last, and always; and their life history, beliefs and attitudes, personality, coping styles, motivations, creativity, and other attributes mediate how they seek help and participate in their care.

The Organization of the Book

This book is divided into three parts:

1. Conceptual Foundations
2. A Clinical Guide
3. Special Clinical Issues

The first section of two chapters presents broad frameworks for understanding mental illness and mental health in later life. Chapter 1 identifies the magnitude of the challenge to meet the mental health needs of a rapidly growing and aging population. It reviews the epidemiology of mental disorders and the demographic impact of the burden of mental illness on a wider range of sociopolitical issues, including the family, the workplace, the community, and health care utilization. Chapter 2 reviews the evolution of geriatric mental health care and presents core concepts and principles about aging and geriatric mental health care that are embedded throughout the textbook. These are intended to provide the reader with a framework for understanding aging and the overall care of older persons and their families.

The thirteen chapters in the second section review the care of older persons who have specific mental disorders or conditions. Chapter 3 reviews the components of comprehensive geriatric assessment, and chapter 4 describes the issues and techniques relevant to interviewing older persons. Chapters 5 and 6 review age-related cognitive changes and cognitive impairment in later life. Chapters 7 through 9 are devoted to Alzheimer disease and other dementias. Chapters 10 through 14 are focused on mood disorders, anxiety disorders, schizophrenia, alcohol and substance abuse, and other mental disorders (eating disorders, somatoform disorders, personality disorders, sleep disorders, and sexual disorders). Each chapter includes an overview of the nature of the disorder, including etiology, risk factors, and the phenomenology in older persons; diagnostic criteria; treatment options; and how to help patients and families access community and social services.

Chapter 15 reviews how to work with family members and balance the needs of older patients and their caregivers, recognizing that the latter are also at high risk for mental health problems. Family members look to physicians and other health professionals for care and support, but it is a challenge for clinicians to deal with the complex needs of family caregivers across the continuum of care. However, to ignore the family and other caregivers is to risk missing data essential for accurate diagnosis and management.

The six chapters in the third section examine specific clinical issues important in mental health practice. Chapter 16 reviews the evaluation of capacity in older persons. It includes an overview of legal and societal views of competence, measurement issues, and specific circumstances that require a clinical determina-tion of capacity. Chapter 17 considers the public health challenge of elder abuse and neglect, including the types of abuse, assessment and intervention, along with legal, forensic, and policy issues. Chapter 18 reviews violent deaths, including prevalence, detection, intervention, and prevention. Chapter 19 examines the needs of older populations in the event of natural and human-caused disasters as well as terrorist attacks, including ways to better prepare for the protection of older adults in the community and long-term care settings.

Although death is not a mental health problem per se, much of the knowledge base in palliative care is in the mental health literature. A great deal can be done to maximize comfort, emotional well-being, and quality of life for people who are dying. The management of depression and psychological distress in older persons who are terminally ill, strategies to promote advanced disease planning or end-of-life care, helping families cope, and hospice care are discussed in chapter 20.

The final chapter, chapter 21, analyzes mental health care for older persons and their families in the context of broader health and human services policy, including health care reform, changes in Medicare, environmental and economic needs, and the importance of reframing perceptions of older adults as real and potential assets rather than as liabilities to society.

Using This Book

We hope that this textbook provides the foundations of geriatric mental health care as well as critical areas of clinical knowledge and skills and that, by integrating principles with Internet resources, the book can serve as a conduit to access updated, authoritative information about relevant topics in the text. We have enhanced appropriate chapters with additional material, ranging from website references to neuroscience pictures, models, and imaging scans, to evidence-based and principle-based clinical guidelines and patient case histories. The sources in the body of the chapters and those cited as references are intended to provide the reader with the tools to stay current with the latest basic, clinical, and health services research as well as educational, clinical, and policy advances. We regret that because of space and cost constraints we were not able to acknowledge many other contributors to the field.

. . . .

Aging is a process we all experience but few of us fully understand. With the rapid aging of the world population, the challenge has been given to us as mental health professionals to help create and perpetuate a caring society in which young and old will grow up and grow old with health and vitality. Only by continued societal investments in care and research as well as a personal commitment to ongoing education and training can we practice the state of our art and science and be armed to provide the quality of care that will best serve the interests of our patients and our professions.

In Appreciation

We appreciate the support and assistance of so many individuals during the long process of writing this textbook. Wendy Harris, thank you for believing in our dream and never giving up on us over the years of production. We are indebted to you in more ways than you know. We also thank the many people who labored with us: Lynn Larsen, for your editing eye, which helped create crisp, accurate chapters; Nicole Graham, Jennifer Greene, and Tiffany Piquet for your tireless efforts with the references; Sharon Purcell, for being the conduit for the revisions between Tampa and Miami.

This text is dedicated to our families, whose love and understanding inspired us to complete this monumental effort. You gave us the time and space to create this book and the strength to prevail when our writing was stalled. The text is also dedicated to the legions of contributors in the many disciplines of geriatric mental health care whose contributions have built the field and continue to advance research, education and training, clinical practice, policy, and the humanity of care.

Finally, our deepest gratitude goes to our older patients and their caregivers, who have taught us so much and are truly heroic individuals.

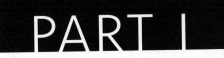

PART I

CONCEPTUAL FOUNDATIONS

Geriatric Mental Health Care in the Twenty-first Century

"One of the essential qualities of a physician is interest in humanity, for the secret of the care of the patient is in caring for the patient." This closing line of Francis Weld Peabody's *The Care of the Patient* (1927) embodies a significant philosophy for physicians and other clinicians in training and practice. Our textbook is dedicated to this way of thinking by describing essential principles of caring, reviewing clinical research and best practices, identifying resources to help professionals remain current with the changing database for optimal geriatric mental health care, and raising ethical issues and dilemmas that occur in clinical practice and research.

Older adults can be exacting clinical challenges precisely because of their age and complexity. Specialized geriatric training is essential for effective clinician-patient/client relationships, productive clinical interviews, accurate diagnosis of clinical disorders and geriatric syndromes, successful treatment and management of patients/clients, effective partnerships with family caregivers, effective heath-promotion and risk-reduction practices for disease prevention, and accurate communication with other professionals across the spectrum of health care and community services.

Older adults have a lifetime of experiences and greater exposure to pathogens, stress, and trauma that contribute to increased vulnerabilities as well as enhanced emotional resilience. Older persons frequently have multiple chronic medical problems that may impair overall functional effectiveness and well-being. A heightened prevalence of co-morbid physical and mental health conditions often complicates clinical care because older people and their family members may be resistant to seeking help and adhering to mental health treatment. Family caregivers, who usually remain dedicated to providing care despite financial, psychosocial, and work stress, may also become patients since they are at increased risk for depression and other psychiatric problems, compromised health, and early mortality.

The Challenges of Geriatric Care

Consider the following case as an introduction to some of the challenges of geriatric care:

ES, a 105-year-old white, widowed female, is in the hospital's skilled nursing unit. Her attending physician requested a psychiatric consultation because staff members were concerned about her recent onset of anxiety, loss of motivation, and morbid thoughts. ES has been on the skilled unit for three months, recovering from right hip replacement surgery and a hospital-based infection in her left leg requiring several surgeries and culminating in amputation below the knee.

ES fractured her hip after a fall at the school where she worked half-time as a volunteer librarian. She had been making good progress in rehabilitation after the hip replacement surgery until complications developed. An undetected infection in her foot proved to be resistant to antibiotics, and after several procedures a decision was made to amputate the leg two months after the hip surgery.

ES had always been a strong-minded individual, and she is insistent that she will walk again and even ride her bike, something she had been doing until her fall. Despite the frustration of the multiple surgeries, ES had been adjusting to her leg prosthesis and building strength in the right hip using a walker, and she was determined to prevail.

Her second husband had died ten years ago, but she had a strong family support system—

3

two children, an 80-year-old son, KS, and a 75-year-old daughter, MB. Both were devoted to her and visited daily. Grandchildren and great-grandchildren and their families also made frequent visits. Although her son and daughter wanted ES to live with them, she was adamant about selling her home and moving into a nearby assisted living residence. ES did not want to be a burden, and several of her friends lived in a nearby senior housing complex.

Over the past four weeks, ES had lost ten pounds and had become increasingly anxious and fearful. She cried easily and lost interest in her favorite activities—reading, eating, watching old movies, and having a little bourbon in the evening. ES had told her son and daughter as well as the physical therapist that she is afraid she will never go home again and that she does not have the strength to go on. Her nurses have reported a reluctance to get out of bed in the morning and a gradual but clear pattern of withdrawal from participating in activities on the unit.

The highlights of ES's history include a normal birth as the second of three children. Her sister died at age 95 of colon cancer, and her brother died at age 92 of a pulmonary embolism following coronary bypass surgery. ES had graduated from college with a major in education, taught English in high school, acquired a master's degree after several summers of classes as a part-time student, retired from teaching at age 80, but continued to volunteer at the high school library until her fall. ES married at age 19 and had two children. Her first husband, who had also been a teacher, died at age 54 from a myocardial infarction. Ten years after his death she married a retired accountant, and he died when ES was age 85.

According to ES, and confirmed by her adult children, she never smoked and she drank alcohol in moderation. She developed diabetes after the birth of her daughter seventy years ago, but she managed it with diet and oral medication until ten years ago, when she was placed on an insulin delivery system for better maintenance. ES has had hypertension controlled with medication for the past twenty years, osteoarthritis managed by nonsteroidal anti-inflammatory

drugs, and occasional episodes of "heartburn" for which she takes over-the-counter medications.

During the interview, ES talked candidly about her anger and frustration with her medical problems and the long hospitalization. She cried several times, admitted feeling anxious, and reported difficulty sleeping, reading, and concentrating. She had no thoughts of suicide but commented that being hospitalized was not living for her. ES became animated when she talked about her family, especially the grandchildren.

The care plan involved clinical and social goals. The clinical issues were the successful treatment of ES's depression and anxiety using an antidepressant, psychotherapy, an exercise regimen, and the active involvement of family and staff to participate in activities that gave her pleasure. The cognitive-behavioral therapy focused on her goals and expectations for the future and adjusting to her limited mobility using a walker and wheelchair. The social issues included decisions about living with family in separate but adjoining quarters or assisted living and the feasibility of part-time volunteer work at the library.

ES may not be an atypical older patient for geriatric mental health professionals in the twenty-first century. Centenarians, 90 percent of whom are women, are the fastest-growing age group in the United States, followed by the population age 85 or older (Shrestha 2006; Rau et al. 2008). The numbers have grown from 15,000 centenarians in 1980 to 65,000 in 2000, and the U.S. Census Bureau estimates there will be 834,000 or more by 2050 (www.census.gov/population/www/socdemo/age/). Although in reality only a small percentage of people live to be 100, about 1 in 10,000 Americans, 25 percent of these are in relatively good health or have some minor level of disability (Calvert et al. 2006), and the rest are cognitively impaired, disabled, or extremely dependent (Hagberg et al. 2001). The latest demographic data can be found at the National institute of Aging Demographic Centers website (http://agingcenters.org).

With biomedical and psychosocial advances, more people will live to 100 and beyond in relatively good health. Centenarians are the latest symbol of the longevity revolution and a metaphor for an attitude shift about what growing old means (www.recordholders.org/en/list/oldest.html). Major studies in the United States include the Georgia Centenarian Study (www.geron.uga.edu/research/centenarianstudy.php) and the New England Centenarian Study (www.bumc.bu.edu/centenarian/). There are also a number of major studies around the world, including the Okinawa Centenarian Study (www.okicent.org; Wilcox et al. 2006) as well as panels in Greece (Stathakos et al. 2005), Sweden (Samuelsson et al. 1997), Denmark (Engberg et al. 2008), Poland (Mossakowska et al. 2008), and many other countries. All have identified a series of variables that promote successful aging and extreme longevity; however, there does not seem to be an empirical consensus about specific single precursors of a long, healthy, and satisfying life. Rather, a combination of genetic, dietary, exercise, and psychological and social factors play a role (Poon and Perls 2007; Poon et al. 2010).

Over the past century, more Americans have been not only living longer but also enjoying better health and spending less time in hospitals and nursing homes (FIFARS 2008, AgingStats.gov). To meet the challenges of the continued rapid aging of society, we will need more geriatric specialists, and geriatric training must become a core component of clinical education (Kane 2002). With proper clinical care as well as lifelong health-promotion practices, older adults, even those who are centenarians and supercentenarians (i.e., persons age 110 or older: www.grg.org/Adams/Tables.htm), should be able to enjoy life and a meaningful existence.

Demographic Changes in an Aging Population

The rapid aging of the population in the United States, indeed, in the entire world, has been a bittersweet success. Although in most countries people are living longer and in better health than ever before, advancing age carries an increasing risk for multiple health problems, chronic diseases, functional impairments, frailty, and a changed quality of life.

Over the next hundred years, we are likely to experience an unprecedented increase in life expectancy. Increasing life expectancy at birth was the gift of time over the last 150 years, with most of the gain occurring from 1900 to 2000 (Kirkwood 1999; Olshansky and Carnes 2002). This was largely the result of improved public health measures, prevention and treatment of infectious diseases, better nutrition, and higher incomes. During the twentieth century, life expectancy at birth of the average American almost doubled, and the number and proportion of persons age 65 or older grew from 3 million (4% of the population) in 1900 to 35 million (13% of the population) in 2000. However, the United States is still a relatively young country compared with other developed nations, where aged people make up 15 percent or more of the total population.

The exponential growth of the aged in the twentieth century will be dwarfed by the increase that will begin in 2011 as the first wave of baby boomers, those persons born between 1946 and 1964, reach age 65. By 2030, one in five Americans (70 million persons) will be age 65 or older, twice the number in 2000, and the population 65 or older will rise to 89 million in 2050. Furthermore, the oldest-old, persons age 85 or older, who are at the highest risk for certain disorders and conditions, will continue to grow more rapidly than any other age group, from 2 percent in 2000 (4 million persons) to 5 percent in 2050 (19 million). If death rates decline in the older age groups, the percentage of the oldest-old population will grow even larger.

The world's population age 65 or older is projected to triple by midcentury, from 516 million in 2009 to 1.53 billion in 2050, whereas the population under 15 is expected to increase by only 6 percent during the same period, from 1.83 billion to 1.93 billion (U.S. Census 2009, www.census.gov/ipc/www/idb/index.php).

Less than 8 percent of the world's population is 65 or older (Kinsella and Wan 2009). By 2030, the world's population 65 or older is expected to reach 12 percent, and by 2050, it will grow to 16 percent. From 2009 to 2050, the world's population 85 or older is projected to increase more than fivefold, from 40 million to 219 million. Because women generally live longer than men, they account for slightly more than half of the older population and nearly two-thirds of the population 85 or older.

Europe likely will continue to have the oldest population in the world, with 29 percent of its total projected to be 65 or older by 2050 (Kinsella and Wan 2009). Sub-Saharan Africa is expected to remain the area with the youngest population as a result of relatively higher fertility and the impact of HIV/AIDS. Only 5 percent of Africa's population is projected to be 65 or older in 2050. Four countries have 20 percent or more of their population 65 or older: Germany, Italy, Japan, and Monaco. By 2030, 55 countries are expected to have at least one in five of their total population in this age category; by 2050, the number of countries could rise to more than 100. Although China and India are the world's most populous countries, their older populations do not represent large percentages of their total populations today. However, these countries do have the largest number of older people: 109 million and 62 million, respectively. Both countries are projected to undergo more rapid aging, and by 2050 they will have about 350 million and 240 million people 65 or older, respectively.

The aging population is characterized by demographic heterogeneity, which will become even more dramatic in the future. In spite of greater prosperity, health, vitality, and well-being with increasing longevity, there are significant gender, racial, ethnic, and economic disparities. These inequalities will challenge us not only to understand the health and socioeconomic needs of a culturally diverse older population but also to prepare and support family members who care for aging relatives.

The feminization of our aging population is particularly salient for several reasons. Older women manifest illnesses differently from older men and may be more vulnerable because of marital status, living arrangements, economic insecurity, and disparities in our knowledge of women's health as compared to men's health. Women account for 58 percent of the population age 65 or older, and 75 percent of the population age 85 or older (www.census.gov/population/www/projections/usinterimproj/). There are 118 women for every 100 men in the age group 65–69, and that ratio increases to 241 women for every 100 men age 85 or older.

Older women are less likely than older men to be married and more likely to live alone. This gender disparity has important implications, because marital status and living arrangements can affect an individual's well-being both economically and emotionally, and being married usually ensures the availability of a caregiver. Older women are more likely to be widowed than older men for several reasons, including a greater life expectancy for women, the tendency for women to marry older men, and higher remarriage rates for widowers.

Of the 35 million persons age 65 or older living in the United States, 16 percent are members of ethnic and racial minority groups, and 11 percent are foreign-born (www.census.gov/population/www/projections/usinterimproj/). In 2000, non–Hispanic whites made up 84 percent of the population age 65 or older: 8 percent were non–Hispanic black, 6 percent were Hispanic, 2 percent were Asian and Pacific Islander, and less than 1 percent were American Indians and Alaskan Natives. However, by 2050, the non–Hispanic white older population will decline from 84 percent to 64 percent, with the Hispanic population increasing to 16 percent, the black population increasing to 12 percent, and Asian and Pacific Islanders as well as American Indians and Alaskan natives growing to 8 percent of the older population. The fastest growth will occur in the older Hispanic population, from 2 million in 2000 to more than 13 million in 2050, and they will outnumber the older black population by 2028.

Racial and ethnic diversity in the United States will increase in the future, and this will require greater knowledge about differences in health and illness behaviors, help-seeking, and patterns of family caregiving as well as greater flexibility in the organization and delivery of mental health services.

Mental Health Care Challenges of an Aging Society

Mental health care for a rapidly aging population is now, and will continue to be, a significant public health challenge. It is estimated that by the middle of this century, 2050, there will be at least 16 million persons who have Alzheimer disease, a significant increase from the 4 million persons who have it in 2000 (Alzheimer's Association 2009). The numbers of persons age 65 or older who have other psychiatric disorders will more than double: from about 7 million in 2000 to more than 15 million in 2030, about 25 percent of the older population (Jeste et al. 1999). Another 10–15 percent will experience significant emotional problems associated with stressful losses in later life. The number of affected older adults will equal or exceed the number of persons age 18-44 who have psychiatric disorders. Mental health is a priority for all ages, but psychiatric disorders in older persons are more likely to go undetected and, if recognized, are less likely to receive adequate or appropriate treatment than in younger people (Bartels et al. 2002b).

The global burden of geriatric mental health care is daunting (www.who.int/whr/2001/chapter2/en/index3.html). The numbers of persons age 65 or older with psychiatric disorders will also more than double, from 106 million persons in 2000 to an estimated 240–300 million in 2025. The number of people who have Alzheimer disease or related dementia is projected to increase from an estimated 37 million in 2000 to 120 million in 2025. Persons age 60 or older have the highest suicide rates throughout the world (Krug et al. 2002).

Estimates are that less than 3 percent of older adults needing mental health care in the United States are seen in outpatient mental health clinics, psychiatric hospitals, and VA medical centers (Olfson and Pincus 1996).

Only one-third of older adults living in the community who need mental health care receive services. Between 65 and 80 percent of nursing home residents have psychiatric disorders, but only 19 percent of them receive mental health services, and the oldest and most physically impaired are least likely to receive care (B Burns et al. 2004).

Unfortunately, the consequences of inadequate treatment include impaired functional effectiveness, excess disability, compromised independent living and quality of life, cognitive impairment, worsened physical health, and increased caregiver strain, among other negative sequelae. Older persons who have mental health problems also have higher use and costs of health care, yet they have inadequate care despite consistent evidence that appropriate mental health services can lead to offsets of health care costs (Unutzer et al. 2003). Without significant reforms in the system of care in the United States, the projected lack of geriatric mental health manpower and inadequate financing will create an unprecedented general health care crisis in the future (Jeste et al. 1999; Borson et al. 2001; Bartels et al. 2002b).

The de facto mental health system for older adults is the primary care network, but the data suggest that a substantial body of primary care physicians usually do not identify or appropriately treat psychiatric illness. This may be the result of lack of interest and training in geriatrics and mental health, too little available clinical time, or limitations imposed within practice patterns (e.g., HMOs). At the moment, 50–80 percent of mental health problems in older persons go undetected and untreated. Older people are at increased risk for inappropriate drug treatment, with a significant proportion receiving unsuitable prescriptions (Bartels et al. 2002).

Older persons may have a broad array of mental health problems, including all those that can affect younger adults. They may have relapses of disorders first diagnosed earlier in life, live with chronic physical illnesses and frailty, survive with persistent severe mental illness, or develop new psychiatric problems in old age. However, the existence of multiple problems and conditions along with atypical presentation of psychiatric symptoms in older people can make diagnosis and treatment a challenge.

Contemporary medical care for this population unfortunately involves the concurrent use of multiple physicians, each prescribing separately with little or no communication between them. As a result, older adults are often taking multiple medications that may impair metabolic functioning and exacerbate problems because of side effects, drug-drug interactions, drug-food interactions, and physiologic changes. Because any of these factors can and often do affect the individual's health status, mental health care requires full knowledge and understanding of the individual's physical, psychological, social, and environmental circumstances.

The public health significance of the unmet mental health needs of a rapidly aging society is consequential in terms of human suffering, premature death, family disruption, and increased health care costs. Undetected and untreated depression coexisting with physical morbidities as well as inadequate medication treatment is associated with poor health outcomes and increased mortality rates (Hanlon et al. 2001; Carney et al. 2002; Yohannes 2006; SK Schultz 2007; Seymour and Benning 2009). Untreated depression in older cancer patients increases the amount of time spent in hospitals, causes poorer functioning, decreases quality of life, and makes pain control more difficult (Williams and Dale 2006). Depression and cognitive impairment independently increase mortality in older persons, but their combined effects appear to be additive (Mehta et al. 2003).

Depression can also be lethal: the population age 65 or older has the highest suicide rate of any other age group, with older men killing themselves in a ratio of 5:1 compared to female age peers (Heisel and Duberstein 2006; Pearson 2006). Although the aged comprised 13 percent of the 2000 population, they accounted for 18 percent of all suicides. More than 40 percent had seen a physician within a week of committing suicide, and 70 percent

within the prior month (Conwell et al. 2002).

Important issues for clinicians include developing an attitude of valuing caring for older adults and appreciating the impact of good mental health on the quality of life. Older people are not "poor and sick old folks" who need help. They are human beings who may or may not have health problems but who have the potential to make important contributions in a complex and rapidly changing society. To dehumanize them or to assume that older people are hopeless and helpless is to place society on a slippery slope toward the future. Indeed, ignoring the mental health needs of a growing population with conditions that are treatable is depriving them of health, vitality, and the right to have meaningful and productive personal, family, social, and work roles.

Individuals are at risk for psychiatric disorders across the lifespan because of a range of factors, including genetic predisposition, multiple life stressors, risky health behaviors, medical illnesses, and multiple medications. Age per se does not cause mental illness. Coping with the vicissitudes of chronic illness, living with Alzheimer disease or related brain disorder, dealing with the loss of peers and family members, and finding a meaningful existence are all challenges to older adults and their families.

Improving mental health care must also involve changing the knowledge and attitudes of older people and their caregivers about growing older. Rather than accepting infirmities as inevitable and avoiding mental health care because of fear and stigmatization, people need to understand the "asset value" of living longer and being active and engaged in meaningful roles. Depression, anxiety, and other psychiatric signs and symptoms are not inevitable consequences of aging. They are treatable conditions in most cases if individuals will seek and obtain appropriate help.

Approaches to Measuring Mental Health

Mental health problems can range from transient adjustments to life stressors, to clinically significant symptoms and full-blown psychiatric disorders that meet the diagnostic criteria of DSM-IV-TR (APA 2000) and ICD-10 (WHO 2007). At least two frameworks are useful to quantify mental health in the population: the epidemiological approach and the impairment/disability model.

Epidemiological Approach

The epidemiological approach to identifying the magnitude of mental health problems in the population is based on a model of diagnosis and treatment in which an individual's presenting symptoms and history are evaluated within a differential diagnostic framework. Consequently, epidemiological surveillance studies report the incidence and prevalence of symptoms as well as diagnostic codes, using standardized taxonomies such as DSM-IV-TR or ICD-10 in subgroups of the population. An understanding of the distribution and patterns of illness by socio-demographic variables (e.g., gender, geography, race, and ethnicity) can lead to important hypotheses about etiology and the roles of genetic or socio-environmental factors. Thus, epidemiological modeling becomes a critical technique not only for assessing need and the burden of illness but also as the basis for policies, including resource allocation.

Population subgroups can also be characterized by other variables, such as a specific site in the continuum of care (e.g., hospital, home, nursing home); risk factors (e.g., life stressor events, medical co-morbidities); treatment outcomes; and mortality. However, information about the number of problems in different subgroups is of limited value unless it is possible to analyze the characteristics and circumstances that can explain what the numbers mean and help clarify the etiologic, clinical, and socioeconomic implications. The mental health care of populations can also be monitored in terms of a wide range of diagnostic and treatment procedures and outcomes, such as drug prescribing practices or the use of medical care across the continuum of care. Measures based on the diagnostic and treatment model lend themselves to socioeconomic analyses of the costs of care, both direct and indirect.

The Impairment/Disability Model

The impairment/disability model is based on the premise that clinical disorders can interfere with an individual's ability to take care of personal needs, thus compromising the person's functional effectiveness and creating a downward spiral of increasing dependency. Functional effectiveness in later life is diminished when multiple illnesses, chronic conditions, and/or injuries interfere with physical and mental functioning. Prevalent chronic conditions in the population 65 or older include arthritis, hypertension, hearing and visual deficits, heart disease, diabetes, cancer, and stroke. Furthermore, emotional distress and psychiatric disorders occur in 25 percent to 50 percent of older persons who have chronic illnesses. The World Health Organization (WHO) now rates depression as the fourth most debilitating disorder and projects that depression will be the second leading cause of disability in 2020 (Moussavi et al. 2007). Individually and collectively, these conditions negatively affect the quality of life and contribute to a decline in functioning and ability to live independently in the community. Therefore, measuring the overall impact of health problems on functional impairment and disability is as essential for care planning as the accurate diagnosis of disease conditions.

Positive trends are also emerging with the decrease in the prevalence of chronic disability in the older population across many national health surveys. The proportion of older Americans age 65 or older with a chronic disability, where disability is defined as the inability to perform tasks of physical, cognitive, and social functioning alone or with assistance, has been decreasing (Costa 2002; Rice and Fineman 2004; Manton et al. 2006). It remains to be seen whether this trend will continue with the increasing prevalence of obesity in younger populations as they age.

The Future of Geriatric Mental Health Care

The prevalence of mental health conditions and symptoms in a rapidly aging society creates many interrelated clinical, research, training, and policy challenges for the future. These include, but are not limited to:

• Low rates of detection, accurate diagnosis, and appropriate treatment in the primary care setting
• Ageism and lack of interest in geriatric care in medical education
• Societal ageism
• Shortage of specialty-trained geriatric mental health professionals
• The increasing proportion of people who have mild or severe dementia as a result of earlier detection, better health care, and increased longevity
• The dehumanization of people who have Alzheimer disease or related disorders
• The increasing numbers of older persons coping with frailty, chronic illnesses, and medical co-morbidities who are at high risk for mental health problems
• Fragmentation of services across the continuum of care and the lack of available, accessible geriatric mental health services
• The impact of the double stigmas—old age and mental illness—on help-seeking behavior and underuse of services by older adults
• Inadequate care for seriously chronically mentally ill people, who account for disproportionate use of services and costs
• High unmet need for mental health care in long-term care settings
• Increasing burden on family caregivers
• Inadequate communication and partnerships with family caregivers and decision makers
• Medicalization of care for older persons and the lack of home and community-based services
• The need to enhance mental health promotion and disease prevention in all age groups
• The need for increased research support to improve mental health care for people of all ages

Trained primary care and specialty clinicians, increased numbers of geriatric mental health specialists, and clinical and mental health services research must be priorities to deal effectively with the growing crisis in geriatric mental health care (IOM 2008). Major reports published in 1999 provided a consensus strategic and tactical plan for our aging population: "Bridging Science and Service" from the National Institute of Mental Health (NIMH 2002), "Mental Health: A Report of the Surgeon General" (1999; www.surgeongeneral.gov/library/mentalhealth/home.html), and a "Consensus Statement on the Growing Crisis in Geriatric Mental Health" from the American Association of Geriatric Psychiatry (Jeste et al. 1999). All emphasized the importance of mental health research, plus the translation of scientific discoveries into practice and policy to meet the special needs of older adults and their family caregivers. Bridging the gap between research and clinical care has been identified by the Institute of Medicine (2001) and the National Institute of Mental Health (2002) as one of the most important priorities in health care. The greatest gap exists in the primary care community, reflecting not only the lack of geriatric training but also the reluctance to assimilate new research findings and the reports of treatment efficacy from evidence-based practice (Bartels 2002).

A Broad Perspective on Mental Health in an Aging Population

Increasing longevity and the continued growth of the aging population bring many challenges beyond the diagnosis and treatment of mental illness in aged people. Although research discoveries have advanced our ability to diagnose and treat cognitive and emotional disorders of later life, research priorities should also include the prevention of disability and the enhancement of individuals' cognitive and emotional capacities to function with increasing longevity.

In future generations we may see the human lifespan stretched like a piece of taffy until it reaches 150–200 years or more. Modern biotechnology offers promising avenues to retard the aging process as well as to extend longevity (President's Council on Bioethics 2003). Life extension may occur in three ways: (1) increasing the numbers of persons who live into old age by decreasing mortality due to major causes of death in younger persons; (2) extending the lives of those who are old by combating the incidence and severity of diseases and functional impairments or by replacing damaged cells, tissues, and organs; and (3) slowing or retarding the aging process so more persons live longer and in better health.

Scientists have already increased the lifespan of a number of nonhuman species, and it is a question of when, not if, this occurs in humans (Carey 2003; Oeppen and Vaupel 2003). As a result, we will be challenged to stretch out the good years for people to live meaningful and productive lives. Research priorities need to go beyond altering the genome to prevent disease and include controlling or retarding aging as well as improving human performance, skills, and temperament in areas such as memory, creativity, cognitive and emotional intelligence, resilience, and healthy decision-making and behaviors.

Although genetic factors contribute to health and quality of life, results of the MacArthur Studies of Healthy Aging suggest that genetic factors are responsible for only 30 percent of what happens in later life (Rowe and Kahn 1997). Studies of centenarians around the world demonstrate that not all persons living past 100 have long-lived relatives. Cognitive abilities, optimism and hopefulness, resilience, being connected to others, meaningful roles and activities, healthy behaviors, and learning how to avoid serious injuries are all important predictors of a long and happy life. However,

to date we have not established that any single factor is more important than any other, and differences among centenarians are greater than similarities.

Aging is not only a personal journey but also a family and community affair. We are living longer, and we are living longer together in our relationships with people—as parents and children, siblings, spouses and partners, and friends. These extended dependencies will affect the distribution of psychological, social, and economic resources across the lifespan. In a society shaped by increasing longevity, sequential generations within the family would grow up and remain vigorous for decades, upsetting the generational interdependencies we know today. Generations within families will be challenged to reshape responsibilities to each other and the roles of succession as everyone lives longer.

Will advances in health and vitality keep up with longevity? Will the onset of chronic conditions and disability be delayed in the future? Will family members be able to absorb the mounting burden of caregiving? How will individuals juggle education, work, play, and retirement with increasing longevity? How will our social, economic, and political structures accommodate to an aging society? Will there be a continuing moral crisis in the valuing of our youngest and oldest members? Will we see a paradigm shift in our attitudes toward aging and older people?

Although there is no crystal ball to accurately forecast the future, one thing is clear: as a society, and particularly among caring professionals, we must be prepared to care for people, regardless of the unpredictable changes in the future.

2

Concepts Underlying Geriatric Mental Health Care

There is a substantial literature in the fields of gerontology, the study of aging, and geriatrics, the study of medical aspects of aging; and research continues to increase our understanding of aging. Many theoretical approaches to aging and mental health have emerged, with hypotheses about aging ranging from the micro- to the macro-level of analysis. However, empirical work derived from these different perspectives is typically interpreted according to the theoretical models and frameworks of specific disciplines.

There is no overarching theory of mental illness/mental health in later life. Instead, there are many hypotheses and models in specialized disciplinary or interdisciplinary areas, and they provide different perspectives for clinical inference and care. A review of the many models and theories is beyond the scope of this textbook. However, this chapter reviews the evolution of geriatric mental health care and a number of concepts that provide a broad theoretical and practical framework for thinking about aging and geriatric mental health care.

Models of Care

Clinical approaches to geriatric mental health care emerged from a traditional disease model: find the cause of the disease, treat it, and the patient should get better if an effective treatment exists. However, for the most part, diseases are not the consequence of a simple causal agent. Disease conditions emerge when an endogenous or exogenous agent(s) alters the body or the host system's adaptive balance. The host-organism relationship can be modified by many different factors that may have additive as well as multiplicative effects on the host. These include biological factors ranging from genes to germs; diet to medication effects;

behavioral and psychological factors such as risky sexual behaviors, sedentary lifestyle, and not recognizing symptoms and seeking help; social and environmental factors such as isolation, poverty, and low educational attainment; or lack of access or ability to pay for services.

Geriatric clinical practice rapidly evolved beyond a simple disease model to a functional model in which the goals are to identify and ameliorate the many possible factors that influence the host-organism relationship and how they affect the person's ability to function in physical, cognitive, emotional, and social domains. It is important not only to correctly diagnose a medical disorder or the existence of multiple co-morbidities but also to identify the extent to which these conditions impair functioning or cause disability. The most effective approach to geriatric mental health care, especially in older and frailer populations, is to focus on the management of geriatric syndromes such as acute confusion, memory loss, suspiciousness, agitation, high bodily concern, anxiety, and depression (Blazer 2006).

Geriatric mental health care embodies the use of multiple approaches to treatment and management, rehabilitation, and health promotion. Combinations of pharmacological, behavioral and psychological, family, and social therapeutic interventions are all necessary to restore individuals to their highest level of functioning and to minimize excess disability. Geriatric mental health care is not just an interdisciplinary field. It is transdisciplinary, transcending the medical model and recognizing the possible cascading effects of disease or treatment that can cause new functional problems and thus need to be part of ongoing assessment. For example, poor dentition may lead to poor nutrition, in turn leading to vitamin deficiency, malnutrition, adverse psychotropic medication effects, and the emergence of cognitive impairment.

Concepts and Principles

The concepts and principles reviewed in this chapter are intended to provide an orientation to aging and mental health, and although deceivingly simple, they provide important perspectives to think about the care of older adults.

Aging is not just about old age; it is a natural process occurring across the lifespan

The way we age is a function of a complex interplay of genetic and environmental factors over the life cycle—from conception through birth, infancy, child development, adult maturation, senescence, and death. Although the phrase "cradle to grave" is commonly used to refer to the life trajectory, a broader view, "from erection to resurrection," more accurately reflects the full range of variables affecting development and aging. "Cradle to grave" is a linear metaphor for lifespan aging, whereas "erection to resurrection" underscores the multiple interacting mediators that affect longevity and health, including, but not limited to, the health of the ova and sperm, our genetic endowment, the role of family and social support systems, religiosity, and numerous other variables.

Aging defines youth as much as it defines old age, because age is essentially a temporal clock marking a trajectory of developmental change that begins with the onset of life but is also influenced over time. What happens early in life can have a profound impact on continuing human development—cognitively, emotionally, and physically—well into later life. Normal or abnormal fetal development is determined by genetic influences as well as by the mother's health, nutrition, and lifestyle. For example, fetal exposure to a mother's influenza has been linked to the development of schizophrenia (Ellman et al. 2009; Brown and Derkits 2010), and a mother's age is related to the risks of Down syndrome and Alzheimer disease (Cohen et al. 1982). Eating

behaviors and food preferences during the first five years of life influence lifelong health, a concept known as metabolic programming (Ismail-Beigi et al. 2006; www.metabolicprogramming .org). Height, which is affected by genetics as well as nutrition, is largely determined by age five. Bone and tooth strength are established by the end of adolescence, which affects risk for osteoporosis in later life. The number and size of fat cells is established in childhood as well, such that children who are obese have more fat cells for the rest of their life.

The health and well-being of children and adolescents is affected by nutrition, exercise, and educational stimulation as well as by the comfort and security of a supportive family and social environment. The results of the Bogalusa Heart study, the longest and most comprehensive study of biracial children in the world, have clearly demonstrated that the major causes of adult heart disease, coronary heart disease, atherosclerosis, and essential hypertension begin in early childhood between ages 5–8 years (www .som.tulane.edu/cardiohealth/bog.html).

Obesity, high blood pressure, hormonal imbalances, stress, trauma, and a universe of other factors, some known and others as yet unrecognized, create a dynamic framework for the evolution of health or illness. Interventions targeting negative risk factors will have a dramatic impact on lowering the risk for strokes and vascular dementias in later life as well as cancer, diabetes, heart disease, and many other health problems.

Aging is more than the number of years a person has lived

Chronological age, the number of years since birth, has important heuristic value, but it does not reflect the full range of biopsychosocial processes that occur during development and aging. While chronological age is associated with an increasing risk for diseases and mortality, age per se is not an etiologic factor for disease or death.

Chronological age is also not a perfect predictor of distance from death. Consider the following scenario.

A set of twins, A and B, were born in 1950. Both enjoyed a happy, healthy childhood, graduated from college and law school, and launched successful careers. However, they had different lifestyles. A never married, and she devoted herself to her criminal law practice, with few outside interests. After a fall, she stopped exercising, worked even longer hours, ate poorly, smoked heavily, and became overweight. B married and had two children shortly after she graduated from law school. She became a successful corporate attorney but also made family activities a priority. B and her husband were avid runners and cyclists, and they enjoyed a wide range of other activities with family and friends.

If A had a heart attack and died in 2000, how old was A when she died? How old was B in 2000? Imagine that B lives until 2050, when she too will have a heart attack. How old will B be when she dies? While both A and B were 50 years past birth in 2000, A was 100 percent old; B was 50 percent old and would be 100 percent old in the year 2050.

This example illustrates several important age-related concepts. Lifespan refers to chronological age at death (50 years for A and 100 years for B). Maximum lifespan is the longest lifespan recorded and verified for a species. To date, the longest human lifespan recorded is Jean Calment, who died at the age of 122 in Arles, France, in 2000. She rode a bicycle until she was 100, entered a nursing home at 115, ate two pounds of chocolate each week, was economically secure, enjoyed an active mind, and had a wonderful sense of humor. Calment celebrated her last birthday with champagne and caviar and released a CD with stories of her life and background rap music.

Distance from death can be defined as life expectancy, the average number of years remaining for a person at any given age, but this assumes that age-specific mortality risks do not change and that patterns of health care and personal activities are unaltered. The 50 percent difference in A's and B's lifespan emphasizes the importance of individual differences that define distance from death and not merely distance from birth.

The older population is best characterized by heterogeneity; they are a diverse group with different values, needs, desires, personalities, and abilities

There is great variability in the aging process across the population. Older people are less alike than any other age group post-infancy. Significant variation is observed in biological parameters, physiological functioning, and cognitive functioning as well as in other psychological and behavioral variables for individuals of the same chronological age. As a consequence, clinicians must guard against overgeneralizations and ageist stereotypes. Beliefs that older adults are isolated, unproductive, and less valuable than younger persons are grossly misleading. Older persons, regardless of chronological age, need to be regarded and treated as individuals.

The heterogeneity in the older population is increasing. People are less functionally impaired, healthier, and more active as each generation ages, and with increasing longevity there is likely to be a postponement of certain disabilities, a phenomenon called the compression of morbidity (Fries 1980; Fries 2002). This transformation is contributing to a new view of aging as a productive period of life as the mix of older persons in the population changes daily.

Neugarten (1975) conceptualized the heterogeneity of the older population using three age groupings: the young-old (persons age 65–74), the old-old (persons age 75–84), and the oldest-old (persons age 85 or older). The young-old are likely to be more active and have fewer health problems. With advancing age the risks for health problems and functional impairments increase, and the highest risks are seen in the oldest-old population, which is increasing in size faster than any other age group.

Aging is not a disease or a disorder

Aging is a natural process mediated over time by biological and psychosocial processes and environmental exposures. The risks for many specific diseases as well as injuries and accidents increase over time, adding trauma to the aging equation. Unfortunately, prejudices about sickness, coupled with ageist beliefs, color our attitudes and expectations about growing older.

Kirkwood (2002) identified two belief systems that are largely responsible for distorting our understanding of adult development and aging: fatalism and ageism. Although fatalism accurately implies that aging must occur because it is a natural process of changes in the body, it is too readily distorted as ageism, an erroneous overgeneralization of inevitable deterioration in later life. This fatalistic nihilism and ageism is illustrated by clinicians who say to a patient: "Well, what do you expect at your age?" Ageism ranks with racism and sexism as a pervasive, destructive, societal force that demeans and devalues human life. However, Kirkwood (2002) argues that ageism has a defining feature that makes it different from other hurtful prejudices. All of us are growing older, and we are all potential victims.

Ageism has had a destructive influence on geriatric health and mental health care

Geriatric mental health care is affected by two of the most damaging aspects of discrimination: the stigma of advancing age and the stigma of mental illness. Mental health problems of later life are largely treatable, but ageist attitudes and health care policies are discriminatory. Services integrating primary care and mental health care are largely unavailable and often inaccessible.

Ageist attitudes color beliefs about the value of older persons as individuals and as members of society, and they have fueled a moral crisis in caring and the valuing of life. Erroneous beliefs that older people inevitably become sick, incompetent, unproductive, helpless, and dependent exist in the health care community. Clinicians without geriatric training not only may see aches and pains, medical problems, fatigue, and depression as normal consequences of growing old, but they may also have nihilistic attitudes about the efficacy or value of treating older people. The result can be a lack of detection, diagnosis, and treatment of illness and excess disability—leading to unnecessary

pain and suffering, poor quality of life, and a tragic loss of vitality.

Discussions about national policy reform are influenced by subtle and not-so-subtle ageism. The rising costs of health care are attributed to the growth of an aging population, leading some to question whether we can afford to pay for the care of older people. The truth is that we cannot afford not to care for the aged because we would cripple the health care system for future generations, including families committed to caring for older relatives. Rationing health care and other resources by basing priorities on age alone is a short-sighted and dangerous approach to investments in our social capital. Furthermore, data now demonstrate that with effective management the cost of caring for the oldest old is not greater than for the younger aged, and we are only just recognizing the contributions being made by older people.

A 2003 report by the Alliance for Aging Research (www.agingresearch.org), *Ageism: How Healthcare Fails the Elderly,* presented the evidence for five major conclusions:

1. Health care professionals are not adequately trained to care for older persons.

2. Older patients receive less preventative care than younger patients.

3. Older patients are less likely to be screened for a wide range of disorders and conditions.

4. Well-established interventions for medical conditions, especially mental disorders, are often not implemented.

5. Older persons are systematically excluded from clinical trial studies, even though they use more drugs than any other age group.

Without a commitment to a national strategy to overcome these biases, everyone in society will be affected. Inadequate care has significant, costly consequences: excess disability, premature and lethal morbidity, increased burden on the family, and increased pain and misery for the aged of today and tomorrow.

Normal aging and pathological aging are interrelated, complex concepts

Normal aging implies an expected or predictable set of changes in all organ systems, such as loss of tissue elasticity, impaired hearing and vision, decreased pulmonary vital capacity, or mild memory and cognitive losses, even in the absence of definable disease. However, losses associated with normal aging do not necessarily mean that older people will always be more physically and mentally impaired than all chronologically younger persons. If we compare the distribution of any number of biomarkers of aging, physical and mental health indices, or performance scores on cognitive and sensory tests, a subset of older persons will perform at levels comparable or better than the mean scores for much younger persons.

If we compare the distribution of biological, psychological, and health variables for several adult age groups in a cross-sectional study, there will be a significant overlap between age groupings. If we compare the scores of age groups followed longitudinally, most persons maintain their rank order relative to others (i.e., individual differences are maintained). A small group will show a decline in their status relative to others, suggesting pathological changes. A rapid decline in cognition and psychological functioning is a better predictor of illness and terminality than age per se.

The existence of a normal aging process also implies that there is a complementary process—pathologic aging. Korenchevsky (1961) first described normal aging as primary aging, or nonpathologic aging, to characterize persons who showed little or no change until late in life, and he attributed marked changes in the mind and body to secondary, or pathologic aging.

Although the normal biopsychosocial changes that occur with aging have an impact on an individual's functioning, it is the effects of disease that markedly impair functioning. The potential impact of diseases and injury can be described with four progressively severe concepts: functional impairment, functional limitation, disability, and handicap. *Impairment* refers to compromised or abnormal functioning; *limitation* refers to restrictions in the ability to think and act; *disability* refers to circumstances in which an individual has difficulty with personal care, work, or leisure activities; and *handicap* refers to situations in which the individual is unable to overcome the disability.

Successful aging is a concept invoked to describe older persons who live long, happy, and vital lives

The story of Ponce de Leon and his pursuit of the fountain of youth in the sixteenth century is well known, but his untimely death at the hands of Indians in Florida at age 47 is less well known (Nieves 2007). Forty-seven was the average age of death of Americans in 1900, but today most Americans live well into their 70s and 80s. These can be successful years of revitalization and reinvestment in personal pursuits, family, and the good of the greater community. The list of world figures making significant social and intellectual contributions in later life is legion.

The concept of successful aging has evolved to describe the increasing population of older persons creating new role models for continued productive and meaningful lives. Havighurst published his seminal article on successful aging in 1961, describing it as adding life to years and getting satisfaction in old age. Although an extensive body of research has developed, successful aging has been defined in many ways (Rowe and Kahn 1998; Depp and Jeste 2009). It remains a confusing designation because "successful" is subjective and ambiguous. Healthy older people may use retirement for civic engagement or creative enterprises, whereas others may spend time in contemplative and generative roles. Chronically ill older persons living at home may feel a sense of accomplishment coping with their challenges. Likewise, some residents in nursing homes and assisted living residences may believe that they are doing the best they can under the circumstances and believe themselves to be successful, even though others may think otherwise.

Successful aging raises aging to a higher esthetic level, with a focus on health and activity rather than decline and infirmity. The results of the MacArthur Foundation Research Network on Successful Aging revealed that a long and happy life is determined less by genetic factors and more by lifestyle—nutrition, exercise, cognitive activity, staying connected to people, and being resilient (Rowe and Kahn 1998). The MacArthur Foundation also supported a Research Network on an Aging Society that led to projections of the economic, health, psychosocial, and policy implications of longevity (Olshansky et al. 2009).

Why people age is not well understood

Throughout history, human survival curves have indicated that the maximum lifespan is relatively constant, a little over one hundred years, even though mean survival is influenced by factors such as wars, famine, accidents, disasters, public health conditions, and other environmental conditions. The maximum lifespan, both between and within species, is probably mostly determined by genetics, but the average lifespan is affected by many health, behavioral, social, and environmental factors (Christensen and Vaupel 1996; Bostock et al. 2009). Life expectancy will vary by socioeconomic status, education, race, and geographic location (Sierra et al. 2009). After the implementation of Medicare in the United States, life expectancy increased significantly for the poor and minorities, demonstrating the potency of social forces on aging (Olshansky et al. 2009).

From an evolutionary perspective, aging is defined as a progressive deterioration in fitness and the ability to survive and reproduce (Kirkwood 2002; Hughes and Reynolds 2005). The evolutionary theory espouses that animals die shortly after reproduction because more life-years would not lead to more surviving offspring. Two genetic theories have been advanced to explain why aging evolved: the accumulated mutations theory and the antagonistic pleiotropy theory.

The mutation accumulation theory, first pro-

posed by Medawar (1952), and the antagonistic pleiotropy theory are based on the notion that the influence of natural selection declines with advancing age (Gavrilov and Gavrilov 2002; Kirkwood 2002). Both theories require the existence of genes that have specific age effects, but the type of age-specific gene effect is different. Antagonistic pleiotropy theory posits the existence of pleiotropic alleles (i.e., alleles affecting several phenotypes) that increase both survival and reproduction early in life but decrease survival and reproduction later in life. These alleles accumulate in the population because the early benefits are greater than the disadvantages in the aged. In contrast, according to the mutation accumulation theory, harmful alleles are more likely to accumulate in the population if the detrimental effects manifest later in life when selection pressures are weak. Both theories assume that the population contains alleles that are harmful to the old but not the young, and although a large number of experiments have tested their theoretical assumptions, results are inconclusive (Hughes and Reynolds 2005).

A third major evolutionary theory, the disposable soma theory, does not rely on genes but explains senescence as the result of the high cost of maintaining cellular functioning (e.g., DNA repair, protein turnover, antioxidant reactions). Because animals in the wild have had a high mortality, fitness for survival evolved from using metabolic resources to enhance reproductive success rather than maintain the body beyond the expected lifetime. The term *disposable soma* is analogous to disposable products—"Why spend money making something better if it will be used for only a short period of time?" (Kirkwood 1999).

A newer theory expands on the classic explanation of aging in terms of natural selection and lifetime fertility. Lee (2003) describes the importance of grandparental care and proposes that mortality at any age in the life cycle is caused not only by how much reproductive life remains but also by the transfer effect, the economist's nomenclature for the ongoing investment of older generations in younger generations. Demographers refer to this as the grandmother effect (Bourke 2007). Species such as dolphins, elephants, primates, and humans that provide nurturing by older members have longer post-reproductive longevity because natural selection will favor genes that contribute to the ongoing protection of the young. This theory explains the reduction in mortality after menopause—women are caring for children and contributing to their survival and well-being. Wade (2003) captured the essence of this new evolutionary theory as follows: "As you write yet another check to cover your child's ruinous college bills, there is definitely a bright side to consider: If you weren't doing this, you'd long since be dead."

Biological theories of aging have been grouped into two general categories

Biological theories of aging fall into two categories: programmed aging, resulting from genetic or internal clocks, and "wear and tear" theories, in which aging is the result of random events and circumstances. The major biological theories, according to Bengtson et al. (2009), include but are not limited to:

• Gene-genetic theories such as the effects of age gene(s), altered proteins, or telomere shortening in chromosomes with successive DNA replication
• The free radical theory, where chronic exposure to highly reactive oxygen free radicals causes oxidative damage (e.g., DNA, protein, and lipid damage) and eventually leads to loss of organ system functioning
• The glycosylation theory, which posits that products from glucose oxidation lead to structural changes (i.e., cross-linking in proteins and nucleic acids), which inhibits protein functioning and damages DNA over time
• Neuroendocrine theories based on the idea that certain hormones, especially those associated with the hypothalamic pituitary adrenal axis, mediate adaptation to stress over time
• Immune theories, where immunological changes affect resistance to stress, cause cell loss, and increase vulnerability to a number of diseases

Psychological theories of aging embrace areas of perception, cognition, moral reasoning and wisdom, emotions and affect, personality, personal adjustment, coping styles, communication, and other behavioral and psychological dimensions

Psychological theories of aging, which address many areas of performance and functioning, are highly diversified (Bengtson et al. 2009). The challenge is to predict normative patterns of change in different aspects of psychological functioning with advancing age as well as to account for individual differences in the population.

Historically, psychological theories have addressed easily observable decrements with advancing age—motor slowing, attentional changes, diminished intellectual performance, cognitive rigidity, and learning and memory problems. Although some cognitive losses occur, in the presence of good health and the motivation to perform, other cognitive areas improve with advancing age. Significant cognitive losses are not a part of normal aging but often signal medical problems. Personality remains relatively stable throughout the lifespan, and in the absence of serious diseases, older people become more like themselves. However, gender, sociocultural factors, and generational influences contribute to personality differences across populations.

Despite significant advances in research, a unified scientific theory of aging and psychopathology does not exist

At the moment, there is no overarching theory that predicts the vulnerabilities of older people to mental health problems. As a consequence, we must be prepared to consider alternative approaches to clinical issues as well as to change our approaches to clinical care as new evidence emerges. Mental health and mental illness are the result of many interactive biopsychosocial and environmental factors across the lifespan.

Drawing a sharp distinction between physical and mental health is artificial and antiquated

Research advances since the classic stress

studies of Walter Cannon (1932) on the "fight or flight response" have increasingly challenged the traditional biomedical model and its reliance on the mind-body dichotomy. Psychological and social factors are interrelated with biological factors that influence physical and mental health. The interactions between thoughts, feelings, and reactions to stressful life events, such as eating, smoking, or drinking, as well as supportive psychosocial relationships with people around us, influence our physical and mental health. This synthesis is largely mediated by processes in the central and autonomic nervous systems and is inseparable from somatic context.

Research discoveries in many fields, ranging from psychoneuroimmunology, endocrine-behavioral relationships, and brain-behavior imaging, to the influence of nutrition, physical and cognitive exercise, and religiosity on health and illness, continue to advance our understanding of the complex and dynamic intricacies of mind-body interactions. It is well known that behavioral factors are responsible for 50 percent of all medical problems, and psychological interventions focused on risk reduction and health promotion are effective in the prevention of many medical disorders and injuries, including HIV-AIDS, cardiovascular disease, depression, suicide, and cancer (Glanz et al. 2001).

Mental health is more than the absence of psychopathology or mental illness

Issues of creativity, productivity, spirituality and religiosity, and quality of life contribute to emotional well-being. The influence of family members, feeling connected to other people, and opportunities for meaningful activities such as work, leisure, and social responsibilities sustain better mental health. Economic security, access to transportation, and desirable living arrangements, as well as the availability and accessibility of health and human services also affect mental health.

Social factors and social institutions influence every aspect of mental health and overall quality of life (Mechanic 2007). The attitudes and beliefs of others around us have a dra-

matic impact on feelings of self-worth, motivations to be active and productive, and personal satisfaction with life. Likewise, the support and effectiveness of psychosocial networks and social institutions reinforce (or undermine) coping abilities and resilience to deal with the vicissitudes of life, encourage (or sabotage) healthy behaviors and lifestyles, and encourage (or inhibit) meaningful participation in the community.

Socioeconomic macro-forces have a decided impact on clinical care as well. The rapid aging of society will create new challenges for upcoming cohorts of older persons, who will need to adapt to shifting social, economic, and political circumstances, including redistribution of resources and perhaps some form of rationing of health care.

Theoretical and empirical approaches to mental health rather than mental illness have only emerged in the past three decades. Vaillant (2007) reviewed the strengths and limitations of six models of mental health: (1) functioning at a level higher than normal; (2) maximizing positive qualities (e.g., self-efficacy); (3) developing maturity, intimacy, identity, generativity, integrity, meaning, and career consolidation; (4) enhancing cognitive and emotional intelligence; (5) developing life satisfaction; and (6) adaptive coping and resilience. Each refers to different dimensions of mental health, but they all inspire creative avenues for research.

More research is necessary for revisions of diagnostic codes (DSM-IV-TR, used in the United States, and International Classification of Diseases, used internationally) to describe geriatric psychopathology accurately

The content of the American Psychiatric Association's *Diagnostic and Statistical Manual of Mental Disorders* has inadvertently led to limitations in certain types of clinical care that could enhance the quality of life of older persons (Blazer 2009). Although there have been many improvements in successive iterations, DSM-IV-TR still has several limitations (First and Pincus 2002). The symptom descriptions and classifications are useful for standardized diagnostic codes, but they do not deal with the personal dimensions and circumstances of geriatric patients such as pain, loss, isolation, loneliness, and disconnectedness. These idiosyncratic factors are not cited in the diagnostic manuals for coding diseases, but they often play crucial roles in a patient's adaptation and help understand the history and circumstances of maladaptive behaviors and symptoms.

One of the advances of DSM-IV and DSM-IV-TR was to develop consensus criteria for age, gender, and specific cultural effects on psychopathology, but rigorous clinical geriatric mental health data were still lacking for older patients. Thus, many of the recommendations for DSM-IV-TR relied on clinical impressions, and more empirical research is necessary to revise diagnoses in the development of DSM-V and beyond. These issues are addressed in detail in the chapters describing the individual psychiatric disorders.

Mortality rates are elevated for older persons who have dementia or depression, but little is known about rates for other psychiatric disorders

The relationship between psychiatric disorders and mortality has relied on the results of death certificate, patient, and community-based studies, all of which have methodological limitations. A number of community-based studies have shown increased mortality for older adults who have depression or dementia compared to age-matched peers who do not have these conditions (Katzman 1976; Blazer et al. 2001; Druss et al. 2001), but little is known about other psychiatric disorders, with the exception of increased suicidality in schizophrenia (Mykletun et al. 2007).

Important questions remain to be answered about the vulnerability of older persons who have psychiatric disorders and the theoretical and clinical implications of increased mortality. Because depression usually goes unrecognized and untreated in older persons, it is possible that aggressive detection and appropriate treatment would be beneficial. For example, the role of depression in heart attacks is well documented, and mortality six months after

a myocardial infarction is higher if depression coexists (Jiang et al. 2002).

Feelings and behaviors that are identified as evidence of psychopathology, or its absence, are often associated with culturally defined perceptions, beliefs, and behaviors

Understanding the cultural background of older patients is essential for appropriate mental health care. Not only may cultural forces create barriers to the expression of pathological thoughts and feelings, but culture and languages also affect manifestations of mental health, mental disorders, help-seeking behaviors, and the use of health care and community services (Kales et al. 2000). For example, a large proportion of the older Hispanic population currently has limited proficiency with English, but relatively few mental health providers speak Spanish or have bilingual staff. Asian Americans and Pacific Islanders often present with more severe psychiatric illnesses because of culturally mediated feelings of shame, embarrassment, and stigma. Alcohol abuse is prevalent among Native Americans, and the suicide rate among Alaskan natives and American natives is 50 percent higher than the national rate.

Substantial differences exist both between and within racial and ethnic groups, making it necessary to understand health beliefs and practices across many Hispanic, African, Asian, Native American, Alaskan Native, Pacific Islander, and other diverse population subgroups. However, socioeconomic factors (e.g., poverty, wealth, occupation, education), family structure and process, residential circumstances (e.g., home ownership, racial segregation), and other contextual variables may influence mental health outcomes more than race and ethnicity.

Older people present complex challenges for clinical care

Disease processes are mediated by many of the same factors among young and old, but many more concurrent factors affect older persons (Kennedy 2001; Blazer 2009). Multiple illnesses, especially chronic diseases, may limit mobility and independent functioning as well as contribute to increased vulnerability to falls, malnutrition, and frailty. Multiple diseases can aggravate each other and increase the risk for the cascading effects of one disease and its treatment on others. Many conditions, such as vascular disease, stroke, and endocrine disorders, are associated with depression, increasing the risk for disability and death. A number of medical disorders precipitate delirium, which often goes unrecognized, increasing a patient's risks for deteriorating functioning, psychotropic medication, dementia, and death. Psychiatric conditions associated with dementia usually lead to disruptive behavioral problems and exacerbate medical conditions. The use of many medications, including treatments for co-morbidities may also have additional side effects as well as drug-drug and drug-nutrient interactions that make treatment a challenge. Furthermore, the high costs of drugs for older patients may affect compliance, unbeknown to the clinician.

Many co-morbidities often lead to common geriatric syndromes that become diagnostic, management, and treatment challenges in clinical practice (Inouye et al. 2007). The lack of coordination among prescribing physicians may lead to serious complications and exacerbate medical problems. Sensory losses, especially sight and hearing, can interfere with the clinical interview and examination and make the older patient appear more compromised than they actually are. Hospitals can be dangerous places for older patients who are at risk for iatrogenic illness, infections, and the negative consequences of bed rest and immobility. Older persons who are extremely ill, and especially nursing home residents, may be vulnerable to a "failure to thrive" syndrome, in which they do not appear to want to recover functioning and want to die. Falls, malnutrition, pressure ulcers, gait disturbances, and sleep disorders are also among the many other serious syndrome risks.

Clinicians' attitudes and beliefs about personal aging, disability, death, and dying affect clinical practice

The way we think and feel about our own aging and the experiences we have with aging parents, relatives, and friends may have profound influences on the way we respond to older patients. Geriatric specialty training will not be successful without early attention to personal beliefs, attitudes, and perceptions of aging, illness and disability, and death and dying. Critical outcomes that often occur as a result of training with seasoned mentors include:

• Increased self-awareness of personal biases that enhance or impair good-quality care
• Changed attitudes about the capabilities of older persons
• Recognition of the continuing roles of older persons
• Greater compassion
• Sensitivity to the complex ethical dilemmas of care
• Increased sensitivity and capabilities in helping older persons and caregivers make complex decisions
• Understanding that the process of caring is tougher than curing

Clinicians need to find ways to communicate and form partnerships with older persons, family caregivers, and other professionals

Ideally, caring for older patients requires an openness and willingness to participate in a collaborative process involving patients, family caregivers, other relatives or designated kin, and professional providers (Levine and Zuckerman 1999). Relatives can be valuable sources of information, but it is important not to infantilize the older patient when a spouse or adult children accompany them. Even when patients are cognitively impaired, it is important to treat them as human beings and, where possible, to ask their permission to involve other family members to collect or disclose information.

Because so many biopsychosocial issues influence an individual's mental health, assistance from other professionals will be necessary, including primary care physicians, internists, medical specialists, nurses, therapists, and social service professionals as well as providers of social and community services, dieticians, financial advisors, and elder law attorneys. Caring needs to transcend a narrow focus on medical care and incorporate psychosocial and environmental approaches to enhance health, functioning, and quality of life.

Personalizing a clinical interview will invite an alliance with older patients and maximize the collection of information

Many attributes are important to establishing and maintaining a therapeutic alliance: honesty, flexibility, trust, respect, warmth, openness, interest, alertness, and confidence. However, these characteristics become even more important in forging effective communication with older patients (Leach 2005; Williams et al. 2007). Older patients may acknowledge a problem but attribute it to normal aging and be unwilling to consider the possibility of an illness requiring treatment. Older persons may also deny that anything is wrong or minimize the presentation of their symptoms to avoid the appearance of needing help because they are fearful of losing their independence or being institutionalized. Even severely depressed and very sick older patients will rally to present themselves as competent and able to care for themselves.

There are several approaches to an effective interview style: sit down near patients; make sure they can hear and understand you; call them by their surnames unless instructed otherwise; ask them to describe what is troubling them but also take a few minutes to ask them about good things happening in their lives. In addition to asking questions about symptoms query them about what makes them happy and listen to the response. Show interest in them as individuals and give verbal and nonverbal clues that you are listening and understanding their concerns and circumstances. Give older patients opportunities to talk about their strengths as well as their medical problems, and be complimentary about their successes. Do not rush the process.

In addition to probing the older person for information, finding ways to personalize the interview with your own thoughts, feelings, and occasional stories can be helpful. This mutual exchange, conducted judiciously, can be an equalizer, especially when the clinician is much younger than the patient. When older persons arrive with adult children, it is critical to maximize the personal relationship with the patient and learn why he or she is the object of attention. The patient must be seen alone to establish confidence in the clinician as "my doctor." Understanding the patient's interpretation of the circumstances of the visit and its consequences is critical. Infantilizing the older patient will deny the clinician the patient's trust, and as a consequence important information will be lost.

The history of the illness or presenting problem(s) is often the key to diagnosis and treatment

A careful history is essential for high-quality clinical care. This is particularly challenging in the care of older persons, whose initial interview(s) may be time consuming and require several informants to piece together the puzzle. Rather than ask open-ended questions, the clinician may need to anchor questions about symptoms to times, events, and major losses in the patient's life. The patient may also be queried about people, activities, and situations that give him or her pleasure, about whether there has been a loss of interest or ability in leisure or work activities, and about the impact of such losses on lifestyle and quality of life.

Psychiatric disorders are illnesses as well as diseases, and understanding the subjective experience of the illness is important for patient care

Older patients, including those who have cognitive impairment, are people first, last, and always! They have a great deal to contribute to the clinical encounter. The way patients conceptualize their illness, respond to symptoms, attribute causation, and plan the future is important information that may affect compliance with the treatment regime. Psychiatric problems can be emotionally distressing and painful, affecting a person's motivations to seek treatment, adhere to treatment, and maintain a constructive, meaningful lifestyle. Indeed, the nature of many disorders is to interfere with thinking, affect, emotions, and the energy to go about daily life.

Kleinman (1987, 1988) articulated eight questions to probe a patient's explanatory model for their illness:

1. What do *you* call the problem?
2. What do *you* think caused the problem?
3. Why do *you* think it started when it did?
4. What do *you* think the sickness does? How does it work?
5. How severe is the sickness? Will it have a long or short course?
6. What kind of treatment do *you* think *you* should receive? What are the most important results you hope to achieve with this treatment?
7. What are the chief problems the sickness has caused?
8. What do *you* fear most about the sickness?

Kleinman's long history of research on the narratives of illness and patients' subjective experience of illness within their personal, cultural, and social context has created a clinically valuable explanatory model to guide clinical practice and optimal patient care (Kleinman 2007).

There is a social etiquette to interacting with chronically ill, disabled, and/or frail older persons

Working with older patients involves social as well as clinical transactions, and the successful clinician will be well served to understand the perspectives and expectations of persons who appear to have significant limitations. In his last years, the poet Robert Frost used a wheelchair and was able to use only one of his hands. When interviewed about how he coped with these circumstances, Frost answered, "When I realized that my mind and my one hand were the only parts of my body that worked, I understood how wonderful they were!"

Living with chronic illness can be a painful and torturous experience—physically and emotionally. However, there are significant individual differences in the ways patients cope with limited functioning, deterioration, acute medical crises, and fatigue, as well as manage boredom, frustration, anger, anxiety, fear, depression, and the uncertainties of the future. There are indignities and stress associated with limited functioning, but human beings still have many strengths, goals, and ambitions; and the human spirit often prevails.

The clinical challenge is to discover individuality in patients and not use superficial information to make inaccurate assumptions about their beliefs, needs, and worldview or what gives them comfort, pleasure, and meaning. Not to acknowledge the identity of what appears to be a crippled, incapacitated human being is to destroy the potential to be—and that is unacceptable in a clinical practice.

An individual's functional status is crucial clinical information

Functional status refers to personal care, what people do around the house, and higher order activities, such as work, personal activities, and social participation in the community. Whereas it is important to diagnose and treat illnesses, evaluating the overall impact of various diseases on an individual's functional effectiveness is essential for developing a care plan. One of the key objectives of geriatric care is to maximize functioning and reduce excess disability.

Drugs are often helpful, but inappropriate drug treatment can have a negative effect on the health and safety of older persons as well as increase health care costs unnecessarily

Annual adverse drug reactions in older patients range from 5 to 35 percent, and adverse drug effects may also cause serious problems, including depression, falls, hip fracture, gastrointestinal distress, confusion, and delirium—all preventable conditions (Wright and Warpula

2004; Hanlon et al. 2006). An Institute of Medicine report estimated that drug-related problems caused 106,000 deaths across the nation each year at an estimated cost of $85 billion (Kohn et al. 2000). However, others have estimated the cost of medication-related problems to be $77 billion for outpatient care, $20 billion for hospital care, and $4 billion for nursing home care (Bates et al. 1997; Bootman et al. 1997). If these medication problems were treated as a disease by cause of death, they would be ranked as the fifth leading cause of death in the United States (Lazarou 1998).

Evidence-based data on older patients' use of medication are limited, but the Beers criteria have been updated for making decisions about medications that should be avoided because they cause severe adverse reactions in older persons (Fick et al. 2003). The Beers criteria identified 48 drugs or classes of medications to avoid regardless of disease or condition. Twenty disease conditions were also evaluated for drugs to avoid, and 66 drugs were identified as having severe adverse effects.

Drug treatment of older patients requires special care, including collecting accurate information from patients and all prescribing physicians

Most prescribed medications have been developed and tested on younger populations, which means that the dose-response curves have been calculated based on patients free from diseases other than the one the drug is targeted to treat. Older persons have more illnesses in general and are more likely to be ingesting prescribed as well as over-the-counter medications, with the increased likelihood of drug-drug interactions and physiological changes that affect the blood levels of specific drugs.

Unless there are specific indications to the contrary, initial drug doses should be low and should be increased slowly because the effects of advancing age, co-morbid medical conditions, other prescribed medications, alcohol, and over-the-counter drugs alter the older patient's ability to metabolize drugs. Impaired kidney and lung functioning also affect drug metabolism.

It is important to do an inventory of all treating physicians and the medications they prescribe and then to follow up with ongoing queries about any changes in medications. Careful and frequent checks on adherence are essential, and blood level assays of some medications are advisable.

Health promotion and risk prevention are important goals

More than 50 percent of health and mental health problems are caused by unhealthy behaviors. Thus, while we will profit by continuing biomedical research, we also have a great deal to gain from developing psychosocial and behavioral interventions to curtail and prevent unhealthy behaviors such as smoking, excessive eating and intake of alcohol, risky sexual encounters, and aggressive and hurtful behaviors as well as to enhance salutary behaviors.

Primary prevention refers to reducing the risks of the onset of disease, such as efforts focused on exercise, nutrition, and psychosocial interventions to maximize functioning and independence. Secondary prevention relies on the screening and detection of early symptoms of psychiatric and physical disorders as well as geriatric syndromes. Tertiary prevention refers to active rehabilitation and interventions with patients who have psychopathology to prevent relapses or exacerbation of symptoms.

Prevention efforts need to be tailored to the individual person based on a number of factors, including age, demographic variables, past medical history, family medical history, current medical status, risk factors for specific diseases and conditions, lifestyle, and social circumstances as well as goals and desires.

Changing health behaviors is a challenge, but Daly and Katzel (2001) suggest several guidelines for working with older patients:

• Make a determined effort to educate patients and family members and use different educational approaches (e.g., classes, videos, written materials, and community resources).
• Do not assume that patients understand the relationship between their behaviors and health.
• Make a written list of behaviors that should

be changed, but let the patient choose the one he or she wants to start to change first.

• Design a specific action plan with explicit tactics and strategies. If possible, set up a buddy program, because partners can reinforce and support each other.

• Monitor progress with telephone calls, visits, or e-mails.

• Be a coach and use your motivational spirit and techniques to compliment and reinforce change.

Older persons are at risk for serious negative outcomes such as abuse, domestic violence, and violent death, including suicide, homicide, and homicide-suicide

In the course of clinical care, it is important to routinely screen patients to detect whether they are being abused by family members and other caregivers or are victims of domestic discord and violence. It is particularly important to spend time alone with the patient because the abuser may be living with the individual and not want to leave him or her alone. Although older persons are a small proportion of homicide offenders, older persons, particularly older men, have the highest rates of suicide and homicide-suicide compared to other age groups. Frequent screens for depression, helplessness, and hopelessness as well as suicidal and homicidal ideation in family caregivers, spouses as well as adult children in a primary caregiver role, are necessary to prevent these violent, unnecessary deaths.

Do no harm, and be advised that anything that can help can also hurt—the patient as well as family caregivers

Any treatment or intervention that can improve an individual's functioning—biologically, psychologically, or socially—from point A to a more desirable point B also has the potential to move that person to point C, perhaps less desirable than point A. Even water, our most critical ingestible substance, can be lethal with an extreme overdose. Frequent and continuing observation combined with an evaluation of changes is essential to good-quality care.

Clinicians need to actively consider ethical sensitivity and sensibility in clinical care and research

Clinicians have a responsibility to examine the ethical principles that affect their daily behavior in clinical, educational, research, service, and advocacy activities. This should be an ongoing concern and a subject for continuing discussions with other colleagues. Health professionals also often have legal responsibilities for their actions, and they therefore need to be familiar with the laws and regulations affecting their practices, to be vigilant about the possibility of conflicts between legal and ethical responsibilities, and to consult appropriate professionals when concerned about the potential legal consequences of decisions.

Four basic principles are at the core of medical ethics:

1. Respect for patient autonomy (the responsibility to be an advocate for an individual's preferences and decisions)

2. Beneficence (the obligation to act in the best interest of the patient and balance those interests and needs with the need to protect the health of the greater society)

3. Nonmaleficence (the obligation to do no harm)

4. Justice (the obligation to participate in the fair distribution of services in health care)

The values underlying these principles should be the framework guiding clinical practice. Respect for patient autonomy is the basis for informed consent in patient/clinician transactions regarding health care decisions. The principle of beneficence embodies the clinician's responsibility to help patients, which may involve taking actions to prevent or remove them from harm. The principle of nonmaleficence, which affirms the importance of medical competence, requires clinicians to meet the prevailing standard of care and not cause unnecessary harm or injury to the patient, either by acts of commission or omission. Medical errors occur, but this principle affirms the fundamental responsibility of health care professionals to do their best to protect patients from harm.

The principle of just allocation of resources (i.e., distributive justice) affects a professional's role as a citizen and a health care provider making decisions about the allocation of resources. The principle of distributive justice requires the fair distribution of health care in society (e.g., people who are equals should qualify for equal treatment). One example is the application of Medicare to all individuals age 65 or older, a population group equal with respect to their age. There are no restrictions regarding the severity of medical needs, disabilities, injuries, or other factors that could affect the allocation of health care to the older population.

The principle of distributive justice mandates the responsibility to try to distribute health care equitably, but exactly how to do this is controversial. The social transformation of health care in the United States, including the growth of managed care, has created a system that does not serve all constituents well, and major reforms are needed. Health care financing is a serious driving force, and the moral values of our society about caring and the value of life will continue to be tested in decisions about resource allocation.

The challenges of geriatric mental health care are daunting but present opportunities

Increasing longevity and population aging herald a future of unknown possibilities, and one in which, we hope, more individuals will be living productive and happy lives. The application of new research discoveries; the evolution of behavioral and genomic health care; an increasing investment in social capital for public mental health; a reversal of the forces that propagate the devaluation of those who are old, sick, and disabled; and policy reforms that cultivate and support healthy people and communities are critical ingredients for societal well-being.

The challenge for mental health professionals is to combat stereotypes of aging and develop the knowledge and skills to intervene thoughtfully and effectively with older persons and their families. Mental illnesses are painful, and the quality of life of afflicted individuals is typically suboptimal. The opportunity to make a difference in the life of a human being is to be cherished as a source of great satisfaction, justifying the years of hard work to become a qualified clinician.

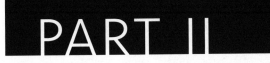

PART II

A CLINICAL GUIDE

3

Comprehensive Geriatric Assessment

This chapter sets the stage for the next twelve chapters describing the major classes of psychiatric disorders. Comprehensive geriatric assessment protocols are the first steps to accurate diagnosis and appropriate care plans. In turn, they can lead to more effective health promotion and risk prevention strategies with a subsequent improvement in functioning and better quality of life. The objectives of a comprehensive assessment are to identify and evaluate the presenting symptoms and their clinical significance; the patient's subjective experience and overall level of functioning; the family and psychosocial supports, strengths, and resources; and the limitations and barriers to care. Assessment relies on an evaluation of the individual from many perspectives, typically using an interdisciplinary team to gather the information needed to derive and coordinate an effective care plan (Gallo et al. 2000; Osterweil et al. 2000).

Multidisciplinary geriatric assessment research began in Great Britain in the 1930s with the pioneering efforts of Marjory Warren (Matthews 1984). The results were institutionalized with the founding of the British National Health System in 1948 (Snowden and Arie 2005). By the 1970s, comprehensive geriatric assessment programs were integrated into most British inpatient and outpatient programs. This approach ultimately resulted in a decrease in hospitalizations and delayed long-term care placement by developing what amounted to strategic health care plans for older persons at risk.

Also in the early 1970s, geriatric assessment programs began to be implemented in the United States and many other countries. However, despite the long-term benefits of this approach, the initial costs and nature of health care funding have limited their use in the United States (Wieland and Hirth 2003). As a result, they usually exist only in academic medical centers with geriatric specialization, and they are almost nonexistent in managed care. However, the outcome of an important study of the effectiveness of a comprehensive geriatric assessment unit in a Veterans Affairs medical center (Rubenstein et al. 1981) led to the existence of these programs in 75 percent of the existing VA medical centers by the mid-1990s (Wieland et al. 1994).

In practice, most geriatric assessment programs target persons who are frail and chronically ill. Consistent with the definition of health as more than the absence of disease and as defined by adaptive capacity, comprehensive assessments have distinct benefits (Osterweil et al. 2000): improved functioning, decreased use of hospitals and nursing homes, and higher ratings of satisfaction with care by patients and family members as well as reduced morbidity and mortality. Evidence that comprehensive assessment reduces overall health care costs is mixed at this time.

The general goals of comprehensive geriatric assessment are to enhance diagnostic accuracy; to inform decisions about interventions and longer-term management, including selection of an appropriate care environment; to identify clinical change; and to predict outcomes. Geriatric assessment can have important outcomes for the short and long term. In the short term, it can be effective in identifying underlying chronic and acute problems that destabilize patient adaptation (e.g., a depressed patient who becomes too impaired to self-manage diet and medication). In the long term, interventions prevent unnecessary admissions to the emergency room or hospital with patients at high risk for a cascading deterioration. The focus is on decreasing excess disability and maximizing functioning through health promotion and risk prevention over and beyond acute medical and psychiatric care. Accurate geriatric assessment is the platinum standard. Any alternative is a compromise and an unacceptable standard of care for which the patient may ultimately pay a price.

The Comprehensive Geriatric Assessment Process

Although primary care practitioners can assess different components of functioning, a core team of geriatric professionals, including a physician, a nurse practitioner, a social worker, and a mental health specialist, are best suited to evaluate an individual's problem (Halter et al. 2009). Ultimately, a wide range of specialists may be needed, including audiology, neuropsychology, dentistry, nutrition, occupational therapy, optometry, pharmacy, physical therapy, podiatry, and speech pathology. At times, clergy, pastoral counselors, elder law attorneys, and financial planners may also need to be consulted. Frequently, the services of other medical specialists are necessary, including neurology, ophthalmology, orthopedics, physiatry, surgery, urology, and others. It is important that a member of the team is designated as the patient coordinator to keep track of referrals to specialists and integrate the information into the care plan.

A number of assessment tools rely on self-ratings or clinician ratings to establish a baseline of symptoms and functioning and communications with other professionals (Gallo et al. 2000). The value of interviews and screening instruments is highly dependent on the examiner's behavior. The best results occur when clinicians show respect for the individual's dignity and personal circumstances, ask thoughtful questions about the patient's experience of their illness or situation, and create a private comfortable environment for older persons who may have sensory, physical, and cognitive impairments. It is necessary to ask permission to involve other family members and informants in the assessment process in order to meet the requirements of

the Health Insurance Portability and Accountability Act (HIPAA), which safeguards the privacy of patient health information (www.aspe.hhs.gov/admnsimp/).

Cultural, racial, and ethnic differences can have a profound impact on patient and family beliefs about the causes of illness and cooperation with a comprehensive assessment. These differences will inevitably alter the perception and reporting of symptoms, help-seeking behavior, cooperation with assessment, communication patterns with health professionals, and expectations for roles and responsibilities of family caregivers as well as decision-making about treatment and management, including compliance with medications, psychological therapies, diet, lifestyle changes, or end-of-life care decisions.

The Components of Comprehensive Geriatric Assessment

The core components of comprehensive geriatric assessment include psychiatric status, psychological status, physical status, family/psychosocial/environmental assessment, elder mistreatment and violence, and end-of-life preferences. This chapter will focus on the mental health evaluation of the patient, briefly review the other components, and conclude with guidelines for developing the diagnostic, therapeutic, and educational care plans.

Psychiatric Assessment

Psychiatric evaluation is an essential part of geriatric assessment for several reasons: (1) primary care physicians and medical specialists who focus on physical symptoms often overlook psychiatric problems; (2) psychiatric treatment has repeatedly been shown to be cost-effective; and (3) untreated psychiatric conditions are painful and disabling to patients and increase caregiver strain and burden.

Psychiatric assessment relies on the mental status examination, which includes an evaluation of the patient's appearance, level of consciousness, mood and affect, perception, and cognitive abilities, including attention, memory, abstract reasoning, judgment, and language (Blazer 2004). It involves a clinical interview and evaluation, often using one or more assessment measures, to identify the history and presence of psychopathology. A mental status examination should be conducted with all patients, and the results need to be integrated with findings from the physical examination and history.

If possible, clinicians should interview patients before using screening measures. Clinical strategies to evaluate individuals who refuse to be interviewed and/or may not have the capacity to understand what is happening are discussed in chapters 4 and 16. After the patient interview, the clinician should ask permission to consult with family members from at least two generations if they are available. Having multiple informed family members provides a broader perspective on the older patient's symptoms and circumstances. If the patient has trouble giving a comprehensible history, the clinician should focus on clarifying what problems the patient believes are the most distressing. Family informants may then provide missing details about the patient's behaviors as well as the psychosocial and medical background.

Several structured psychiatric interviews have been developed to diagnose patients in research programs and clinical settings to maximize diagnostic reliability (Blazer and Steffens 2009). The Structured Clinical Interview for DSM-IV (SCID) is the most frequently used structured interview in the United States (First et al. 1997), and it can be easily adapted for DSM-IV-TR. However, many of the questions are irrelevant for older adults (e.g., detailed questions about psychosis). The Diagnostic Interview Schedule (DIS) is a detailed, structured, computer-scored interview (Robins et al. 1981) that can be useful with older patients. Structured interview protocols require more time than semistructured psychiatric interviews to elicit the older patient's history and current mental status, and they minimize opportunities to elicit valuable information from older patients who may be anxious, uncomfortable, embarrassed about their symptoms, and slow to disclose personal details.

The components of the geriatric psychiatric interview are reviewed below, and guidelines for conducting a clinical conversation and establishing a therapeutic alliance are described in chapter 4.

The history of the patient should cover:

- Temporal history of the presenting problem and life stressors that may be contributing to the chief complaint
- Psychiatric history, including current and previous diagnoses, inpatient and outpatient encounters, psychotropic drug use, suicidal ideation or attempts, and alcohol and substance abuse
- Medical history of acute and chronic conditions
- Medications, including over-the-counter drugs, alcohol, herbal remedies, and illicit drugs
- Family history of psychiatric disorders and symptoms
- Psychosocial history of educational attainment, occupations, marriage(s) and relationships, family and psychosocial supports
- Current living situation and available caregivers

The mental status examination should include:

- General appearance and behaviors
- Type and range of affect
- Mood
- Thought processes, including language and speech, associations, flight of ideas, echolalia, perseveration, and frame of reference of self to the world
- Thought content, including the presence of hallucinations, delusions, illusions, and suicidal or homicidal ideation
- Insight
- History of childhood abuse or significant adult trauma
- Judgment, based on recent life decisions
- Cognition, including level of consciousness, orientation, and performance on mental status screening tests

Psychological Assessment

Psychological assessment includes neuropsychological testing when cognitive impairment is suspected, evaluations of functional abilities, other psychometric evaluations of psychological functioning, and evaluations of family caregiver distress (Molinari et al. 2003). The American Psychological Association has published reports regarding the competencies of geriatric psychologists (APA 2003) and multicultural competencies for geropsychologists (APA 2009).

There are many different mental health screening instruments, including brief mental status examinations, cognitive tests and scales, clinical global assessments, behavioral rating scales, and functional activity ratings. Several of the most frequently used measures are cited here, but omissions do not reflect a lack of appreciation for other screening instruments.

Cognition

Cognitive screening instruments are intended to guide the choice of more cognitive and neuropsychological evaluations to determine the nature of impairment(s) and identify specific strengths and weaknesses of the individual's abilities. The most commonly used standardized clinical tool is the Mini-Mental State Exam (MMSE), which tests orientation, memory, attention, naming, comprehension, praxis, and visuospatial skills (Folstein et al. 1975). It is used primarily for screening but may also be a general proxy for progression of illness in persons diagnosed with dementia. There are different cut-off scores by age and educational level, and there are cultural variations. The MMSE has been criticized because it ignores certain cognitive areas (e.g., executive functioning) and is insensitive to early stages of dementia in individuals who have high intelligence.

A number of other screening tests can be used to supplement the MMSE or in place of it. The Mini-Cog Test, which consists of a three-item memory registration and recall test as well as the Clock Drawing Test, is useful in the emergency room and primary care settings because of its brevity (Borson et al. 2006). The Alzheimer Disease Assessment Scale (Rosen et al. 1984), which takes a little longer that the MMSE, is a standardized instrument measuring the severity of cognitive and noncognitive impairments. It includes tests of word recognition, word recall, naming, commands, constructional and ideational praxis, orientation, spoken language, and word-finding. The Montreal Cognitive Assessment (Nasreddine et al. 2005) taps many of the same domains but also includes a more comprehensive screen of memory and executive functioning (www.mocatest.org).

The Severe Impairment Battery (Saxton et al. 1990) is used to evaluate functioning in severely impaired patients using single words, short commands, and gestures for nine areas: social interaction, memory, orientation to name, orientation, attention, language, praxis, construction, and visuospatial skills.

Brief Psychiatric and Behavioral Scales

The Brief Psychiatric Rating Scale (BPRS: Overall and Gorham 1962), which is completed after an interview by an experienced clinician, rates the presence and severity of somatic concern, anxiety, depression, suicidality, guilt, hostility, elevated mood, grandiosity, suspiciousness, hallucinations, unusual thought content, bizarre behavior, self-neglect, disorientation, conceptual disorganization blunted affect, emotional withdrawal, motor retardation, tension, uncooperativeness, excitement, distractibility, motor hyperactivity, and mannerisms and posturing.

The Behavioral Pathology in Alzheimer's Disease Rating Scale (BEHAVE-AD: Reisberg et al. 1987) and the Neuropsychiatric Inventory (NPI: Cummings 1997) are useful for rating the presence and severity of psychopathology in people who have dementia. The BEHAVE-AD assesses behaviors in seven areas: paranoid and delusional ideation, hallucinations, aggressivity, depression, anxiety, phobias, activity, and circadian disturbances. The NPI consists of a brief series of questions directed to caregivers to evaluate twelve neuropsychiatric disturbances: delusions, hallucinations, agitation, dysphoria, anxiety, apathy, irritability, euphoria, disinhibition, aberrant motor behavior, night-time behavior disturbances, and appetite and eating abnormalities.

Several brief depression and anxiety measures are useful for screening. The Cornell Scale for Depression in Dementia (CSDD: Alexopoulos et al. 1988) assesses 19 signs and symptoms of major depression in dementia on the basis of a semistructured interview of a qualified informant as well as observing and interviewing the patient. The Geriatric Depression Scale (GDS: Yesavage et al. 1983) is a 15-item self-assessment of mood, feelings, and activities over the past 24 hours. The Center for Epidemiological Studies Depression scale CED-D (CES-D: Radloff 1977) is one of the most common self-report screening instruments, with 20 items that measure mood, feelings, behaviors, and activities over the past week. The Geriatric Anxiety Scale (GAS: Pachana et al. 2007) is a 20-item self-report or nurse-administered scale to identify dimensions of anxiety.

Physical Assessment

A standardized medical protocol is useful for the long-term follow-up of patients. The physical examination, accompanied by laboratory tests and a review of medications, is essential to assess changes in medical status. The physical exam should include a review of systems, an assessment of overall hygiene, nutrition and hydration, falls/gait and balance problems, signs of injury, and/or suspicious bruises that may suggest abuse or neglect.

Other important components of the physical assessment are queries about health practices: alcohol use, recreational drug use, smoking, eating habits, exercise, sleep, exposure to toxicants, work habits, pleasurable activities, and attitude toward life. It is important to probe the patient's fears and beliefs about illness and expectations for appropriate treatment. These attitudes and beliefs affect the older person's readiness to disclose information and adherence to treatment.

The physical examination process may need to be modified for very old, frail, and impaired patients (Williams 2008): interviewing patients and family members separately, scheduling two or more sessions because of fatigue, and relying on the results of the physical examination when a complete and accurate history is not available.

Medication Assessment

A comprehensive drug history should include:

- A complete list of all medications (ideally having the patient bring in all drugs at the time of evaluation), including prescription drugs, over-the-counter drugs, topical medications, drops for the eyes, nose, and ears, and self-prescribed herbal and home remedies
- Contact information for prescribing physicians and pharmacies as well as whether drugs are borrowed from friends or neighbors
- The purpose, dose, and directions for each drug
- How the patient is actually taking the drugs and who is administering them
- History of allergies and adverse reactions
- Name and phone number for the patient's prescription drug plan, if the patient has one

Frequent, regular follow-up of drug use is important as a basis to consider whether each drug is still necessary, whether it is being administered correctly, whether the patient is complying with directions, whether interventions are necessary to minimize drug hazards for high-risk patients and to review possible interactions when new drugs are added (Hajjar et al. 2005). Bergman-Evans (2006) published evidence-based guidelines for medication management in older adults.

Noncompliance with the physician's drug treatment plan is a serious problem in all age groups, but there are special problems with older patients who may not be able to afford their medications, may have cognitive and functional impairments, or may not understand the purpose and importance of the drug. Older persons may stop taking a drug because of uncomfortable side effects or because they obtain symptomatic relief and do not believe they need it anymore. Noncompliance also takes many forms, such as forgetting, intentional or unintentional overdosing, incorrect administration or dosing frequency, and using drugs prescribed for others.

Anything that can help can harm, and older patients are at high risk for adverse drug reactions. Medical and pharmacy practices as well as patient characteristics and circumstances can increase the risk for negative drug reactions. Physician risk factors include incorrect dosing for age, duplication of drugs, unclear directions, poor drug history, and inadequate monitoring. Risk factors associated with pharmacy practice include automatic refills, prescription errors, not reviewing medications, and failing to provide materials to educate patients and caregivers. Patients heighten their risk by giving an incomplete drug history, abusing alcohol, or obtaining drugs from more than one source.

Older patients are at increased risk for drug-drug, drug-food, and drug-disease interactions when they have co-morbidities and because age-related and disease processes change sensitivities to drugs (Hanlon et al. 2000). Several strategies in addition to those mentioned earlier are useful to minimize risks:

• Knowing the pharmacological properties of the drugs
• Using computer-based resources to check medication interactions
• Consulting a geriatric pharmacist, if available, to review the medication regimen
• Simplifying complex therapeutic plans whenever possible
• Taking time to educate the patient and caregivers about drug storage, drug usage, drug side effects, and the use of pill boxes and other aids
• Requesting the patient and/or caregiver to create and update a medication calendar, including each medication, dosage, and time of administration
• Asking about untoward reactions on a regular basis

Functional Assessment

Although older persons may have many different health problems, the impact of medical conditions, injuries, and frailty on overall personal functioning is as important as an accurate diagnosis (Kresevic 2008). Activities of Daily Living (ADLs) and Instrumental Activities of Daily Living (IADLs) have become a standard component of geriatric assessment that is often done by nurses, social workers, occupational therapists, or physical therapists. To live independently, one must carry out personal activities effectively on a regular basis. Changes in ADLs and IADLs are often an early warning, or a late warning if ignored, that there are significant untoward changes that mandate scrutiny.

Personal ADLs refer to basic personal care activities such as dressing, eating, toileting, and transferring. Instrumental ADLs, or IADLs, refer to a range of activities such as medication management, meal preparation, and many other daily life transactions as well as work-related and leisure activities. Having ADL capacity means that the person is able to perform an ADL independently, and ADL-ability means that the individual is able to perform the ADL even though it may be difficult, painful, or take more time. When assessing functional status, the foremost questions are "Does the patient perform the activity or not?" If not, or if the patient has difficulties, "What are the physical, mental, or psychosocial reasons?"

Many standardized assessments of functional status exist (Asberg 2002; Wells et al. 2003). Among the most frequently used instruments are the Katz Index of ADLs (Katz et al. 1963); the Lawton-Brody assessment of ADLs and IADLs (Lawton and Brody 1969); Barthel's Index (Mahoney and Barthel 1965); the FIM instrument, which is based on a modification of the Barthels Index (Pinholt et al. 1987); and a brief ADL assessment adapted from the Older American Research and Service Center instrument (Fillenbaum 1988). Evaluations of specific functions include gait and balance: the timed get up and go (TUG) test evaluates how well the patient gets out of a chair, walks, and turns back to sit down again (Podsiadlo and Richardson 1991); and the Berg Balance Scale (BBS) assesses stability during several common everyday movements (Berg et al. 1989).

The results of these evaluations are not only valuable for treatment and care-planning decisions but are also used to determine eligibility for services, including community-based services, rehabilitation, nursing home admissions, and other long-term care services.

Assessment of Pain

Pain is defined as an unpleasant sensory and emotional experience or simply whatever the patient says it is, whenever it occurs. Many older adults have injuries and medical conditions that predispose them to pain, such as falls, vascular diseases, cancers, herpes zoster, osteoporosis, osteoarthritis, and rheumatoid arthritis. The routine assessment, evaluation, and treatment of pain has finally been acknowledged as an important component of patient care for people of all ages, and guidelines have been published by several professional aging health care organizations. These include the American Geriatrics Society (2002; www.americangeriatrics.org/education/ manage_pers_pain.shtml), the Hartford Institute for Geriatric Nursing (www.hartfordign .org/resources/education/tryThis.html), and the American Association of Pain Management Nurses (www.commercecorner.com/aspmn/ productlist1.aspx). Professional organizational guidelines for the assessment and treatment of pain in people who have dementia, are nonverbal, or are residents in long-term care include the American Medical Directors Association (www.amda.com/tools/cpg/chronicpain.cfm), the City of Hope (www.cityofhope.org/prc/ elderly.asp), and the American Association of Pain Management Nurses (2005; www.aacn .org/AACN/practice.nsf/vwdoc/PainAssmt).

The routine use of pain screens is essential to elicit an individual's experience and use responses to gauge the impact of treatment interventions to reduce pain. An American Geriatrics Society (AGS 2002) panel recommends that all older patients be screened for pain, including chronic and persistent pain, at the time of initial evaluation, whenever they are admitted to the hospital, as well as at regular intervals.

The following strategies are recommended to screen for pain in older adults who are not cognitively impaired (AGS 2002):

· Asking patients to quantify the pain on a scale ranging from 0 (no pain) to 10 (excruciating pain)
· Asking patients to describe the type of pain, such as burning, needlelike, tingling, aching, or throbbing, and where it occurs
· Asking patients about activities associated with pain
· Asking patients to identify remedies they have tried for relief
· Observing the patients' nonverbal behavior when discussing the pain

When evaluating patients who are cognitively impaired, the clinician should repeat questions several times and give them time to answer, observing carefully as they walk, talk, moan, and respond to various requests. Pain should be suspected whenever a patient who has dementia shows a sudden change in behavior.

Nutritional Assessment

Nutritional assessments and interventions are essential procedures to achieve optimal health and functioning (Chernoff 2006; Morley and Thomas 2007). The Nutrition Screening Initiative (NSI), a ten-year initiative consisting of a broad coalition of health care organizations led by the American Dietetic Association and the American Academy of Family Physicians, was the first major national effort to target specific goals to improve the nutrition of older adults (American Academy of Family Physicians: www.aafp.org/x16081.xml). These included the development of several nutrition screening measures, guidelines for nutritional interventions, professional and public educational programs, successful advocacy forums, and federal policy initiatives.

Nutritional approaches have been shown

to promote healthy aging in the prevention and management of chronic diseases and their consequences, and they are a cost-effective and desirable alternative to drug therapy (White et al. 2003; Chernoff 2006). It is estimated that nutrition intervention could save $168 million for older adults who have hypertension, $132–$330 million for those who have diabetes, and $54–$164 million for those who have high lipid levels.

Involuntary weight loss, which occurs in 13 percent of older persons seen in outpatient settings and more than 50 percent of nursing home residents, is usually an indication of a serious decline in health (Evans et al. 2005). Involuntary weight loss may not always be clinically apparent, and there are many causes, making it a clinical challenge, but it can be identified by a systematic evaluation of physical, psychological, and social status (White et al. 2003; Chernoff 2006).

The DETERMINE Nutrition Checklist, developed by the NSI, is a 10-item questionnaire to screen for risk of poor nutritional health by staff in all settings from senior centers to outpatient offices (www.aafp.org). DETERMINE targets the following warning signs: *D*isease, *E*ating poorly, *T*ooth loss/mouth pain, *E*conomic hardship, *R*educed social contact, *M*ultiple medicines, *I*nvoluntary weight loss or gain, *N*eed for personal care assistance, and *E*lder years above age 80.

WAVE and REAP are two brief practical tools to help physicians and other health care providers assess nutritional health and counsel patients (Gans et al. 2003). They were developed under the auspices of the Nutrition Academic Award Program, an initiative to improve nutrition training across a network of U.S. medical schools. The WAVE acronym and instrument is intended to stimulate provider/patient discussions about the patient's *W*eight, *A*ctivity, *V*ariety, and *E*xcess, and it can be done in 5–10 minutes. REAP (Rapid Eating and Activity Assessment) is a tool to assess diet and physical activity, and it adds about 5 minutes to the clinical interview. REAP includes questions about whether the individual has trouble shopping or cooking, follows a special diet, and is willing to make changes to eat healthier.

Assessment of Oral Health

Oral health refers to healthy teeth, gums and surrounding tissues, the palate, lining of the mouth and throat, tongue, lips, salivary glands, chewing muscles, and the jaws. It means being free from oral-facial pain, oral and throat cancers, soft tissue lesions, and other conditions that affect the craniofacial area. The Surgeon General's Report on Oral Health (USDHHS 2000) emphasizes that oral health is integral to overall health at all ages, "allowing us to speak and smile; sigh and kiss; smell, taste, touch, chew, and swallow; cry out in pain; and convey a world of feelings and emotions through facial expressions." Oral tissues and structures reflect nutritional deficiencies, systemic diseases, psychiatric diseases, infections, immune functioning, and injuries.

Older persons face some serious oral health risks, making a thorough dental evaluation essential to geriatric assessment (Ghezzi and Ship 2000). Two-thirds of all oral and pharyngeal cancers occur in persons age 65 or older, and poor oral health is related to cardiovascular disease and aspiration pneumonia. About 25 percent of persons age 65–74 have severe periodontal disease, and those at the lowest socioeconomic levels are a higher prevalence. Only 7 percent of persons age 75–84 have healthy periodontal tissues. Periodontal disease in older adults is affected by medical conditions, immune functioning medications, decreased saliva flow, and diabetes as well as cognitive and functional impairments. Older persons are at risk for dental caries on the tooth crown and roots. With more people living longer with more of their teeth, older persons will have the largest increase in risk for cavities. National data show that 47 percent of persons age 65–74 and 56 percent of persons age 75 or older have decayed or filled roots. Risk factors for root caries include poor oral hygiene, decreased saliva flow, partial dentures, gingivitis, and cognitive deficits. Many medications, both prescribed and over the counter, are associated with decreased saliva flow that adversely affects oral tissues as well as the ability to speak, taste, chew, and swallow.

Sexual Functioning

A sexual history and discussion of current sexual functioning are important, although some physicians are uncomfortable talking with older patients about these issues. Older persons, like younger persons, may have sexual dysfunction due to boredom, fear, fatigue, and grief, but sexual problems in older adults are also often associated with health problems, depression, and drug effects (Arena and Wallace 2008).

Older people may also be uncomfortable discussing sexual functioning. Having an available partner is often an issue, especially for older women, who outlive and outnumber men. Older people and health care professionals may be even more uncomfortable discussing unprotected sex and the risk of HIV/AIDS and other sexually transmitted diseases, masturbation, alternative sexual activities, homosexual relationships, or transgender changes. However, not everyone chooses to exercise her or his rights to be a sexual human being, and clinicians need to respect this position. Openness and respect, coupled with reassurance and information, may help patients talk more freely about their sexual needs, desires, and activities as well as treatment for sexual dysfunction.

Sleep Assessment

There are normal age-related changes in sleep patterns (see chapter 13). They include frequent arousals during the night, increased sleep latency, early morning wakening, decreased time spent in deep sleep, and a small drop in body temperature. However, more than 50 percent of older people in the community and more than two-thirds of long-term care residents have significant sleep disturbances that may be caused by illness, medications, lifestyle changes, lack of exercise, and loss of interest in activities as well as by bereavement and major losses (Brannon et al. 2009).

Among the numerous factors likely to be causing sleep disturbances are painful conditions such as arthritis, heart disease, emphysema, gastrointestinal disorders, and gastric reflux. Sleep disruption, especially early morning wakening, is often a symptom of depression. Older men in particular also have an increased incidence of sleep apnea and myoclonic activity. Poor sleep hygiene may lead to problems including excessive daytime napping, evening use of alcohol, caffeine, and nicotine, and spending too much time in bed. Nighttime use of diuretics leads to multiple awakenings and trips to the bathroom. Many drugs have stimulating effects that disrupt sleep: decongestants, bronchodilators, selective serotonin reuptake inhibitors, and some antihypertensives. The inappropriate and extended use of hypnotic medications is one of the most significant causes of impaired sleep.

Several screening questions need to be asked about sleep satisfaction, interference of sleep problems or daytime fatigue on activities, and partner observations about unusual sleep behaviors (e.g., snoring, kicking). If sleep problems are present, several diagnostic strategies should be incorporated into the psychiatric and/or physical examination: (1) taking a complete sleep history; (2) instructing the patient to keep a 24-hour sleep log for 4 days; (3) asking the bed partner, if available, to make notes about sleep patterns; (4) asking about sleep disorders in family members; and (5) referring the patient for a specialized sleep evaluation if there is evidence of serious sleep apnea, narcolepsy, or periodic limb syndrome. Sleep disturbances not only affect quality of life but are associated with increased risk for cognitive impairment and mortality.

Family/Psychosocial/Environmental Assessments

Evaluation of the patient's family and social support system and living situation is also important for care planning. Family members provide for most of the care needs of older relatives, and assessing family caregiver resources, competencies, and vulnerabilities and forming an alliance with the family are as important as evaluating the identified patient. This assessment can be done by psychologists, social workers, and other staff in health care and community settings using a checklist described in chapter 15.

A visit to assess the patient's home and community environment is worth a thousand words, revealing a great deal about the patient's world. This includes their living conditions, ability to care for themselves and maintain their home, availability of neighbors and friends, fire safety, safety of the neighborhood and home security, potential for falls and accidents, and proximity to available health and community services.

Assessment of Elder Mistreatment and Violence

Mistreatment of older adults refers to physical abuse and neglect, psychological abuse, sexual abuse, financial exploitation, and violation of human rights. Abuse is a serious problem affecting about 2 million older people, and unfortunately it is often overlooked by clinicians (chapter 17). Diagnosis is based on evidence of suspicious injuries and behaviors, a detailed history from the patient and family caregivers, and a comprehensive physical examination. Risk factors include cognitive impairment, poor health or disability in patients as well as caregiver, alcohol abuse, and a history of domestic violence. Most states have mandatory reporting laws, and when elder mistreatment is suspected, it should be reported to the state adult protective service agency.

The Hwalek-Sengstock Elder Abuse Screening Test (H-S/EAST) is useful in clinical settings (Hwalek and Sengstock 1986; Neal et al. 1991):

1. Do you have anyone who spends time with you, taking you shopping or to the doctor?

2. Are you helping to support someone?

3. Are you sad or lonely?

4. Who makes decisions about your life—like how you should live or where you should live?

5. Do you feel uncomfortable with anyone in your family?

6. Can you take your own medication and get around by yourself?

7. Do you feel that nobody wants you around?

8. Does anyone in your family drink a lot?

9. Does someone in your family make you stay in bed or tell you you're sick when you're not?

10. Has anyone forced you to do things you didn't want to do?

11. Has anyone taken things that belonged to you without your OK?

12. Do you trust most of the people in your family?

13. Does anyone tell you that you give them too much trouble?

14. Do you have enough privacy at home?

15. Has anyone close to you tried to hurt or harm you recently?

Assessment of Advanced Disease / End-of-Life Preferences

Many health professionals have shifted the emphasis from end-of-life planning to advanced disease planning while a person is healthy. Instruments to help patients and families identify their wishes and desires include the Values Questionnaire (Dubler and Nimmons 1982) and Five Wishes (Towey 1997). The Values History questionnaire has two sections: a review of legal documents, wishes about specific medical procedures, and special concerns; and attitudes and beliefs about health, life, and death as well as perceptions about the role of physicians, family members, and other people.

There are several mechanisms for individuals to specify wishes and preferences if and when they become incapacitated (chapter 16). A living will is a written statement of an individual's health care preferences in the event of a terminal illness or permanent vegetative state. A living will does not become effective until a person is incapacitated, does not specify who makes decisions, and requires certification by a physician. A durable power of attorney (POA) is a written legal document authorizing a surrogate named by an individual to make financial and legal decisions. A POA can be general in scope or limited to specific decisions and actions. A durable power of attorney for health care, also known as an advance directive, authorizes a proxy specified by an individual to make health care decisions including terminal care.

Beginning advance disease planning as early as possible provides ample opportunities for individuals to reflect and make plans rather than to be caught in an emergency and unable to make decisions. These issues should also be dealt with if a person is in the early stages of dementia, while the patient still has the capacity to make these decisions.

Using the Results of Geriatric Assessment for Care Plans

Comprehensive geriatric assessment is a coordinated, iterative process, the results of which are used to formulate diagnoses, to create a list of patient strengths and problems as well as family strengths and problems, and, for each problem, to create a care plan with diagnostic, therapeutic, and educational components. The diagnostic component may include referrals to medical specialists and recommend other assessments (e.g., physical therapy, additional laboratory studies, home visits). The therapeutic element may include decisions about what conditions to treat or when to provide palliative care, decisions about pharmacotherapy, surgery, psychotherapy, and family interventions as well as decisions about home and community-based services, home-assisted devices, and physical and occupational therapy. Other care options to be considered may be the need to move to another care setting, legal decisions regarding a durable power of attorney, and decisions about end-of-life care. The educational component focuses on helping patients and families understand and deal with the nature and course of problems as well as treatment, management, and rehabilitation interventions.

An essential clinical skill in the care planning process is the effective communication of risks (Burkiewicz et al. 2008). The results of geriatric assessment and diagnostic examinations may not always clearly establish the certainty of a particular disorder or condition, and the treatment and management options carry risks as well as benefits that need to be explained clearly and accurately. Clinicians frequently use words such as "There is a chance," "It is unlikely," and "Probably." However, there is wide variability in the way clinicians ascribe these attributions of probability. Probability is a statistical concept, and it is important to clearly communicate numbers in words, to be aware of different ways to communicate the probability of a disease condition or adverse outcomes, and to anticipate the impact on patients. Taking the time to ensure that the message is understood is essential, because an ambiguous message may be a source of anxiety and distrust by patients and family members.

Appreciating the Complexity of Older Patients

The examiner's appreciation of what data are important for an individual patient is a critical part of the care plan formulation. Men who have recently seen a physician because of a change in health or who have received an undesirable prognosis are at heightened risk for suicide, if they are seriously ill, or for homicide-suicide, if they are caring for a dependent spouse. Among the other populations vulnerable to mental health problems are caregivers, relocated patients, persons who have had a recent stroke or heart attack, those who have a prior psychiatric history, and those who are in a stressful situation without social supports. These are only a few examples of persons for whom the examiner should take special care to explore mood, thinking, and beliefs about the future in greater depth. The more the examiner brings to the assessment, the better the assessment and the more valuable the resulting data for clinical inference.

4

Interviewing and Developing an Alliance

Effective communication between patients and clinicians is important for health outcomes in all age groups. Patient satisfaction with a physician's communication style is associated with better adherence to treatment, increased psychological well-being, better health outcomes, and fewer formal malpractice complaints (Williams et al. 1998; Hickson et al. 2002; Stelfox et al. 2005; Clever et al. 2008). Poor patient-physician communication has costly, and sometimes deadly, consequences (Hickson et al. 2002; Wissow 2004).

Interviews are the cornerstone of clinical care because they are the bridge to communication and provide elemental information for diagnosis, treatment, management, rehabilitation, and prevention. The time and effort invested in effective interviews and an appreciation of critical psychosocial and environmental factors in a patient's life lead to the highest standard of geriatric mental health care.

This chapter examines issues relevant for interviewing and developing a clinical relationship with older persons. Verbal and nonverbal interpersonal communication is a science as well as a fine art, and it is essential for optimal health care (Travaline et al. 2005). However, clinical interviews with older patients, which are often complicated by unique physical, cognitive, psychological, social, and generational factors, may be a challenge (Blazer 2004).

Ethical Issues

Interviewers encounter several ethical issues with older patients and family members in clinical and research settings: consent, confidentiality, beneficence and autonomy, and fidelity (APA 2002; Mueller et al. 2004).

Consent

Because older persons are often accompanied and sometimes are pressured by relatives to seek help, clinicians need to determine whether the older adult independently consents to the interview. Unfortunately, it is common for interviewers to join the family in urging the patient to participate when he or she does not want to consent. The clinician's responsibilities are to educate and inform the patient in the consent process, and this commitment to the older patient's consent is a critical aspect of building rapport and trust. If family members are at odds with a patient's refusal, the interviewer has at least two options: (1) support the patient and refer the family for help to deal with their concerns, and (2) educate the family about the legal issues involved in privacy and confidentiality.

Cognitive impairment does not by itself preclude an individual's right to consent to an interview, test, or clinical procedure. Criteria for ascertaining whether patients who have dementia have the capacity to give consent are not clearly established, but guidelines are discussed in chapter 16 and several other articles (Vass et al. 2003; APA 2004). The guiding principle is to carefully evaluate the individual patient for cognitive strengths and weaknesses, desire to participate in interviews, clinical needs, and previous statements about preferences.

Confidentiality

Family members frequently ask about previous discussions the interviewer has had with the patient. Clinicians must not violate the patient's confidentiality. However, when appropriate, interviewers may ask patients if they want to share information with specific family members. Clinicians also need to obtain consent to contact other health professionals. This consent should be in writing, and most clinics, hospitals, and other health care institutions have standard forms for patients and witnesses to sign.

In situations in which patients are at risk of being a danger to self, are deteriorating in health status, are self-neglecting, or are at risk for other dangers, contacting appropriate professionals is important. Some states have laws about the clinical responsibility to report these situations (e.g., elder abuse, involuntary commitment). Balancing the individual's wishes with the risk of harm can be challenging.

Many professional organizations, federal and state agencies, state licensing boards, and state and federal laws regulate confidentiality standards of practitioners. The federal Health Insurance Portability and Accountability Act (HIPAA) mandates how patient information and health care records are to be managed, shared, and protected. The use of electronic transmissions was the original stimulus for HIPAA, which requires health care providers and payers to meet standards set by the Department of Health and Human Services to protect privacy in the exchange of health and billing information during transactions such as health care claims, payment, remittance advice, eligibility, and inquiries about claim status.

Professionals must comply with three rules: the transaction rule, the privacy rule, and the security rule. The HIPAA transaction rule is a set of regulations that standardizes the electronic transmissions, including codes, between health care providers and payers. The privacy rule, enforced by the Office of Civil Rights (www.hhs.gov/ocr/privacy/), protects the confidentiality of Protected Health Information (i.e., personal identifiers). The clinician must obtain the patient's consent before using Protected Health Information for treatment, payment, or health care organization operations. The security rule specifies high standards to protect the security of Protected Health Information and the implementation of patient education procedures and materials explaining patients' rights. These standards are enforced by the Centers for Medicare and Medicaid Services (www.cm.hhs.gov).

Autonomy

Autonomy refers to an individual's right to make decisions, act for him- or herself, and not be constrained by controlling influences. However, respect for autonomy does not mean that clinicians merely permit patients to make their own decisions. Clinicians have the responsibility to respect an individual's right of self-determination and to construct the conditions for people to make autonomous choices. This means that clinicians are obligated to educate patients to understand their health issues and circumstances, including explaining available options as well as the risks and benefits; to deal with denial and emotions that may interfere with a patient's ability to make decisions; and to counsel patients about difficult, complex, and upsetting choices. Respect for autonomy also includes confidentiality, obtaining consent for medical treatment and procedures, discussing information about a medical condition with patients, and maintaining privacy.

Beneficence and Nonmaleficence

Beneficence refers to actions that are taken for the benefit of others, either to help prevent or remove harm or to improve their circumstances. Clinicians have responsibilities for obligatory beneficence (i.e., to use their specialized knowledge and skills to enhance the health and welfare of patients) and nonmaleficence (i.e., to do no harm). Specifically, clinicians are obligated to consider and balance potential benefits against possible risks. Beneficence may include protecting and defending the rights of patients when family members have opposing concerns about what should be done.

Balancing Autonomy and Beneficence/Nonmaleficence

Clinicians will encounter a number of ethical issues when an older patient's autonomous wishes and decisions are contrary to the clinician's beneficent responsibility to provide for the patient's health and welfare. For example, patients may not want to take necessary medications or continue seeing a clinician or may refuse to refrain from health-threatening behaviors such as smoking or drinking heavily. Interviewers will frequently find themselves in situations in which the patient's right to autonomy conflicts with the family's or a long-term care facility's desires to help the patient. Conflicting situations frequently occur when patients are cognitively impaired or have other psychiatric disorders that impair insight.

In situations in which the patient's autonomous choice conflicts with the clinician's duty of beneficence, clinicians face a tough challenge. As long as the patient understands the decision(s) at hand and is not making decisions based on distortions resulting from psychiatric problems, clinicians must respect these decisions and continue trying to convince the patient otherwise.

Fidelity

Fidelity, that is, faithfulness to the responsibilities attendant in a therapeutic relationship with the older client, may become a concern, especially when others, such as family members, physicians, other health professionals, and long-term care staff, refer older patients. Although the intent of the referring agent is to help older persons, clinicians may find themselves being asked to do what the referring source wants, something that may not be in the patient's best interest or that violates the patient's autonomy.

The ethical issue is to identify whether responding to a referring agent's request is inconsistent with the fidelity of the clinician-patient relationship. Such requests commonly include scheduling surgery or a medical procedure when the patient's competence is questionable or prescribing medications to treat agitated or aggressive behavior, to make a patient stop complaining about nursing home staff, or to prevent wandering by sedating the patient. Clinicians are well advised not only to know and communicate what they can and cannot do clinically, legally, and ethically but also to find more clinically appropriate methods to address the issue.

Interviewing to Understand Presenting Problems and Patients

The clinical psychiatric interview is affected by the interacting biases of older adults and clinicians (Blazer 2004). Patients not only have diseases but also experience diseases as illnesses, and these are very different. Clinicians attend to signs and symptoms to diagnose diseases, but patients experience the symptoms subjectively, challenging the clinician to look beyond the diagnosis to the person.

Patienthood has been conceptualized as a social state of being less functional and desirable, causing individuals to feel less valuable (Eisenberg 1977). Older adults, who are often influenced by family and friends, develop a self-diagnosis and make attributions about their problem(s) and the extent to which they believe they are perceived as a problem. These illness beliefs as well as the social and cultural background of older patients affect attitudes and beliefs about the nature of their condition and the potential for recovery (Kleinman et al. 2006).

An individual's beliefs—especially those of patients who attribute their mental health problems to aging and have multiple, different, and shifting complaints—can be challenging obstacles (Blazer 2004). It is important to listen to patients who blame age for their problems but not to accept attributions of age for emotional distress. Patients' statements that "I guess I'm just getting old and there's nothing really to worry about" or "Most people slow down when they get to be my age" can be countered with comments such as "Yes, many people do get upset with being older and having these problems, but what other things have happened to you?" or "Often there is something we can do to compensate for these age-related changes."

Older adults who present with new and distressing symptoms or demand immediate relief over a series of office visits can test the clinician's patience and even disrupt the diagnostic process. The expression of many somatic complaints or insistence on obtaining a prescription for drugs advertised on television challenge the relationship, but clinicians should not be threatened by a patient's need to assume control and obtain quick relief. This attitude, when expressed by patients or caregivers, needs to be evaluated in the context of lifestyle, expression of unmet needs, or anxiety about current or future problems. Anguish about problems such as sexual functioning, chronic pain, and feeling depressed may also devastate older patients and may, if clinicians are seen as indifferent, lead to self-medication with alcohol and drug abuse or, in extreme cases, to self-destructive behaviors, including suicide.

Older patients, like most patients, are usually anxious about being interviewed. Ideally, anxiety diminishes as a trained interviewer takes the history and identifies why the interview is necessary. Casting questions broadly, with an affirmative, optimistic tone will reduce anxiety and stimulate conversation: "How can I help you today?" or "What has brought you to see me today?" If the patient does not relax, the interviewer should check his or her hearing and visual acuity as well as probe more directly into the basis for the anxiety, particularly the patient's beliefs about the role of the clinician and the motivations of others making the referral.

An essential component of the initial interview involves direct questions and answers, but these are best done after a period of assessing the strengths and weaknesses of the patient as well as the patient's perceptions of the implications and confidentiality of the interview process. Experienced interviewers do not apologize for asking specific questions, such as the mental status examination, but carry out the evaluation in a matter-of-fact manner.

The chief complaint is the prologue to the history of the illness, and many older persons are able to adequately relay the development of their symptoms. If interviewers are tactful and flexible, patients will discuss personal and sensitive issues relevant to the current situation, but more than one interview may be necessary. Clinicians should focus on understanding the current level of distress and the major complaints: "What is bothering you? When did your symptoms begin? How long have they lasted? Has the severity changed over time? Are there physical, family, social, or environmental events that precipitate the symptoms? What have you done to deal with the symptoms? Have any of these interventions proved successful? Do the symptoms vary during the day, week, or season of the year? Do you have several problems or symptoms that you would like to talk about? Are there any other issues you want to discuss?" During the review of symptoms, it can be useful to identify a time frame with specific reference events over the past year (e.g., holidays or anniversary of the death of a loved one). This technique allows clinicians to anchor symptoms in time because older patients often focus on the immediate distress. It may also provide clues about the etiology of problems or anniversary reactions.

Interviewers need to probe patients' beliefs and fears about their problems.

LL, a 90-year-old nursing home resident, was referred for a consultation because of a recent onset of screaming throughout the night after going to bed. A review of her medical record indicated that she likely had a mild anoxic encephalopathy following cardiac bypass surgery. LL was cooperative throughout the interview but became agitated when the interviewer left the room momentarily to take a phone call. When questioned about the agitation, LL replied that she did not like being alone. During the remainder of the interview, LL said she yelled at night when she could not hear the nurses because she was afraid of being isolated and dying alone.

Interviewing about History

Older persons are generally experts in the "remembrance of things past." Many have a great need to share their memories, and the clinician is frequently given a great deal of material about the individual's early history. This can be time consuming, despite the interviewer's attempts to structure the interview within the allotted time. There are several strategies to encourage the flow of information, respect the individual's stories, and also control the interview. Sit relatively close to the patient, if acceptable, and face the person. If the answer begins to ramble, touch the patient's hand or arm, maintain a smile and eye contact, and interrupt, saying something like, "Please forgive me for interrupting. I appreciate what you are saying, but right now we need to cover other parts of your life." An interruption with touching, clear cues that you are interested, followed by redirection can be effective, but monitor the patient's reaction to this approach. Long narratives may reflect the loneliness of older persons who have not had opportunities for social contact. The attentive interviewer creates an attractive opportunity to talk. The patient with loose associations and a desire to be heard is often a challenge. In these circumstances, it is important to inform patients that what they are saying is important, but to listen to the patient for a few minutes before redirecting the focus.

Clinicians should query patients about the occurrence of similar problems or episodes in the past, how long these lasted, when they occurred, and the frequency of such occurrences throughout their life. Patients may become irritated when asked such specific questions. However, clinicians need to emphasize the importance of this information to understanding the current problem and to reassure the patient that the interview is confidential. Clinicians should also review any history of previous hospitalizations, physician visits, and medications. They should ask older patients specific questions about the occurrence of serious illnesses or trauma in childhood or young adulthood because patients may not volunteer this information as relevant to their present problems.

A good history uncovers important insights about current symptoms, and sometimes, as this case illustrates, issues in early adulthood are associated with disturbances in later life:

JK, a 77-year-old woman who had terminal breast cancer, was seen in the hospital's intensive care unit. The consultation request indicated that JK was expected to die very soon, but she was angry and agitated, screamed frequently even though her pain was controlled, and cried that she did not want to die. The referring oncologist wanted advice about how to calm JK and eliminate her screaming. When JK was interviewed, she was extremely weak, but she was able to communicate that in her younger years she had had an abortion. She had never thought much about the abortion until the cancer was discovered at a late stage and she had returned to her early Catholic faith. She was terrified of her punishment in the afterlife because of the abortion, and that screaming was the only way to express her awful feelings. JK accepted the clinician's suggestion that she speak with a priest, and she died peacefully the day after the visit.

Interviews in Long-Term Care Settings

Communicating with residents in long-term care facilities presents technical and ethical challenges due to the frailties of the population as well as facility characteristics and operations. Nursing home residents by definition require 24-hour skilled care and are attended by shifts of staff employees, clinicians, and consultants with varying competencies in mental health. Individuals residing in assisted living facilities require assistance with health care and daily living needs by employees and health care providers. Daily life for residents therefore involves a mix of routine personal care activities, medical treatments and interventions, and maintenance and preventive care as well as social interactions, all occurring in an institutional environment where privacy and choices are often limited.

As many as 60 percent of nursing home residents have cognitive impairment, and at least 85 percent have unmet mental health needs (Snowden et al. 2003). Therefore, clinicians need to assess patients' capacities to communicate effectively, understand information and the alternatives available to them, and make informed, voluntary decisions reflecting their preferences. Issues that are of paramount importance involve respect for an individual's rights and dignity; appreciation of their inner experience; informed knowledge about their condition, including strengths and deficits, cognitive competence, and emotional functioning; sensitivities to personal circumstances, sensory limitations, expressions of pain, emotional distress, and boredom; knowledge about how staff perceive and interact with the resident; and sensitivity to the possibilities of neglect and the risk of abusive and hurtful staff behaviors.

Successful interviews require knowledge about long-term care, a comfort level with the institutional environment, and patience to communicate with human beings who are disabled and impaired. Interviewers should find the most comfortable spatial proximity with a resident, adjust the content and pace of the interview without demeaning or infantilizing the person, listen actively and reflect understanding, use appropriate therapeutic touch, and be understanding and helpful when problems occur (e.g., incontinence, loose dentures, sexual overtures). Many residents need affirmation that they are still interesting, attractive people despite their disabilities, and it must be genuine affirmation, not an artificial attempt to be cordial.

Protecting a resident's confidentiality is essential, and this can be complicated, given the numbers of other people working in the facility who believe they have a right to know. At the beginning of the interview the interviewer should have a discussion with the resident about the communication practices of the facility, such as progress notes and care plan meetings, and agree about what information will be communicated and what information can be shared with family. Communication with staff should be in general terms and should focus on information essential to the health and well-being of the resident.

Communication between Clinicians and Patients

The patient's age is precisely what makes clinical interviews an interesting experience. The life history of older patients typically surpasses that of the health professionals, who are usually younger. This age differential may affect

the interviewer's ability to understand and communicate with a patient, despite clinical training. Many generational and historical circumstances influence the patient's behavior and readiness to participate in the diagnostic and treatment process, including acute or chronic traumatic experiences; military service, including exposure to death; the death of a spouse or children; immigration and cultural factors; refugee experiences; natural disasters or terrorism; and abuse and domestic violence.

Patients' attitudes toward health professionals will vary across generations and racial and ethnic groups as well as among individuals (Barry and Beital 2008). The current population of older persons, especially those over age 75, may appear more passive and less assertive about asking questions, motivated by fears of being perceived as disrespectful. Some patients also rely on spouses or children as surrogates for communication. Younger, healthier older persons, who are armed with information and resources from the Internet, may be active, challenging, and even assertive participants in the interview. Many older patients are reluctant or unwilling to talk about personal issues such as sex, economic security, abuse or exploitation, memory, or family issues, particularly on the initial interview. Older men, in contrast to older women, have greater difficulty asking for and accepting help.

Communication styles need to be tailored to the individual. Interviews usually proceed easily with older persons in good physical and mental health who participate readily once they feel a sense of trust and comfort with a clinician. Indeed, keeping the interview flowing but focused can be a challenge when older patients find someone they can confide in and who is interested in them. Frail, very old, and chronically ill patients often require more time and a less formal approach to establish rapport.

The interview process requires expressions of respect, compassion, interest, and support for the older patient. Although the clinician needs to structure the interview to gather appropriate information within a reasonable time frame, it is also important not to dominate the conversation in the interest of speed so as to be unresponsive to themes of concern to older clients. Clinicians who do most of the talking will miss a great deal of relevant information. Clinicians should practice empathic listening and speak to redirect the focus, to clarify specific points, or to support and reassure, as needed.

Nonverbal behaviors such as eye contact, smiling, or nodding are helpful because they are signals of the clinician's attentiveness to the patient. However, some minority groups, such as Asian Americans, avoid eye contact with health professionals. The clinician needs to actively consider older patients' cultural beliefs, behaviors, and practices (Cegala and Post 2006).

Sensory and cognitive impairments are barriers to the clinician's ability to elicit and discuss findings and recommendations. Many older persons present with multiple medical comorbidities and medications that may require more complicated interventions, and the care plan needs to be explained carefully. Clinicians should ensure that older persons and caregivers understand the issues, using techniques such as asking them questions about what was discussed and giving them written materials.

Clinical encounters are often associated with emotional distress, fear of the unknown and known, and anxiety about appearing sick, frail, or weak. Some older persons, even those who are very sick or terminally ill, wish to present themselves as proud, strong, and in control of their problems. Many are fearful of being hospitalized or sent to a nursing home, even if only for rehabilitation, because they may fear that once being admitted, they will never leave.

It is usually helpful to let older patients know that you sense their anxiety, that these feelings are natural, and that almost everyone has them. Letting patients know you understand their fear about seeing a mental health professional and reassuring them that they are not "crazy" and do not need to be "put away" can significantly alter the course of the interview. Clinicians need to be clear about how the clinical interview can be helpful and to emphasize that the patient's privacy will be respected.

Emotional Development in Later Life

Human development and aging are associated with gains and losses. However, in later life, the years ahead are fewer than the years past, and older persons may dwell on lost opportunities rather than future options. Clinicians need to avoid over-empathizing with their patients about their complaints and instead probe for information to understand their strengths and accomplishments. Many older persons remain vital and engaged in personal, family, community, and work activities and remain optimistic, resilient, and satisfied in spite of life changes, illness, limitations, and losses. A significant percentage of older persons support their families financially and instrumentally, for example by caring for grandchildren. The interviewer's challenge is to appreciate the productive roles and responsibilities patients have and can continue to have with good care.

Emotional Well-Being

Clinicians are often surprised when older people report feeling satisfied with life even in the face of significant health concerns. Physical and psychosocial changes may be distressing, yet with help, many older persons are able to shape their environments to fulfill the goals they value most highly and maintain a high level of emotional well-being. Many continue to make productive contributions to their families and community. Older adults frequently maintain a high sense of emotional comfort and life satisfaction because of perceptions that more time is behind than ahead of them (Wade and Frazier 2003). For some, it is this sense of anticipating an end that influences them to derive emotional meaning, savor the present, and spend time with those closest to them. Younger clinicians are often more anxious about the nearness of death than their older patients.

The Ageless Self

Older persons know they are chronologically old, but many perceive themselves as decades younger, what Sharon Kaufman (1994) referred to as having the "ageless self." This psychological state of mind is not a denial of growing older but rather a reflection of a coherent sense of self. Even in advanced age, many older persons regard themselves as the same person they have always been, and this self-perception needs to be appreciated in the clinical setting.

This information allows clinicians to implement two tactics: (1) acknowledge or compliment the individual, creating a positive personal alliance; and (2) structure the conversation to inquire about the specific problems that have adversely affected the patient and precipitated a visit for help. It is not uncommon for patients to deny problems and indicate that they are seeing someone only to appease an insistent spouse or child. Therefore, it is appropriate to inquire why the individual is seeking help and ask what the person believes has upset family members. This approach, demonstrating respect for the patient's strengths while addressing the individual's problems, helps create an atmosphere of trust and empowers the patient to create a therapeutic alliance with the clinician, as the following case illustrates.

MK, an 82-year-old married woman, reluctantly visited her physician, Dr. F, accompanied by her oldest daughter. MK denied that anything was wrong with her and believed that a visit to a psychiatrist was a waste of time because she was old. She had lost 10 pounds in two weeks, stopped her volunteer activities, slept much of the day, and refused invitations to spend time with her daughter and grandchildren. When Dr. F asked MK to describe how old she was in her mind's eye, MK replied: "When I look at myself in the mirror, I cannot believe that wrinkled old woman is me. Until recently, I have always felt like a 40-year-old woman, even though I am 82."

Dr. F encouraged MK to talk about some of her accomplishments and future goals. MK described how proud she was of her family, her career as a high school teacher, and her volunteer work in the county juvenile detention center. Dr. F complimented MK, emphasizing how she admired her emotional strength to work with troubled children. MK replied: "These kids aren't all bad. There are reasons they got into trouble. They are wounded souls who need help, and I think they respond to me because I care about them." When Dr. F praised her ability to relate to these children, she answered "I haven't been very good at it recently. Since I started feeling so tired and down, I don't have the energy to be with them, and I feel old, useless, and empty. Maybe I am the one who is wounded."

Dr. F continued the interview, and MK talked more openly about her depression and the loss of her cat, who had been her cherished companion for more than 18 years. MK also wondered if she would get better so she could go back to helping the kids again. Fortunately, MK was treated successfully for depression and resumed volunteer work at the juvenile detention center.

The Identity Crises of Later Life

Later life is characterized by developmental changes that threaten the integrity of even the most adaptive individuals. Erik Erikson (1956) proposed that the fundamental challenge of old age was the achievement of integrity over despair. Integrity refers to the acceptance of changes, in one's self and in others, with the passage of time. Well-adapted older persons adjust to life changes as they grow older, maintaining or enhancing their identity and capabilities. When ego defense mechanisms wall off painful emotions, they can alter an individual's relationship with others, leading to social isolation.

Erikson proposed that during adolescence there is a gradual process of identity formation as children strive to develop autonomy, but that identity formation also continues in later life. There are vulnerabilities to identity formation in younger years as individuals grow up, but there are also identity crises in later life related to losses, sickness, physical limitations, and other problems.

These assaults on an individual's sense of self may have profound effects on an individual's thoughts, feelings, and actions. The maintenance and preservation of a person's narcissism, a sense of self and ability to validate self-esteem and self-worth, is a major task in coping with ongoing losses in later life. Recognizing and accepting the physical signs of aging and the depletion of physical vigor, even in physically active older persons, can be painful as individuals face changes in work and leisure roles, which may have been pleasurable and fulfilling earlier in life.

Because adapting to these changes is usually associated with threats to body image, self-identity, and self-esteem, changes in the individual's emotional dynamics and interpersonal relationships are likely to occur. It is important for clinicians to discriminate between realistic feelings about growing older and those that are self-destructive. Older people who have coped well in the past often continue to function well, whereas poorly functioning individuals frequently regress and lose adaptive capacity. If this is coupled with developing physical and emotional limitations, such regression results in behaviors and the need for gratifications not previously expressed. Clinicians may observe patients who were once vigorous and independent alternate between a pattern of refusing help and expressing unrealistic denial to becoming dependent and helpless. This regression can also be seen when patients become preoccupied with eating, toileting, and loss of sexual functioning, focusing their energy on those areas of loss that alter and threaten their self-perception.

Clinicians may also discern unusual behaviors such as hoarding what may seem to be meaningless objects. Individuals can invest enormous emotions in the items collected because they have significant symbolic value or because these collections have the ability to comfort, similar to a blanket or stuffed animal retained for years past childhood. Hoarding may also indicate a serious mental health problem, usually one associated with obsessive-compulsive disorder that needs treatment (Matais-Cols et al. 2005; Levin 2008).

Regression may also lead to the manifestation of more primitive behaviors, such as becoming overly demanding, resistant, or aggressive, which would have been uncharacteristic in an earlier period. When these behavioral regressions are observed, interviewers need to identify the person's current underlying needs, conflicts, and cognitive and emotional status, as the following case illustrates.

RD was a cognitively intact 93-year-old nursing home resident who was referred to a psychiatrist by the medical director because the staff could no longer tolerate RD's incessant complaints about his bowels. RD insisted that he had to have a bowel movement at frequent intervals to relieve his constipation, and if this did not occur, he demanded digital rectal examinations. Although his many gastrointestinal examinations did not show any basis for his problems, RD also demanded frequent enemas from the nursing staff. If they were not responsive, RD yelled, complained of bowel pain, stayed in bed, and refused to eat. An interview revealed that he had had a liaison with a female resident in the home with whom he enjoyed frequent sexual gratification, and discussions with staff indicated that the onset of his bowel obsession coincided with her death.

To cope with the emotional pain associated with the deaths of loved ones and perceived losses, older persons may become emotionally isolated and compartmentalized in their thinking. What emerges is an apparent lack of concern about making new friends or replacing tennis or golf partners who have died. When the clinician is discussing painful losses, the older person may become emotionally unavailable and appear resistant or negative during the interview. This behavior may reflect an adaptive way of walling off painful emotions and anxiety. If the interviewer does not recognize this defensive mechanism and encourage the older person to deal with the emotional impact of losses and fears, the interview will become unproductive.

Establishing a Relationship: Transference and Countertransference

The success of any interview depends in large measure on the quality of the relationship that develops between the clinician and the patient (Morgan 2003). The initial objective is to help the patient talk freely about personal concerns and focus on understanding what needs to be done to foster the optimum clinical relationship. Without this alliance, the interviewer may not be able to elicit the information needed to identify the patient's problem(s) and feelings, formulate a diagnosis, and develop a therapeutic strategy. This, in turn, may lead the clinician to rely too heavily on information from informants.

Transference, an unconscious process through which the patient responds emotionally to the interviewer, plays a powerful role. Patients will not only experience the clinician as an individual in the here and now but also will respond with attitudes and emotions stemming from prior relationships with others. The origin of transference feelings may come from any part of an older person's life and be stimulated by any number of clinician-associated variables, including their name, personal appearance, attitude, and affectations as well as verbal and nonverbal responses to the patient. It is common for patients to react to the clinician in positive and negative ways that developed in relation to a child, younger sibling, parent, grandparent, spouse, an erotic object, a business associate, friend, or authority figure. This process also occurs in individuals who have dementia. The cognitively impaired patient may see the interviewer as a long-dead parent or child. A retired business executive who has mild cognitive impairment may react to the clinician as a subordinate and behave in ways that are not appropriate for the interview but would have been in the individual's previous work role.

Many interviews with older persons flounder in the beginning if clinicians are not aware of the transference dynamics. The interview may also begin smoothly but collapse at a later point as these unconscious misidentifications are exacerbated by the clinician's attitude and questions, in turn affecting the patient's thoughts and feelings and eroding her or his ability to have confidence in the interviewer.

With so little known about transference in older persons, interviewers should be guided by a clinical understanding of their clients and may wish to ask questions, such as "I wonder if I remind you of someone?" It is helpful to understand what the patient has been led to expect, and one way to do this is to ask the family what the patient has been told about your professional role (e.g., psychiatrist, internist, and psychologist). Patients will judge the clinician's behavior in the context of their expectations.

A reciprocal unconscious mechanism, countertransference, is also operating during the interactive process in the clinician. Countertransference refers to the process in which the clinician projects personal feelings onto the patient. It is all too easy to experience the older person as a parent, grandparent, or a projection of the older person the clinician is afraid to become. Interviewers need to understand their own reactions to each client. These may include feelings of discomfort or sadness with frail, chronically ill patients, anger toward difficult or hostile clients, repulsion because clients are unattractive, indifference, and other ageist attitudes. Without an understanding of countertransference, it may be difficult for the clinician to engage in a productive interview.

Much closer to consciousness are adverse reactions to patients who are severely ill, emaciated, disfigured, or unkempt as well as noncompliant patients who are obese, are chronically ill, or abuse alcohol. Foul odors from bad breath, poor hygiene, or incontinence, especially in nursing home residents, may be difficult to overcome and may impair the clinician's ability to relate effectively. Even hospitalized older persons can provoke negative reactions, and clinicians may distance themselves because of sights, smells, and sounds (e.g., drooling or cracked lips, caked food on face). Unless interviewers find ways to deal with their reactions, the relationship is threatened. Some circumstances are easy to deal with, for example, by washing the patient's face, while others require clinicians to come to grips with their responsibilities to comfort and care for patients who have significant unmet needs.

Patients, including those who are very sick, can usually sense an interviewer's discomfort and distancing, which increases the fear of rejection and emotional abandonment precisely at the time they need to feel connected. Patients deserve genuine and objective contact and communication. Clinicians who find themselves too emotionally enmeshed, positively or negatively, are well served to discuss their feelings with an experienced colleague. Identifying and sympathizing with the patient's children can also create clinical and ethical problems that require careful self-examination.

Older persons become exquisitely sensitive to the slightest verbal and nonverbal nuances of the interviewer. This sensitivity often relates to the patient's underlying sense of poor self-esteem or fear of being placed in an institutional setting or a more restrictive environment. It is important to avoid comments that may be perceived as critical, intrusive, or overly familiar. A condescending attitude (e.g., using the patient's first name without her or his permission, yet expecting the patient to call you Doctor) establishes an unbalanced power relationship in which patients may be reminded of their powerlessness and respond with anger.

As a patient becomes aware of the interviewer's genuine interest and respect, the initial distance usually melts away. Many older persons have a genuine desire for contact and communication but report a sense of being devalued, ignored, and separated from the mainstream of life. Others may express guilt over being a burden on others or feel so chronically impaired and in pain that death is welcome. Empathic clinicians provide the environment in which such life issues can be discussed.

The interviewer's sense of acceptance, understanding, and concern, coupled with empathy, not pity, communicate clearly to patients. Older people are usually sensitive to artificial involvement and will not participate effectively. This attitude is especially important with cognitively impaired older patients, who usually retain intact nonverbal skills. Interviewers need to understand the patient's use of language as much as possible. This often means using short phrases and simple direct questions, nodding when answers are incoherent, and showing interest in the individual's responses. It is important to give them time to answer, insert words carefully when necessary, repeat or rephrase questions carefully, maintain gentle eye contact, and let the patient know you care about their answers, even when they are nonsensical. These interactions require practice, but when mastered, they foster communication with the full range of cognitively impaired patients.

5

Age-Related Changes in Cognition in Later Life

Age-related changes in cognition have been recognized for about as long as physical aging, and they remain the subject of intense investigations (Salthouse 2004). Some cognitive abilities change while others do not, but little is known about why cognition changes, where this happens in the nervous system relative to other functions, and how it occurs. This is unfortunate, because cognitive functioning is central to optimal aging as a fundamental mediator of meaningful engagement.

Cognitive impairment is not the inevitable consequence of aging after maturity. Some changes in cognitive processing and performance are likely to occur across the lifespan, but aging per se does not cause cognitive losses that significantly affect an individual's ability to function. Declines in cognitive performance may be caused by a variety of factors, including poor nutrition, medical conditions, substance abuse, and trauma. Many such problems may be partially or completely reversible, including those secondary to medications, infections, metabolic and endocrine alterations, malnutrition, isolation, or depression. However, cognitive impairments associated with Alzheimer disease and related dementias are not yet reversible.

Comprehensive reviews of theoretical models of cognitive aging, age-related changes, and the many biopsychosocial and cultural mediators of cognitive aging are covered in excellent references (Craik and Salthouse 2000; Park and Schwarz 2000; Hofer and Alwin 2008). This chapter has three major objectives: (1) to present principles and a conceptual framework for understanding cognition in later life; (2) to review age changes in several aspects of cognition, including intelligence, sensorimotor functioning, memory, and executive functions; and (3) to examine the prospects for cognitive enhancement. Subsequent chapters will review cognitive impairment (chapter 6), Alzheimer disease (chapter 7), and other dementias (chapter 8).

A Framework for Understanding the Aging Mind and Brain

Myths concerning cognition and aging still exist among the general public and health professionals alike. Comments such as "You cannot teach an old dog new tricks" abound. The renowned English historian Arnold Toynbee wrote that two things are inevitable in life—senility and death—but he was only half right. Mild cognitive impairment (MCI) and cognitive losses severe enough to impair functioning, the hallmark of dementia, are not the inevitable consequence of aging. However, erroneous beliefs fuel negative stereotypes about cognitive abilities, treatability, and, however subtle, the value of older persons. These beliefs have also had the unfortunate consequence of normalizing dysfunction, with comments such as "What do you expect at your age?"

The aging brain and mind change, but until recently most research has focused on cognitive deficits and not on cognitive growth, strengths, or the potential for developing compensatory abilities to optimize functioning. Cognition involves many different components that show different trajectories of change over time (Hedden and Gabrieli 2004; Salthouse 2004), and although declines occur in some areas, performance on many measures is characterized by increasing heterogeneity (Martin and Hofer 2004). Individual differences in most cognitive domains are larger among the older population than among younger adults. Many older persons are proficient and accomplished and maintain mental acumen and productive potential throughout life (Fillit et al. 2002; Schaie 2008).

Research advances are improving our understanding of cognitive changes during aging, and the evidence is clear that there are many ways to help older persons maintain and/or improve cognitive acuity (e.g., physical and mental exercise, good nutrition, and cognitive enhancement strategies) (Bielak 2009; Depp et al. 2010). The concept of brain plasticity and the value of cognitive exercise are recent developments and represent a shift in the long-standing belief that the brain loses neurons, limiting the ability of older adults to profit from cognitive training.

A pioneering multisite study demonstrated that certain mental exercises can offset some of the expected decline in cognitive skills and may maintain cognitive abilities needed to do everyday tasks. The Advanced Cognitive Training for Independent and Vital Elderly (ACTIVE) Study is the first randomized, controlled trial to demonstrate long-lasting, positive effects of brief cognitive training in older adults for five years (Ball et al. 2002; Willis et al. 2006; Langbaum et al. 2009). However, training had a limited effect on participants' ability to tackle everyday tasks, with reasoning training leading to less functional decline. The results of ACTIVE also showed that improved cognitive functioning was associated with decreased medical care expenditures (Wolinski et al. 2009).

That it may be possible to enhance cognitive performance for a significant proportion of the population is essential information for clinicians doing preventive care counseling. Indeed, continuing discoveries in the cognitive neurosciences may well eventuate in prescriptions for exercises to strengthen mental resiliency and capacity in later life, exercises paralleling the role of physical exercises for cardiovascular health.

Age-affected cognitive processing reflects changes in specific brain regions (Raz et al. 2005, 2009). Although cognitive performance is usually stable when associated with areas of the brain resistant to age changes, it is also possible that age-related changes in parts

of the brain can lead to a reorganization of functioning that promotes new or enhanced compensatory abilities. For example, functional neuroimaging studies have demonstrated that when older adults performed tasks involving memory systems, different brain regions were activated as compared to younger adults performing the same tasks, and older persons were more likely to show significant bilateral activity in the prefrontal areas (Reuter-Lorenz and Lustig 2005; Dennis and Cabeza 2007). These results suggest new ways of thinking about mechanisms underlying age-related cognitive changes, including the possibility for some brain plasticity across the lifespan.

Neuropathologic and imaging studies have documented a number of other changes in the aging brain, including decreased brain weight, expansion of the sulci, enlarged ventricles, and decreased cerebral blood flow (Raz 2009). However, such changes may be modest, and the functional consequences are unclear. The sensory cortices and the cerebellum show few age-related changes, and no changes are documented in the lower brain areas. The most significant regions of brain changes are the prefrontal cortex, the neostratum of the basal ganglia, and the hippocampus. Although the mechanisms underlying these brain changes have yet to be identified, it is likely that interacting biopsychosocial factors are causative. For example, chronic psychological trauma (e.g., depression, physical abuse) and genetic variables have been implicated in hippocampal thinning (Bremner 2004; Ystad et al. 2009). Age-related changes in neurotransmitters, the distribution of intercellular calcium ions, micro-cerebrovascular changes, and other factors have also been implicated (Raz 2009). The challenge is to identify and clarify the dynamic interrelationships of brain changes, strategies that affect cognitive and behavioral performance, and life history variables as well as psychosocial and environmental influences.

The Institute of Medicine Commission on Behavioral and Social Sciences and Education (Stern and Carstensen 2000) published a comprehensive report about the aging mind, including the presentation of a conceptual framework which posits that the performance of cognitive tasks by older persons is dependent on three interactive systems: healthy neurons and functional connections, the integrity of cognitive structures and processes, and the individual's behavioral, psychosocial, cultural, and environmental context. The aging mind refers to cognitive structures, processes, and content used by older adults, and the use of the term *mind* transcends brain changes and psychometric tests to include cognitive aspects of personal reflections and attributions, behavior, personality, and social interactions.

The commission's framework is based on several postulates:

1. *It is important to identify how individuals function effectively in daily life, not just to clarify factors that alter cognitive performance.* Not only do intelligent thinking and behaviors depend on the exercise of cognitive abilities, including perception, attention, learning, memory, judgment, problem-solving, executive functioning, and language, but also on competency in the performance of life skills, socially appropriate and responsible behavior, and competent work performance.

2. *Many biopsychosocial factors affect the aging mind over the course of an individual's lifetime.* Although healthy neurons are critical for a keen mind, so are social and cultural supports, personal control of decision-making, economic security, a comfortable and safe living environment, adequate nutrition, restorative sleep, and good health. Intellectual and cognitive performance is influenced by an intricate, interactive array of biopsychosocial and environmental factors. The individual's performance, competency, and productivity are the joint expression of growth and declines, and they vary according to differences in individual abilities, personality, life experiences, flexibility, openness to new experiences, personality, and resilience.

3. *The aging mind is adaptable and flexible.* One of the most remarkable characteristics of the aging mind is its plasticity in responding to various environments. Therefore, contextual modifiers affecting development and aging are critical to understand cognitive functioning.

Contextual modifiers refer to biological factors, cultural practices, attributions, power hierarchies, gender bias, patterns of communication, and technologies.

Cognitive Changes in Later Life

Over the years, there have been many studies of the stability and/or decline of cognitive functioning (Craik and Salthouse 2000; Hofer and Alwin 2008). Cross-sectional studies of different age groups have shown a characteristic bell-shaped curve of cognitive performance scores for most abilities, whereas longitudinal studies have revealed maintenance or increases in some abilities and decline in others. Both approaches have been criticized, however, because various age groups or cohorts of older persons included in the study populations have different educational backgrounds, psychosocial and environmental characteristics, historical experiences, medical histories, exposure to trauma, and other experiences. To remedy this, cross-sequential age-cohort designs using overlapping age cohorts followed longitudinally have been used, and the results of numerous studies show a mixed profile of age-related changes in cognition.

Age differences in cognitive performance may be explained by several cohort effects: educational attainment of an age group; length of time since completion of education; test-wiseness more characteristic of younger populations; involvement in stimulating leisure activities, lifetime experiences, and health. Health status may include a wide variety of chronic conditions as well as the longer-term unrecognized brain changes resulting from exposure to diseases (e.g., measles, mumps, and chicken pox) experienced by older cohorts but not by immunized younger cohorts.

The rapid increase in the incidence and prevalence of Parkinson disease and other neurological conditions years after the influenza pandemic of the post–World War I era, 1918–1919, is a prominent public health illustration of an age cohort exposure. Infection and cell destruction from a neurotoxic strain of the influenza virus, coupled with age-related dopaminergic cell loss and other factors, led to increasing numbers of people who had Parkinson symptoms years later (Maurizi 1985; Toovey 2008). When the outbreak of Parkinson disease cases first occurred, it was identified as an age-related increase. Only after the relative incidence of new cases declined decades later was the etiologic role of the pandemic influenza virus on this age cohort identified, refuting the hypothesized direct link between aging and Parkinson disease.

A number of other factors affect cognitive performance throughout development and aging. Early childhood experiences (e.g., nutrition, emotional support, poverty, trauma, enriching and educational activities) as well as diseases and medications, play a role in the manifestation of the cognitive and emotional functioning of middle-aged or older adults. Some experiences may have an immunizing effect, increasing adaptability and resilience, whereas others may be sensitizing, increasing vulnerability in later life. Still other experiences may have a dormant phase and emerge years later with little phenomenological similarity to earlier phases (e.g., general paresis secondary to syphilis). Genetic vulnerabilities may not present until later in life, while others are detected at birth or early in development.

Age-Associated Changes in Selected Cognitive Domains

Cognition is a broad construct encompassing many mental abilities, and recent overviews of cognitive aging have focused on specific components: speed of information processing; explicit memory (i.e., memories of a specific event); inhibition of attention; sensorimotor deficits; executive functioning (e.g., decision-making, planning, and judgment); language and praxis; adaptation and optimization of functioning; expertise and wisdom. A comprehensive analysis of intelligence and cognition as well as intellectual and cognitive changes with aging is beyond the scope of this book, but many excellent references were cited at the beginning of this chapter.

Intelligence

Intelligence batteries usually include tests of vocabulary skills, spatial reasoning, abstraction and judgment, short-term memory, long-term memory, and perceptual motor skills. Intelligence testing is based on a century-old model that was designed to predict scholastic performance (Wechsler 1944). A child's mental age (MA) was defined as the score on a standardized intelligence test using age norms, and the ratio of MA and chronological age (CA) was calculated to derive the child's "intellectual quotient (IQ)," where a score of 100 plus or minus 10 was considered average or normal. Assuming a bell-shaped curve for the distribution of IQ scores, deviations above the norm were identified statistically as lying in the following ranges: High Average, 110–119; Superior, 120–129; and Very Superior, 30 points above the norm or higher. Deviations below the norm included cut-off points for Low Average, 80–89, Borderline, 70–79, and Retarded, 69 or lower.

The concept of mental age was discarded when intelligence tests were developed for adults (Wechsler 1944). Age-related normative scores were created after testing thousands of community subjects of all ages, but the normal distribution curve with statistical cut-off points was retained to identify an individual's age-adjusted IQ. The IQ score has remained as a description of ability, or perhaps more accurately, the ability to succeed academically, although some subtests have been criticized for sociocultural and linguistic biases.

Despite such criticism, intelligence tests are valuable for estimating overall cognitive performance during clinical evaluations (e.g., diagnosis of dementia, capacity evaluations) because intelligence tests involve a cluster of subtests that tap into various abilities with differential vulnerabilities to change. When intelligence tests are administered appropriately, the pattern of test scores will identify changes from premorbid levels of overall cognitive functioning to the current level of assessed intellectual functioning.

Although IQ scores remain relatively stable into later life in the absence of serious health problems, several studies have described a steady terminal drop in IQ scores, averaging five years before death, with wide variability in the length of terminal decline, ranging from 1 to 14 years (Rabbit et al. 2006; Wilson 2008). It is not clear whether this is a general decline or whether selective components are affected.

There are many causes of terminal decline. Different medical conditions could mediate differential losses in the period before death, and it is possible that there may be a generalized effect of aging. However, marked and often rapid intellectual deterioration signals biological and psychological changes leading to death. The results of a prospective study from the Kungsholmen Project in Stockholm (Fratiglioni et al. 2007; www.kungsholmenproject.se) showed that much of the terminal decline in cognition was associated with preclinical dementia.

Numerous studies have reported consistent age-associated changes in two broad domains of intelligence, crystallized and fluid intelligence, first described by Horn and Cattell (1967; Cattell 1987). Crystallized intelligence describes skills that are well learned as a result of being practiced frequently throughout life, and these skills reflect mastery of social and cultural knowledge. Tests of vocabulary, general information, verbal analogies, and verbal memory are examples of measures of crystallized intelligence, and performance scores remain stable or improve in later life. Fluid intelligence relies significantly on information processing abilities, including the ability to detect relationships among items, the speed of analyzing information accurately, and the capacity of working memory. Test items that reflect fluid intelligence include spatial visualization and reasoning, perceptual speed, picture sequencing, and number series, and these scores are more likely to change in older persons over time, likely reflecting brain changes and adverse biological and psychosocial factors.

The crystallized/fluid intelligence model has proved to be useful for identifying the components of age-associated change as well as testing interrelationships of cognitive domains as performance improves or declines (Kaufman et al. 2006). Although factors most reliant on fluid intelligence may decline in middle age, the decreases in information processing may not be significant enough to influence many crystallized skills until late in life. The more a specific ability depends on fluid intelligence, the earlier it begins to decline. However, the maintenance of crystallized intelligence in accrued knowledge, experience, and expertise can offset losses in fluid intelligence. Likewise, many mixed crystallized/fluid factors may not be significantly affected in later life, especially in adults who have high educational attainment and stay intellectually and physically active. Finally, older persons who maintain high levels of intellectual performance use "selective optimization with compensation," a process of focusing on specific, personally meaningful goals and finding new ways to use their strengths to compensate for losses (Baltes and Smith 2003).

Even with age-related changes in some cognitive skills, there is no clear relationship between age and work performance across various jobs (Charness 2008; Fisk et al. 2009). Many older persons perform well in the workplace, reflecting years of experience using the strategies and skills required for a particular set of job-related responsibilities. However, older persons working in jobs that rely heavily on fluid intelligence skills (e.g., learning new computer programs) may have performance problems. Older persons do well in self-paced tasks compared to tasks that must be completed quickly. Changed work tasks and responsibilities may be more difficult for some older persons when phenomenological aspects of the new setting are similar to the old but new and different responses are required.

Sensorimotor Functioning

Age-related changes in sensory perception and motor functions are well documented, and they may influence measured cognitive performance if not detected and corrected (Lia and Lindenberger 2002). Decrements in visual, auditory, olfactory, and kinesthetic senses occur over time, but significant individual differences are observed in the rate of change (Spirduso et al. 2005).

Vision

Visual changes usually occur after age 40, and the vast majority of older persons over age 65 have corrected visual acuity in at least one eye. Impaired vision results from a reduction in light reaching the retina caused by yellowing of the lens, shrinking of the pupil, clouding of the vitreous, and cell loss in the retina and optic nerve. Dark adaptation is more difficult, and depth perception can be problematic due to impaired binocular vision. Presbyopia (i.e., blurred near vision when doing tasks such as reading or writing) stems from changes in the proteins in the lens leading to a gradual decreased flexibility. It usually begins in the 40s and is a correctable condition with reading glasses or eye surgery.

Visual difficulties have an impact on the confidence and daily performance of older adults in almost all daily activities (Rudberg et al. 1993). Visual impairments severe enough to significantly hinder daily living occur in about a third of persons age 85 or older (Congdon et al. 2004). This means that older persons are more dependent on the environmental context (e.g., level of illumination, size of an image, time to recognize people and places).

Hearing

Hearing impairment is caused by stiffening of the eardrum and other membranes as well as cell death and cerebrovascular changes in the inner ear and auditory cortex. High frequencies are most affected, and complex tone discrimination becomes more difficult. Impaired speech perception is common after age 70, and the inability to perceive the content and emotional context of speech adversely affects life satisfaction.

Exposure to very loud noises over the lifespan or during some period earlier in life may cause subsequent hearing impairment. This may lead to permanent deficits that are not readily perceived by the individual, as would be the case with visual loss, resulting in problems with interpersonal communication.

Hearing aids may be useful but are not always completely effective in restoring comfortable hearing. Many older persons find hearing aids undesirable for various reasons: they may deny having hearing loss, find the devices uncomfortable, or report that hearing is even more distorted. Hearing aids may improve hearing in a low noise environment but make it worse in high noise environments. Microelectronic instrumentation has improved the effectiveness of hearing aids by reducing extraneous noise through the use of focused microphones and programming devices specific to a person's auditory needs. Surgical interventions that bypass the middle ear may improve hearing in some people when hearing aids are not effective.

Because hearing loss may result in the raising of the absolute threshold for sound, individuals who have this form of recruitment deafness barely hear, but when they ask others to "speak up," they may experience being admonished for shouting. The result is often a reluctance to communicate, resulting in a feeling of isolation. Clinicians need to establish the general level of hearing ability during each examination. One way to do this is to ask permission to stand behind the person, talk softly near each ear, have him or her repeat what was heard, and increase speech volume as necessary.

Touch

Sensitivity to touch changes significantly in the hands, especially the fingertips, but alterations are not as great in other areas of the body. Decreased touch sensitivity is due to the loss of touch receptors and decreased blood circulation in the extremities. Visually impaired adults who rely on Braille will have trouble with the spacing of letters and therefore their ability to understand.

Motor Functions

The speed of responses—spoken or manual—can be used to assess motor performance. Age effects are negligible for simple reaction time, but slowing occurs in choice reaction time tasks as well as the planning and execution of complex movements. An individual's physical fitness and health status may also affect motor performance. Musculoskeletal changes account for only a small amount of the slowing seen in motor activities.

Memory

The literature on cognitive aging has focused on memory impairment and the neural substrate of age-related memory changes. However, measuring the impact of aging on memory is a challenge for at least four reasons: (1) there are many dimensions of memory that are affected by different factors; (2) apparent declines in memory may be secondary to age-related psychomotor and sensory changes that affect assessment but are unrelated to memory per se; (3) many biopsychosocial and environmental variables affect memory functioning; and (4) there is a large range of variability in what is considered normal performance.

Memory is the mental mechanism by which we store information to be used at a subsequent time. Various parts of the brain are responsible for different memory functions, and the integrity and interactions of all parts of the brain's memory systems are required for normal memory functioning. Because memory is complex, it is important to review its various components to understand what parts of the brain are involved in effective processing and to appreciate what brain areas are vulnerable to pathology.

Information is processed through working memory for immediate use. The encoding phase of the memory process does not seem to deteriorate with age nor does the ability to store information briefly. Remote or long-term memory for material that is overlearned and procedural memory for well-rehearsed motor tasks are also relatively stable. Secondary memory (i.e., memory for recent events) is more vulnerable to age effects, especially when a large quantity of information needs to be mastered.

Budson and Price (2005a, 2005b) reviewed four memory systems that are clinically signifi-cant for understanding the diagnosis and treatment of memory disorders: episodic memory, semantic memory, procedural memory, and working memory. Some systems (e.g., episodic and semantic) are experienced consciously (i.e., are explicit), and recall is a conscious process (i.e., declarative). Other systems (e.g., procedural) are manifest by a change in behavior (i.e., are implicit) and are usually unconscious processes (i.e., nondeclarative).

Episodic Memory

Episodic memory is an explicit and declarative memory system used to recall personal experiences in the world (e.g., how to change a tire, remember a news story). Successful episodic memory performance depends on the integrity of the medial temporal lobes, including the hippocampus and the parahippocampus, the frontal lobes, and other parts of the brain (Tulving 2002). Abnormalities in any of these structures may impair episodic memory functioning.

The subtypes of episodic memory deficits reflect the location of brain lesions (e.g., damage to the frontal lobes versus damage to the medial temporal lobes). Budson and Price (2005) described a clinically useful heuristic framework. The frontal lobes, which are important for attending to and encoding information sent to the medial temporal lobes, can be conceptualized as the "file clerk" of the episodic memory system. The medial temporal lobes are analogous to the "recent memory file cabinet," and other cortical regions function as a "remote memory file cabinet." Thus, although patients diagnosed with either depression or Alzheimer disease may have impaired episodic memory, the former have a dysfunctional file clerk and the latter have a dysfunctional recent memory file cabinet.

Semantic Memory

Semantic memory is a declarative and explicit memory system, which refers to a person's overall knowledge of the world, not related to specific episodic memories (e.g., the last president of the United States). The inferolateral temporal lobes are core structures for semantic memory, although other cortical areas may be involved, depending on the types of knowledge being accessed (Chao 2001). Alzheimer disease is the most common disorder disrupting semantic memory, but semantic and episodic memory decline independently in patients who have this disease. Any disorder or condition that damages the inferolateral temporal lobes (e.g., strokes, tumors) can impair semantic memory.

Procedural Memory

Procedural memory refers to the ability to learn behavioral and cognitive skills as well as algorithms that are processed at an automatic, unconscious level. It is nondeclarative, but when skills are being acquired, they may be explicit (e.g., learning to drive a motorcycle) or implicit (e.g., learning a sequence of numbers on a cell phone without conscious effort). Functional imaging studies have revealed that the supplementary motor area, basal ganglia, and cerebellum, all core areas in procedural memory, become active as a new task is being learned (Ullman 2004). Because the cortical and limbic areas of the brain are affected in early stages of Alzheimer disease but not the basal ganglia and cerebellum, patients manifest impairment of episodic memory but have intact procedural memory performance.

Working Memory

Working memory refers to the ability to momentarily preserve and control information (e.g., remembering a new phone number). It is an explicit and declarative memory system that relies on the prefrontal cortex as well as a network of cortical and subcortical areas of the brain, depending on the task at hand (Haxby et al. 2000). For example, if a person is listening to driving directions, the posterior visual-association areas would be coupled to form a circuit with the prefrontal regions. More regions on the left side of the brain are activated during phonologic tasks, whereas spatial working memory involves more regions on the right side (Fletcher and Henson 2001). However, bilateral brain activation occurs when more complex spatial or verbal tasks are

being processed in working memory, and the number of activated regions in the prefrontal cortex increases with the increasing complexity of the task (Rypma et al. 2001).

Alzheimer disease, related dementias, and any disorder that interferes with frontal lobe functioning and connections to the posterior cortex and subcortex impair working memory. Other psychiatric disorders that impair attention (e.g., obsessive-compulsive disorder, schizophrenia, depression) may also affect the working memory system.

Executive Functioning

Executive functioning is involved in controlling or organizing other cognitive operations; however, there is no consensus about what executive functioning is and how it is measured (Salthouse 2005). Definitions of this construct assume that executive functions consist of a set of distinct skills that include choosing and initiating goals, understanding consequences of goals, producing multiple response options, monitoring and changing behaviors when circumstances change, and functioning well with distractions. Executive functions are frequently regarded as the most complicated cognitive abilities focused on the planning and organization of purposeful, goal-directed behaviors. Because many aspects of executive functioning appear to be affected in individuals who have frontal lobe damage, these abilities have been associated with frontal lobe functioning.

Many investigators have hypothesized that executive functioning and fluid intelligence are closely related, and Salthouse (2005) demonstrated that tests of executive functioning are associated with tests of reasoning and perceptual speed. It remains to be seen whether executive functioning skills are a distinct group of cognitive skills. In spite of the theoretical and empirical questions, a number of neuropsychological tests can be used to evaluate the executive functioning abilities of persons who have Alzheimer disease or related dementias. These tests may include tests of judgment, verbal fluency, sorting, alternation tasks, and proverb interpretation.

The Future of Research in Cognitive Aging

At least three groups of hypotheses have been advanced to explain declines in cognitive functions with advancing age (Hofer and Alwin 2008): psychological theories about common mediators of cognitive decline such as slowing and sensory acuity; biological models, which focus on changes in the brain and other organ systems; and socioenvironmental theories about how social and environmental factors account for cognitive and health disparities as well as differences in rates of change. These disciplinary approaches are related to one another, and therefore interdisciplinary approaches to the study of cognition and aging are needed.

The magnitude of the increased number of older people in the United States and the rest of the world makes the study of how population dynamics affect cognitive aging a global priority (Hofer and Alwin 2008). Most of the research findings about cognitive aging are based on studies of populations born in the early part of the last century, and it is reasonable to question whether what is known about previous historical influences on cognitive performance applies to later cohorts.

The inevitability of cognitive decline is controversial, and this is another priority research area. As discussed earlier, a considerable body of research documents changes in a number of cognitive domains, substantial heterogeneity in the patterns and extent of change, and stability and growth in other cognitive areas. Some argue that the concept of normal cognitive aging has little value and that cognitive decline reflects a non-normal process that may be subject to intervention. This viewpoint is consistent with evidence that populations showing certain types of cognitive declines may be at increased risk for dementia.

Scientific research reflects values and biases as well as theoretical and empirical rigor. Many clinicians and investigators have contended that priorities should be shifted from cognitive decline to cognitive success and successful aging, and the NIA established a Cognitive and Emotional Health Project to examine the biopsychosocial predictors of cognitive and emotional health with advancing age (Hendrie et al. 2006; Laditka et al. 2009). Interdisciplinary longitudinal studies are essential to tackle the complex challenges of understanding the interrelationships of brain health, physical health, behavioral health, environmental health, and cognitive functioning. Our aging global populations' vitality and productivity depend on new advances in cognitive aging research.

Cognitive Impairment in Older Persons

Older persons who complain of mild cognitive problems may be experiencing a transient problem due to stressful circumstances, the adverse effects of medications, or an anxiety or depressive disorder. They may also be in denial about significant cognitive losses or in the early stages of a condition that will ultimately lead to a dementia. This chapter provides an overview of cognitive impairment ranging from mild deficits to more severe but reversible conditions, including delirium, and then reviews clinical approaches to assess and diagnose cognitively impaired individuals.

Kral (1962) first described a condition called benign senescent forgetfulness, but relatively little research was done, perhaps because it was identified as benign. Other terms were subsequently used to identify mild cognitive problems, including age-associated memory decline or memory deficit, age-related cognitive decline, and age-associated memory impairment (AAMI). AAMI has prevailed as the most commonly used description of mild losses attributed to age since the NIMH consensus conference in 1986 (Crook et al. 1986). AAMI is defined as a mild decline in memory that is not progressive but presents with a measurable deficit in concentration, attention, learning, thinking, or use of language. However, the measured memory deficit is not more than one standard deviation below the mean performance of a younger adult population.

With increasing clinical and research interest in dementia, including the prospect of treatment and even prevention on the horizon, a focus on diagnostic markers for early stages of Alzheimer disease and related disorders or of milder forms of cognitive problems has emerged as a significant research priority. The results of brain imaging studies indicate that subtle biological changes underlying Alzheimer disease and other dementias may occur decades before the cognitive symptoms become manifest (Nestor et al. 2004; Desikan et al. 2009). The clinical value of early detection lies in the possibility of preventing or treating cognitive impairment by ameliorating its biologic substrate.

Mild Cognitive Impairment

The belief that "senility" is a normal consequence of aging has been discarded, spurring greater interest in the pathology of cognition, including the construct now widely referred to as Mild Cognitive Impairment (MCI). The term MCI was coined in the 1980s by the New York University Medical Center group, and it has been studied intensively since then (Petersen 2003). There is growing consensus that MCI is not a "normal" condition, nor is it dementia, but it is characterized by subjective complaints of cognitive problems and objective evidence of cognitive impairment greater than expected for an individual's age and education. There are two subtypes of MCI: *amnestic,* which is characterized by memory impairment, and *nonamnestic,* which is characterized by deficits in one or more cognitive domains (Petersen and Morris 2005). An individual whose only complaint is memory loss would be described as having "amnestic MCI, single domain," and a person with memory deficits and complaints of other cognitive problems would be classified as having "amnestic MCI, multiple domains." If an individual complains of cognitive problems in areas other than memory, that person would be categorized as having "nonamnestic MCI," with either single or multiple domains. The deficits of both amnestic and nonamnestic MCI are not severe enough to interfere with functioning (Ganguli et al. 2004; Artero et al. 2006).

There is significant variability in the criteria used for the various types of MCI (Petersen and Morris 2005; Portet et al. 2006). Different clinical trial and laboratories use differing neuropsychological tests and statistical cut-off scores, but it is generally accepted that persons who have MCI show performance scores of at least 1.5 standard deviations below the mean on one or more cognitive tasks as compared to age-matched control populations.

The prevalence rate for MCI varies considerably, depending on the criteria used to define it. Prevalence estimates range from 3 to 20 percent (Ganguli et al. 2004; Portet et al. 2006). Results from a population-based sample showed that the prevalence of MCI was 19 percent in adults over age 75, and incidence rates were 1–1.5 percent each year, with depression, increasing age, and lower education implicated as risk factors (Lopez et al. 2003).

Clinical Evaluation for Mild Cognitive Impairment

Because so many factors can adversely affect cognitive performance, a careful clinical assessment is essential to rule out contributing problems (Petersen and Morris 2005; Gauthier et al. 2006; Chertkow et al. 2009). If a clinician thinks a patient meets the criteria for MCI, the patient should be monitored longitudinally with measures of functional effectiveness and neuropsychological tests. The Quality Standards Subcommittee of the American Academy of Neurology recommended guidelines for evaluating and monitoring individuals who have MCI (Petersen et al. 2001). Several screening instruments and specific cognitive tests were recommended, including the Mini-Mental State Examination (MMSE, Folstein et al. 1975), the Kokemen Short Test of Mental Status (Kokemen et al. 1991), the Memory Impairment Screen for Dementia (Buschke et al. 1999), and the 7-Minute battery (Solomon et al. 1998). Other informant-based instruments were recommended, including those useful with illiterate and non-English-speaking persons such as the Informant Questionnaire on Cognitive Decline in the Elderly (IQCODE, Fuh et al. 1995), the Blessed-Roth Dementia

Scale (Blessed et al. 1988), and the Clinical Dementia Rating (CDR, Morris 1997). A short neuropsychological battery of tests provides a profile of deficits to make the distinctions between amnestic and nonamnestic, single and multiple-domain, MCI.

The research findings from multicenter national and international clinical trials since the 1991 guidelines have led to a consensus that new guidelines are necessary to disaggregate MCI subtypes (Moreira et al. 2008). The Alzheimer's Disease Cooperative Clinical Trial on MCI used very precise criteria, and 212 of the 214 participants who progressed from MCI to dementia were diagnosed with probable or possible Alzheimer disease (Grundman et al. 2004).

Mild Cognitive Impairment as a Transition Syndrome for Dementia?

Some investigators believe that MCI is a precursor to Alzheimer disease because between 40 and 80 percent of persons who meet the criteria for MCI develop Alzheimer disease over a five-year period, a rate of up to 10–15 percent a year compared to a rate of 1–2 percent in age-matched controls (Fischer et al. 2007; Chertkow et al. 2009). Others suggest that the conversion rate is much lower and cite the finding that a subgroup of persons who met the criteria for MCI at one point in time was normal at follow-up 12 years later. A meta-analysis of 19 longitudinal studies published between 1991 and 2001 showed an average rate of conversion of 10 percent, but there was significant variability (Bruscoli and Lovestone 2004). Two patterns of conversion emerged: (1) patients in outpatient medical clinics had higher conversion rates than studies using volunteer community residents; and (2) baseline cognitive performance scores were much lower in persons who converted from MCI to dementia than in those who remained classified with MCI.

Although the high rate of conversion may be interpreted as evidence that MCI is a prodromal stage of Alzheimer disease, the lack of 100 percent conversion suggests that a subtype of MCI, as yet undefined, may represent people who have a developing dementia. The pathophysiology of MCI has yet to be determined, and it is not clear that there is a single pathway for its expression and progression (Petersen 2003).

Treatment

The importance of MCI as a possible precursor of Alzheimer disease has been fueled in large measure by the increasing availability of cognitive-acting medications that have limited effectiveness in slowing the progression of Alzheimer disease. If it turns out that some forms of MCI (e.g., the amnestic type) is early Alzheimer disease, neuroprotective drugs may modify its progression and prevent or postpone decline. However, to date, there is no proven pharmacological treatment for MCI (Chertkow et al. 2009; Weiner and Lipton 2009). In a large study of patients who have MCI and controls, vitamin E had no effect on conversion rates from MCI to Alzheimer disease (Petersen et al. 2005). In the same study, donepezil was associated with a lower rate of progression to Alzheimer disease during the first year of treatment, but after three years, the rate of conversion was similar to patients treated with a placebo. There are also no clinically tested nonpharmacologic interventions for MCI despite the body of research supporting the value of cognitive and physical exercise to improve cognitive functioning in older populations (Chertkow et al. 2009).

A systematic review of randomized trials of the effectiveness on MCI of three cholinesterase inhibitors approved for use in Alzheimer disease (see chapter 7)—donepezil, rivastigmine, and galantamine—showed slight but marginal improvement in cognition and functioning (Raschetti et al. 2007; Raina et al. 2008). Furthermore, there are safety risks associated with the use of these medications in the MCI population. The uncertainty about MCI as a clinical syndrome has raised clinical and ethical questions about the value of drug trials (Karlawish 2009). At this time there is no consensus about clinical value of MCI, but further biopsychosocial research may clarify its clinical utility (Allegri et al. 2008). Ellison

(2008) urged the importance of developing evidence-based evaluation and treatment of MCI, including the management of co-morbid disorders and lifestyle behaviors.

Diagnosis of Dementia

Dementia refers to a loss of memory and other aspects of cognition from a previously higher level of functioning leading to functional impairment in an individual who is not acutely ill or delirious. Dementia and Alzheimer disease are not the same, although the general public and many clinicians often confuse the two terms. Alzheimer disease is a disorder with dementia as its hallmark feature, and it is the most prevalent of the late-life dementias, perhaps contributing to the confusion in terminology.

The two most commonly used classification systems to diagnose dementia are the American Psychiatric Association's DSM-IV-TR criteria and those established by a scientific task force of the National Institute of Neurological and Communicative Disorders and Stroke and the Alzheimer's Associations—NINCDS-ADRDA—Work Group (McKhann et al. 1984). The DSM-IV-TR and NINCDS-ADRDA criteria have been validated using neuropathological criteria with diagnostic accuracies ranging from 65–96 percent, but the specificity of these criteria with regard to other dementias is 23–88 percent (Dubois et al. 2007).

Both criteria are outdated in the light of the unprecedented growth of scientific knowledge. There are now reliable biomarkers of Alzheimer disease using structural magnetic resonance imaging (MRI), molecular neuroimaging with positron emission tomography (PET), and cerebrospinal fluid analyses. This progress was the basis for an international consensus paper that revised diagnostic criteria were necessary to identify the earliest stages and the full spectrum of the illness (Dubois et al. 2007). The criteria proposed include measures of early and significant episodic memory impairment and the presence of at least one or more abnormal biomarkers among structural neuroimaging with MRI, molecular neuroimaging with PET, and cerebrospinal fluid analysis of amyloid β or tau proteins. Clinical studies are necessary to evaluate these criteria and test their sensitivity, specificity, and accuracy.

Several excellent clinical resources describe criteria for the differential diagnosis of the dementias, including the clinical examinations and laboratory tests:

• American Psychiatric Association Practice Guidelines: www.psychiatryonline.com/pracGuide/pracGuideTopic_3.aspx
• American Academy of Neurology Guidelines: www.aan.com/professionals/practice/pdfs/gl0071.pdf

The American Geriatrics Society website has a list of tools for assessing and managing memory loss in primary practice (http://dementia.americangeriatrics.org). These tools include guidelines for patient evaluation, screening instruments, detailed forms to record results, and resource materials for patients and caregivers.

Because detailed accounts of the examinations and tests for differential diagnosis are specified in the consensus guidelines, the basic components of the diagnostic procedures are described briefly below. Most of these clinical evaluations and screening tests and measures areas are also reviewed in chapter 3.

Physical Examination

A comprehensive physical examination should include a review of all organ systems and an assessment of overall hygiene, nutrition and hydration, falls/gait and balance problems, signs of injury, and/or suspicious indications of possible elder abuse or neglect.

Blood Chemistries

Laboratory tests should be done with follow-up if abnormalities are identified: blood cell count and cobalamin to exclude infections, including HIV/AIDS and hematological diseases; liver enzymes to rule out hepatic disease; blood cortisol to exclude adrenal disease; thyroid stimulating hormone to exclude thy-

roid disease; rapid plasma reagent to rule out syphilis; and vitamins B_6 and B_{12} to exclude vitamin deficiencies.

EEG Studies

An EEG may identify tumors, seizures, and other causes of dementia such as encephalopathies and prion-related disorders.

Cerebrospinal Fluid Tests

A lumbar puncture may be done when the clinician suspects conditions such as normal pressure hydrocephalus, syphilis, cryptococcosis, or other central nervous system infection.

History

A personal history as well as family medical and lifestyle histories are valuable to identify health status, genetic vulnerabilities, risk factors, exposure to toxicants, exposure to head trauma due to occupational or recreational activities, and health practices that contribute to illness patterns. The history of the problem should be documented to identify the time of onset of recent memory losses, especially disorientation and confusion, as well as other symptoms, including language, visuospatial, motor problems, and personality changes.

Medications

An accurate history of current and recent prescription medications, especially pain and psychotropic medications, and over-the-counter medications, herbals, and vitamin supplements, as well as the use/misuse of alcohol and other substances is important.

Neurological Examination

A neurological examination is necessary to evaluate the integrity of the central nervous system. Some of the tests used in the mental status exam may overlap with the psychiatric evaluation.

Psychiatric Examination

A structured psychiatric examination focuses on mental status, which includes an evaluation of the patient's appearance, level of consciousness, mood and affect, perception, and cognitive abilities, including attention, memory, abstract reasoning, judgment, and language. It involves a clinical history and interview, usually using one or more assessment measures, to identify the history and presence of comorbid psychopathology.

Mental Status Tests and Neuropsychological Tests

Mental status screening assessments, psychological testing, and neuropsychological testing are essential to document cognitive impairments. The screening instruments reviewed in chapter 3 are frequently used to determine the presence and severity of overall deficits. The results of additional psychological testing are important for differential diagnosis as well as to identify the profile of a patient's cognitive strengths and weaknesses. A battery of neuropsychological tests is valuable to identify specific cognitive domains related to functioning in specific areas of the brain. Although neuroimaging techniques inform about structural and metabolic changes in the brain, only neuropsychological testing describes how the brain is functioning in specific cognitive domains.

At a minimum, the neuropsychological battery should include premorbid intellectual functioning estimated from level of educational and occupational attainment, current intellectual functioning assessed using an intelligence test, perceptual and motor skills, attention, visual and semantic memory, susceptibility to interference in learning and memory tasks, executive functioning, and language skills. In addition to the cognitive assessment, certain aspects of personality need to be evaluated to identify symptoms of personality disorders.

Functional Assessment

A comprehensive functional assessment of impairments in activities of daily living (ADLs) and instrumental activities of daily living (IADLs) will identify personal limitations resulting from the dementia as well as other medical disorders and conditions (see chapter 3). Direct assessment of functional performance (McDougall et al. 2001) as well

as detailed interviews with caregivers provides valuable information.

Imaging Studies

Routine imaging studies should include computerized tomography (CT) scans and magnetic resonance imaging (MRI). MRI imaging reveals changes in brain volume as well as brain chemistry. Many dementias that appear clinically similar to Alzheimer disease have different images and characteristics on the MRI (e.g., frontal lobe dementias, Lewy body dementia). Although functional MRIs are not routinely used at this time, they are likely to be increasingly valuable.

Positron emission tomography (PET) studies have shown a significant reduction in glucose metabolism in different regions of the brain of patients who have Alzheimer disease, and patients in early stages show decreased glucose metabolism in the posterior temporoparietal region. However, patients who have arteriosclerosis of the brain show a similar pattern of glucose metabolic changes, so the differential diagnostic value awaits further specification. A clinical tutorial using the PET scan in Alzheimer disease as well as detailed information about PET scan can be found at www.radiolog.ru/pet/lpp/clinpetneuro/alzheimers.html.

Imaging modalities reveal the structural and metabolic condition of the brain, but only a neuropsychological test battery will show the brain's functioning. Correlations between experimental behavioral tasks as well as neuropsychological test scores and functional brain imaging in laboratory settings are a source of important new information about precise areas of the brain affected with specific cognitive dysfunction.

Potentially Reversible Dementias

Approximately 30 percent of patients who see a physician for the first time with concerns about serious memory problems have a reversible or partially reversible cause for their complaints. The major causes are listed below.

Infections

Infections, especially urinary tract infections, change the body's metabolism, cause pain, and influence the way an individual behaves. Older individuals who have even a modest infection may become confused and lethargic, even delirious, eat sparingly, and find little pleasure in social activities. They may refuse to answer questions and become angry or aggressive. Because older persons may have problems regulating body temperature, they may show only a small rise, or no rise, in body temperature, even with serious infection.

Metabolic and Nutritional Disorders

Many physical disorders cause intellectual and emotional problems. Patients who have hypothyroid dysfunction may feel fatigued, have difficulty concentrating, and become forgetful and depressed. A disturbance in the body's electrolyte balance, resulting from dehydration or too much fluid consumption, kidney problems, or the use of drugs like diuretics, may cause a change in mental state. Poorly controlled diabetes may also lead to behavioral disturbances and mimic dementia.

The nutritional health of older persons may be compromised by many factors, including economic circumstances, social isolation, or dental health problems. Older people may have difficulty purchasing or preparing food because of poor access to transportation, limited mobility, physical frailty, or mental health problems. Eating is also a social activity. The same meals eaten night after night following the loss of a spouse or the death of close friends are lonely occasions. Under the influence of depression and dysphoria, tea and toast can become just tea, with significant long-term negative consequences.

Poisoning

Poisoning may cause cognitive problems in older persons, and certain occupations are at particular risk (e.g., farmers, miners, and painters). Pesticides such as arsenic used in gardening, particularly indoor gardening, can have toxic effects as can other substances containing lead or other heavy metals in the home. High consumption of seafood may be problematic because of high levels of mercury in certain fish.

Cardiovascular and Pulmonary Diseases

Cardiovascular and pulmonary disorders may contribute to cognitive losses, apathy, and other behavioral changes. Because the cardiovascular system plays a central role delivering oxygen and nutrients to the body, eliminating carbon dioxide, and maintaining a constant body temperature, a decrease in the working performance of the heart and blood vessels or impaired oxygen exchange in the lungs will affect the amount of oxygen and other nutrients that reach the brain, compromising neuronal integrity.

Many vascular problems, such as high blood pressure, arrhythmias, severe heart disease, and arteriosclerosis in the cerebral blood vessels, affect memory and learning. Although not everyone who has cardiovascular disease develops intellectual deficits, the potential vascular basis for a change in mental status deserves a careful evaluation. Some of these conditions can be treated successfully, thereby partially or completely reversing the cognitive changes.

Medications

The side effects of prescribed medications are probably the most common cause of reversible cognitive impairment in older adults. If they are identified early, the disturbances can usually be corrected. Diuretics used in the treatment of high blood pressure may cause an electrolyte imbalance and subsequent cognitive difficulties. Long-term use of drugs such as digitalis, thyroid, and insulin can lead to problems because they have side effects which cause losses in cognitive abilities in some persons.

Visual and/or Hearing Loss

Older persons who have sensory impairment, especially very old and/or frail persons, may appear unable to answer questions. Clinicians should evaluate sensory functioning to avoid the erroneous conclusion that failure to respond appropriately indicates the existence of a major memory problem. Hearing loss, which is common, particularly among older men, is often subtle and difficult to detect. Indeed, while individuals can see that they have visual problems, those who are hearing impaired may be unaware of the extent of the dysfunction. Older persons who have known hearing loss may not use their hearing aids or may fail to replace batteries as needed and appear more cognitively impaired than is actually the case.

Depression and Emotional States

A range of emotional disorders may impair thinking and intellectual performance, and it can be a diagnostic challenge to determine whether a severely depressed or anxious person has an irreversible brain disease causing dementia or a severe, but reversible, emotional condition. Depressed individuals may be apathetic and unresponsive, while others are restless and agitated. In most cases, memory is affected and activities of daily living are performed with greater difficulty. Persons who are suspicious or paranoid are usually concerned about the purpose of an examination or interview, and they may respond with no answers or describe stories of being poisoned, sexually manipulated, or visited by aliens.

Isolation and Sensory Deprivation

Older persons who live alone, are homebound, or are institutionalized may experience deprivation of human touch, activity, and excitement. This lack of meaningful human interactions has a potent effect, and the individual may become unresponsive, forgetful, or confused.

Patients who have hearing deficits and live in relative isolation may become suspicious, and indeed paranoid, with the result that they do not cooperate during an interview. They may not answer questions because they do not understand them or because they distrust the examiner and/or fear that the purpose of the examination is to "put them away."

Structural Damage in the Brain

A thorough psychiatric and neurological examination, including a CT scan or MRI, may be needed to determine whether structural damage is causing dementia. For example, older patients admitted to the emergency room at night with confusion and disorientation often have a history of falling and sustaining a subdural hematoma, but they do not recall the incident or their family may not have observed it. Following a fall, a subdural hematoma can cause increasing pressure inside the skull with concomitant confusion and delirium. However, if the blood leakage is slow enough, cognitive impairments may occur.

Tumors are another potential cause of structural damage to the brain. Tumors may be insidious and remain undetected for a long time. The first sign may be subtle cognitive losses and personality changes as reflected in poor emotional control and agitated behaviors.

Normal-pressure hydrocephalus (NPH), first described by Hakim and Adams (1965), has received much attention because it is sometimes reversible (www.allaboutnph.com; www.emedicine.com/NEURO/topic277.htm). NPH is rare: only about 5,000 cases are diagnosed annually in the United States. Although it is unusual in persons over age 65, it reportedly occurs in 5 to 6 percent of those with dementia under age 65.

There are two major forms of hydrocephalus: primary and secondary. In secondary hydrocephalus, the pressure of the cerebrospinal fluid within the ventricles of the brain is increased as a result of some problem inside the skull cavity such as a brain hemorrhage, head trauma, or meningitis. A number of conditions, including head trauma, can block the natural flow of the cerebrospinal fluid, increase pressure within the skull, and cause brain damage. The pressure can sometimes be relieved by a neurosurgical procedure called shunting. A tube is placed in the brain, allowing the fluid to drain into other areas of the body, where it may be absorbed without harm and thereby reduce intracranial pressure.

Primary hydrocephalus is difficult to diagnose. When cerebrospinal fluid circulating down the spinal cord is blocked above the spinal cord, cerebrospinal fluid pressure builds up in the ventricles of the brain where it is formed, but the pressure down the cord, where lumbar punctures are routinely done, may appear normal. In such instances, primary hydrocephalus is also called normal-pressure hydrocephalus. The spinal fluid pressure appears normal, but the CT scan shows that the ventricles located in both sides of the brain are enlarged. People who have primary hydrocephalus also usually show three specific clinical symptoms: (1) walking with difficulty, appearing to have forgotten how to do so, and exerting great effort to move their arms, legs, and feet; (2) urinary incontinence; and (3) relatively rapid intellectual deterioration.

When a patient shows this clinical triad with a relatively rapid onset, a careful neurological/neurosurgical workup is necessary before a decision about a shunt is made. Neurosurgery involves placement of a shunt to transfer cerebrospinal fluid from the brain area into a body cavity, such as the gut. It has been reported to be effective in about 65 percent of patients who have secondary hydrocephalus, but only 40 percent of patients who have primary, normal-pressure hydrocephalus show some improvement. The mortality rate associated with this procedure has been reported to range between 6 and 10 percent, and surgical complications and infections reportedly occur in more than 40 percent of patients. In the latter instance, another operation is usually indicated and a new shunt inserted. This decision needs to be carefully considered with a knowledgeable neurosurgeon prepared to educate and support patients and family members.

Delirium

Delirium is a clinical state with a rapid onset in which patients exhibit an acute fluctuating change in mental status and an altered level of consciousness. Patients have difficulty focusing and are unaware of their environment. If detected and treated appropriately, delirium is a reversible condition, but if unrecognized and untreated, patients are at serious medical risk (Saxena 2009). Older persons in the hospital who have delirium have a worse prognosis than older hospitalized patients who do not have delirium, including extended hospital stays, poorer functional effectiveness, higher rates of institutionalization, increased risk for cognitive decline, and higher mortality rates (National Guidelines for Seniors' Mental Health 2006; Voyer et al. 2007; Koster et al. 2009).

There are three types of delirium, classified by the patient's level of psychomotor activity: hyperactive, hypoactive, and mixed. The hyperactive patient, who appears agitated and may yell and scream, flail his or her arms, and pick at clothes or skin, is the easiest to recognize. The hypoactive patient, who is quiet and withdrawn, may be misdiagnosed as having depression. Mixed delirium is characterized by oscillating hyperactivity and hypoactivity.

Delirium is inevitably associated with medical disorders and conditions that can range from a mild condition to a life-threatening emergency (Gupta et al. 2008). Unfortunately, delirium is frequently undetected, and estimates are that 70 percent of patients who have delirium are not identified and treated appropriately (Alagiakrishnan and Blanchette 2009). As a result, serious medical problems may develop, including significant morbidity, permanent dementia, and death. It is also associated with more frequent hospitalizations and extended hospital days, poor functioning, increased health care costs from the hospital to home care, and increased caregiver strain (Ouimet et al. 2007; Young and Inoyue 2007).

Delirium may be caused by a wide range of conditions, including post-anesthesia, bladder catheterization, physical restraints, infections, drug toxicity (prescribed or otherwise), intentional or accidental drug overdose, metabolic disturbances (dehydration, hypoxia, renal dysfunction), acute illnesses (infections, fractures, malnutrition, alcohol withdrawal), severe cardiac conditions, and overstimulation in intensive care (Young and Inoyue 2007; Rockwood 2008).

Delirium most frequently presents on admission or early in a hospitalization, but the prevalence varies by patient population and clinical setting. Siddiqi and colleagues (2006) reported that delirium occurred in 42 percent of hospitalized older patients. The prevalence is higher in people who have dementia (Cole et al. 2002; Boettger et al. 2009), and it may be as high as 58 percent in nursing home residents (Lyons 2006). In the community the occurrence is low, about 0.5 to 1 percent (Andrew et al. 2006).

Cole and associates (Cole 2005; Cole and McCusker 2009) reported that 79 percent of patients who have delirium recover in six months, but many do not. Delirium is not always a bimodal phenomenon, and partial recovery as seen in subsyndromal delirium (SSD) may persist for a long time after the initial onset of delirium. Patients who have SSD and do not recover fully may experience cognitive impairment and heightened risk of mortality, but their prognosis is better than that of patients who do not recover.

Several standardized assessment measures are available, including the Delirium Rating Scale (Trzepacz et al. 2001), the Confusion Assessment Method (Inouye 2003; Wei et al. 2008), the Confusional State Evaluation (Robertsson et al. 1997), and the Delirium Symptom Interview (Albert et al. 1992). The CAM is particularly useful because it has integrated the DSM criteria for confusion into five defined criteria: evidence of acute onset, fluctuating behavioral changes during the day, disrupted attention and ability to focus, disorganized thinking, and altered level of consciousness. The diagnosis of delirium requires the co-occurrence of acute onset and fluctuating course, as well as inattention and either disorganized thought or altered level of consciousness.

Nonreversible Dementias

When delirium and reversible causes of dementia have been ruled out, the next step is the differential diagnosis of the nonreversible dementias described in the next several chapters. Alzheimer disease is the most common disorder, affecting about 50 percent of the dementia population, followed by vascular dementias, affecting 15–20 percent of patients. Mixed dementias (i.e., the co-existence of Alzheimer disease and vascular dementia) account for another 20 percent. The prevalence of Lewy body dementias, including Alzheimer disease with Parkinson symptoms and the dementia associated with Parkinson disease, may be as high as 25 percent of late-life dementias. The relative prevalence is greater than 100 percent because of differences among studies.

7

Alzheimer Disease

In 1901 a 51-year-old woman, Auguste D., became the patient of Dr. Alois Alzheimer, who followed her until her death in 1906. Alzheimer presented the case at a psychiatric conference in Tubingen in 1906, where he reported his clinical findings of significant dementia and paranoia, coupled with postmortem findings of neuronal loss, a high density of neuritic plaques and tangles, and glial proliferation. Although he noted that some of Auguste D.'s symptoms were different from those of other dementias he had studied, Alzheimer did not appear to recognize that he had discovered a new disease (Berrios and Freeman 1991).

Emil Kraepelin (1910) named this dementia "Alzheimer's krankheit" in his revised psychiatric textbook, in which he reclassified senile dementia as two diseases, presenile and senile, with presenile dementia labeled "Morbus Alzheimer." Although Alzheimer disease (AD) became widely accepted, Alzheimer himself originally questioned the distinction between the presenile and senile dementias (Alzheimer 1911).

Almost sixty years later, a team of British scientists published a series of papers replicating Alzheimer's findings of a high density of postmortem plaques and tangles associated with clinical dementia among older patients presumed to have dementia secondary to atherosclerotic cerebral arteries (Roth et al. 1967; Blessed et al. 1968). These findings were repeatedly confirmed, and since then AD has been regarded as a distinct neuropathologic disease associated with aging (Katzman and Bick 2000).

AD has emerged as an urgent worldwide public health priority. It is 1.5 times more common than stroke or epilepsy and as common as congestive heart failure. There are several authoritative websites continually updated with the latest breakthroughs in AD research: The Alzheimer's Disease Education and Referral (ADEAR) Center of the National Institute on Aging (www.nia.nih.gov/Alzheimers/); the National Institute of Neurologic Disorders and Stroke (www.ninds.nih.gov/disorders/alzheimersdisease/alzheimersdisease.htm); and the Alzheimer Disease Forum (www.AlzForum.org).

Overview of the Prevalence and Impact

The 2009 Alzheimer's Association Report estimates the number of Americans who have Alzheimer disease as 5.3 million Americans, with 5.1 million age 65 or older (Alzheimer's Association [AA] 2009). That number is expected to increase to between 11 million to 16 million by 2050 (Hebert et al. 2003). The 2009 World Alzheimer Report estimated that the global prevalence of dementia, predicted to be more than 35 million in 2010, will almost double every 20 years, to 65.7 million in 2030 and 115.4 million in 2050.

About 60 percent of individuals who have dementia live in low- and middle-income countries, but this percentage will rise to 70 percent by 2050 (AA 2009). The growth figures forecast are 117 percent for East Asia and 107 percent for South Asia, 134–146 percent in parts of Latin America, and 125 percent in North Africa and the Middle East. The report projects an increase of 40 percent in Europe, 63 percent in North America, 77 percent in southern Latin America, and 89 percent in the developed Asia Pacific countries.

These projections have serious health care, psychosocial, and financial implications for families and societies around the world (AA 2009). In the United States, an estimated 40–75 percent of caregivers have significant mental health problems, and 15–32 percent have clinically diagnosable major depression. The economic cost of dementia across the globe is estimated at $315 billion annually. In 2008, at least 9.9 million unpaid caregivers in the United States provided about 8.5 billion hours of care, with an estimated economic value of $94 billion. The direct costs to Medicare and Medicaid for the care of persons who have AD or a related dementia in 2005 were $91 billion and $21 billion, respectively. The indirect costs to businesses for employees who were caregivers were estimated at $36 billion in 2005.

AD and other dementias slowly destroy a person's ability to take care of personal needs. Indeed, the nature of progressive dementias has been described as the "loss of self" (Cohen and Eisdorfer 1986). Patients struggle to cope with the uncertain course of an illness with an inevitable end. Although the course is progressive, there is enormous variability in the rate of change of different cognitive abilities and skills, emotional and affective responses, and personal functioning in the patient population.

Whitehouse and George (2008) emphasize the need to transcend the biomedical model and "re-imagine" the disease to focus on the humanity of the individual-turned-patient. When cognitive losses are viewed as simply a pathological disorder, the emphasis is on the disease and cure rather than on the people who experience the illness and quality of their care. The label is socially stigmatizing for people who are immediately seen as inept and socially useless, a belief system that disconnects them from others. Individuals who have dementia are people actively coping with losses in their own way, and they deserve a psychosocial process of care that enhances a sense of identity, connectedness, and feelings of usefulness.

The Subjective Experience of Alzheimer Disease

AD and related dementias affect the subjective experience of patients throughout the illness, and these "individuals-turned-patients" have much to inform clinicians about their beliefs,

perceptions, emotions, thoughts, and desires. To the extent possible, patients want to be empowered and involved in their care, which preserves their dignity and enhances well-being and comfort. This is true early in the illness when cognitive skills are less impaired and patients can participate in economic, legal, medical, lifestyle, and family discussions and decisions. It may be just as true when they are profoundly demented and others are making decisions for them. Investing time to understand and respond to the personal and social needs of patients will enhance comfort and quality of life and may ease the burden of caregiving.

It is important to understand people who have dementia in the context of their personal history and family as well as their needs and aspirations. Every patient has a history, including food preferences, lifestyle activities, diurnal cycles, accomplishments and failures, and relationships with other people as well as their dreams and ambitions, however limited. Professionals and family members, including teenagers and children, need to respond to them in human ways, even in the later stages of dementia.

Coping with dementia is a process involving a series of psychological adaptations as the disease imposes significant limitations on the person. Cohen and colleagues (1984) described six phases of the subjective experience:

- Recognition and concern: "Something is wrong."
- Denial: "Not me."
- Anger, guilt, and sadness: "Why me?"
- Coping: "To go on, I must do . . ."
- Maturation: "Living each day 'til I die."
- Separation from self

Not every patient experiences these phases in the order described, but they provide a guide to understanding and responding to patients' needs during different stages of the illness. The insidious onset makes the period before diagnosis confusing and frustrating for patients and family members. After the diagnosis, some patients deny the disease, while some become angry and depressed. Coping with the disease is difficult because dementia by definition impairs cognitive abilities and skills necessary to adapt and communicate effectively. However, most people in the early and middle phases are capable of responding to cognitive rehabilitation and learning to cope with the limitations of some of their deficits.

The maturation phase may last for years, and people need increasing structure and supervision. They may be difficult to deal with, but they are still human beings with needs to feel a sense of worthiness, intimacy, and acceptance as well as to be active and mobile. In the separation from self phase the personality is all but gone. People react to sights and sounds, but their behavior seem reactive rather than proactive. The major needs are comfort, security, and activity.

Diagnosis

Although the definitive diagnosis is based on a neuropathological examination at autopsy, the clinical diagnosis is currently based on evaluations of the onset and history of symptoms; a combination of physical, neurological, and psychiatric examinations; cognitive testing; and the course of illness. The preliminary presence of dementia is usually established from patient and family informant reports about a history of progressive cognitive and behavioral changes and a mental status examination. Screening instruments such as those described in chapter 3, may be administered during the mental status examination to identify the presence and severity of deficits. These measures are not diagnostic but rather signal the need for a careful assessment. Mental status screening tools also have limitations because scores are affected by education, advancing age, visual and auditory impairments, and culture as well as by disorders and conditions that impair speech, writing, and attention.

When clinicians suspect serious cognitive problems, clinical diagnostic evaluations should be done to establish the nature and severity of cognitive and functional impairments and the existence of reversible or par-

tially reversible causes of dementia. Differential diagnosis of AD is based on an analysis of the characteristic clinical features of the disorder as well as consideration of the occurrence of related dementias. The diagnostic guidelines of the American Psychiatric Association, American Academy of Neurology, and other professional organizations afford a diagnostic accuracy of 65–96 percent (Dubois et al. 2007). The consensus criteria for the clinical diagnosis of AD, known as the National institute of Neurological and Communicative Disorders and Stroke—AD and Related Disorders Association (NINCDS-ADRDA) criteria for probable and possible Alzheimer disease (McKhann et al. 1984), have generally stood the test of time (Raginwala et al. 2008). A diagnosis of probable AD reflects the highest degree of clinical certainty, and a diagnosis of possible AD indicates the possible involvement of other contributing causative factors.

Diagnostic guidelines acknowledge that AD presents with a mild, slowly progressing history of memory impairment deficits in two or more areas of cognition, age of onset between 40–90 years, and exclusion of other testable causes of cognitive dysfunction. Psychiatric symptoms and disorders as well as behavioral disturbances are usually present. Progressive aphasia, agnosia, and apraxia may also occur. Over time, more cognitive skills are affected, and functional effectiveness is impaired. AD is an unlikely diagnosis when the onset is sudden, and/or focal neurological findings, gait disturbances, and seizures occur early in the course of illness.

As introduced in chapter 6, an international work group met in 2005 to examine the need to develop a research diagnostic framework to revise the NINCDS-ADRDA and the DSM-IV-TR diagnostic criteria (Dubois et al. 2007). The recommendations reflected current findings about prodromal symptoms, biomarkers, and patterns of impaired cognitive domains in AD as well as diagnostic guidelines for non-Alzheimer dementias. The proposed clinical diagnostic criteria for probable AD include core diagnostic criteria, supportive features, and exclusion criteria. Core diagnostic criteria include the presence of objective evidence of episodic memory impairment that is gradual and progressive over more than six months and objective evidence of impairments in other cognitive domains. Supportive features include positive results from one or more biomarker studies: MRI evidence for the presence of medial temporal lobe atrophy; abnormal cerebrospinal markers (e.g., low beta-amyloid, increased total tau concentrations, or increased phosphor-tau concentrations, or combinations); positive results from functional imaging with PET (e.g., reduced glucose metabolism in bilateral temporal parietal regions, other ligands such as Pittsburg compound B or FDDNP), or evidence of an Alzheimer autosomal dominant mutation in the immediate family. The exclusion criteria are similar to previous criteria with regard to history, clinical features, and other medical disorders.

Definitive laboratory tests may soon be available to positively diagnose AD (Sunderland et al. 2006; Dubois et al. 2007; Craig-Schapiro et al. 2008). For example, Sunderland and colleagues (2003, 2004) confirmed the value of potential markers using analyses of cerebrospinal (CSF) fluid. The CFS levels of two protein fragments, beta-amyloid and tau, distinguished patients who had clinically diagnosed AD from controls with 89–92 percent accuracy. Beta-amyloid was lower and tau higher, and the two markers together had a sensitivity of 92 percent and a specificity of 92 percent.

The introduction of amyloid imaging with living human beings is a significant research breakthrough because it detects the early stages of cerebral amyloidosis, a key pathologic component of AD, using Pittsburgh Compound B with positron emission tomography (Klunk et al. 2005; Price et al. 2005; Bacskai et al. 2007). This technology will likely permit earlier diagnosis of AD if research demonstrates that positive amyloid scans predict deterioration in mildly impaired individuals and tracks the efficacy of antiamyloid therapeutic agents. Although early results are encouraging, the findings need to be interpreted cautiously

because the cerebral amyloidosis occurs early and does not equate with either clinical or pathologic criteria that define AD.

Risk Factors

A number of other risk factors have been implicated, including advancing age, family history, gender, education, maternal age, depression, type I and type II diabetes, total serum cholesterol, apolipoprotein alleles, and a history of head trauma and multiple concussions.

Age

Age is far and away the most significant risk factor (Prince et al. 2004). The occurrence of AD is rare before age 65. The prevalence is about 2.5–3 percent at age 65, and it roughly doubles every five years, until age 85–90, when the prevalence approaches 50 percent and appears to plateau. Although some international studies yield lower rates, the age-associated pattern persists (Ferri et al. 2006).

Family History

Individuals with a family history of early-onset AD have a greater risk than those with no family history (Bertram and Tanzi 2005). Early-onset familial AD accounts for about 5 percent of all cases. Genetic factors also likely play a role in the susceptibility to later-onset AD, probably accounting for another 5–10 percent of cases.

Education and Childhood Cognitive Capacity

Lower educational and occupational attainment, especially in women, have been consistently linked to AD (Katzman 1993). This finding has been interpreted as an indication that reduced cognitive capacity or reserve makes the aging brain more vulnerable. Results of the well-publicized "Nun Study," indicated that nuns found to have less cognitive capacity as young women were at higher risk for dementia later in life (Snowden et al. 1996; Snowden 2003).

Gender

The differential vulnerability of women may be due in part to the fact that women have a significantly longer life expectancy compared to men as well as the result of lower estrogen levels after menopause.

Maternal Age

Older maternal age and Down syndrome in later life have been implicated as risk factors for AD. Several studies have shown that persons born to older mothers are at increased risk (Cohen et al. 1982; Rocca et al. 1991).

Cognitive Exercises

Cognitive activities appear to be related to a reduced risk in prospective studies, but the mechanism is not well understood (Wilson et al. 2002). Participation in engaging leisure activities (e.g., board games, knitting, gardening, traveling, dancing, playing musical instruments) has also been linked to a reduced risk of dementia (Eggermont et al. 2006; Arkin 2007). The mechanism of how these activities enhance cognition is unknown, but they may have an impact similar to that of educational attainment (i.e., enhancing brain reserve through ongoing cognitive exercises) (Katzman 1993; Wilson et al. 2002).

Race

Racial factors appear to play a role but are not well understood. Differing prevalence rates suggest the interplay of genetic and environmental factors (Burchard et al. 2003). Palistinian Arabs living in the Wadi Ara community in Israel have the highest reported rates of Alzheimer disease in the world—with a prevalence of 20 percent in persons 60 or older and 60 percent in persons 85 or older (Farrer et al. 2003). The prevalence of AD is lower than the prevalence of vascular dementia (Ineichen 2000), and the prevalence in African Americans in the United States appears to be twice as high as that observed in Africans living in Nigeria (Hendrie et al. 2001). The prevalence in China, Japan, and Korea is lower than observed in the United States, but the prevalence of vascular dementia is higher (Zhang et al. 2004; Jhoo et al. 2008).

Diabetes

Diabetes mellitus is strongly associated with cognitive decline and an increased risk for AD, vascular dementia, and other dementias, although the mechanism is not clear (Arvanitakis et al. 2004). Recent epidemiological studies have shown that diabetic patients have a 30 to 65 percent higher risk of developing AD compared to individuals who are not diabetic. The increased risk applies to both type I and type II diabetes, which share hyperglycemia as a common pathogenic factor (Luchsinger et al. 2004).

It is possible that the diabetes-dementia link is associated with Alzheimer changes in the brain, vascular changes that may mediate vulnerability to AD, or insulin resistance in the central nervous system (Rönnemaa et al. 2008). Recent evidence indicates that hyperinsulinemia resulting from poor glycemia control is implicated in amyloid beta plaque deposition (Biessels and Kapelle 2005; Burdo et al. 2009). The risk is especially high when people have borderline diabetes mellitus coupled with severe systolic hypertension (Azad and Power 2008). A Swedish population-based study found diabetes was associated with a higher risk for vascular dementia, not AD (Hassing et al. 2002).

Cardiovascular Health

Cardiovascular problems are a powerful mediator of cognitive decline and dementia (Whalley et al. 2006). There is mounting evidence for the protective effects of cardiovascular exercise, a heart healthy diet, and cognitive exercises. Persons who are physically and mentally inactive between the ages of 20 to 60 years are four times more likely to develop AD than those who are active.

Cholesterol

Total serum cholesterol is one of several cardiovascular risk factors for cognitive impairment and dementia (Panza et al. 2006). A meta-analysis of prospective studies showed a consistent relationship between high midlife total cholesterol levels and AD and other dementias but no relationship between high late-life total cholesterol levels and dementia. Neither high-density lipoprotein nor low-density lipoprotein was associated with Alzheimer disease or any other dementia. The co-occurrence of high cholesterol and high blood pressure are also associated with increased risk (Kivipelto et al. 2002).

Head Trauma

A number of studies indicate a relationship between head trauma and risk for AD (Fleminger et al. 2003). A study of World War II veterans compared the number of veterans who had AD or other dementia and a head injury to those who had no head injury (Plassman et al. 2000). The risk of dementia increased about twofold among those who had moderate head injury, and the risk increased with the severity of the injury. Veterans who had severe head injury and had been hospitalized and were unconscious or amnesic for 24 hours or more had a fourfold greater risk.

Multiple concussions in retired professional football players have been associated with the occurrence of MCI and subjective reports of memory impairments (Guskiewicz et al. 2005). A study conducted by the Center for Retired Athletes of more than 2,500 retired professional football players in their mid-50s showed that retired players who had three or more concussions were five times more likely to have significant memory problems as those who had no concussion (McKee et al. 2009; G Miller 2009).

Etiology

The etiology is best understood at several levels: pathogenetic processes leading to the production of amyloid plaques and neurofibrillary tangles; the role of mutations on at least 5 genes on 4 chromosomes; amyloid-derived diffusible ligands; inflammatory immunological processes; free radical formation; diminished production and transmission of acetylcholine; neuronal dysfunction and death; and perhaps microvascular circulation in the brain.

Amyloid Plaques and Neurofibrillary Tangles

Amyloid plaques and neurofibrillary tangles in the brain are characteristic markers of AD. Researchers have focused on the processes that lead to their formation and have targeted two families of proteins: beta-amyloid proteins (BAPs) that lead to plaques and tau proteins that form tangles. Both processes are part of the pathogenesis of dementia (Hardy and Selkoe 2002), and there is evidence that these pathological entities are functionally linked (Gamblin et al. 2003).

Amyloid plaques form before neurofibrillary tangles, and they first occur in parts of the brain most involved with learning and memory. BAP is a protein segment created when it is snipped from the larger amyloid precursor protein (APP) (Hardy and Selkoe 2002). BAP is believed to damage brain cells in several ways: creating inflammation or free radicals that cause cellular damage; causing nerve cells to be more vulnerable to ischemic injury; interfering with nerve cell connections around the plaques; and increasing the amount of intracellular calcium.

APP, which is essential for the growth, maintenance, and repair of injured neurons, is produced in the brain and attaches to the neuron's cell membrane, looking like a needle penetrating a swatch of fabric. Because APP sticks out of the membrane, it is vulnerable to being cut into tiny pieces that leave the cell and accumulate outside the membrane. Two protease enzymes snip the APP in two places: beta-secretase cuts APP to form BAP, and alpha-secretase snips the APP at another site so it cannot form BAP. Thus, the BAP created when APP is cleaved has two lengths. The shorter BAP is soluble and aggregates slowly, and the longer BAP, known as "sticky" BAP, quickly forms insoluble clumps.

The clumps of "sticky" BAP grow into long, insoluble filaments outside the cell membrane, known as diffuse or preamyloid plaques. They are considered precursor lesions because they lack the pieces of dead and dying neurons as well as the microglia and astrocytes that form the amyloid plaques characteristic of AD. Precursor lesions as well as pieces of alpha-beta proteins are produced naturally in the brains of people who do not have AD, and they accumulate with age in persons who do not show cognitive impairment.

Although scientists once believed that the number of plaques increased as the disease progressed, this does not appear to be the case. The amount of BAP appears to be relatively constant over time. Laser scanning microscope studies show that the plaques are not solid but are peppered with small holes, suggesting that beta-amyloid is in a dynamic process of equilibrium. This research has fueled optimism that it may be possible to find ways to break down the insoluble plaques after they have formed.

Neurofibrillary tangles (NFTs) are structures formed from paired helical filaments, which are composed of abnormally phosphorylated tau proteins, wound together in a double helix (Delacourte and Buee 2000). The formation of NFTs follows closely but independently, of Aβ-peptide production and deposition, but the processes appear to be linked in a way not yet understood (Cotman et al. 2005). Tau proteins are an essential part of the neuron's cytoskeleton and play a critical role in intercellular transport. In normal neurons, cyclin-dependent kinase 5 (Cdk5) is regulated by a p35 protein to maintain healthy tau protein activity. However, in AD, Cdk5 forms a complex that causes hyperphosphorylation of tau proteins. This destabilizes the cytoskeleton, and the altered tau proteins wrap around each other, forming tangles that eventually fill the neuron's cytoplasm causing degeneration and death of the nerve cell.

Amyloid-derived diffusable ligands (ADDLs) are tiny clumps of amyloid protein called oligomers, and although they may initiate the pathogenesis of AD (Lacor et al. 2004), the process by which they block memory functioning may be reversible (Gong et al. 2003). ADDL formation likely occurs when specific inflammatory proteins are present in the brain.

One protein, Apo J, which is elevated in the brains of persons who have AD, is believed to make the amyloid protein toxic but prevent the formation of amyloid fibrils (Harr et al. 2002).

The small ADDLs cross the blood-brain barrier and bind to nonspecific proteins on cell membranes, in contrast to the large amyloid beta peptide fibril, which cannot pass through the blood-brain barrier. Although both are amyloid beta peptide fragments, ADDLs differ significantly from amyloid fibrils (Catalano et al. 2006). ADDLs are found in large amounts in the Alzheimer brain and are made up of about 12 or 24 amyloid beta proteins clumped together. ADDLs are soluble and easily diffuse between brain cells until they find vulnerable synapses. They have a high binding affinity for proteins residing mainly in the hippocampus and frontal cortex. Toxic ADDLs disrupt synaptic transmission, leading to cellular dysfunction but without killing neurons. ADDLs cause functional changes that interfere with nerve impulses and affect memory storage and learning. They impair a process known as long-term potentiation in the hippocampus, which is necessary for information storage for short-term memory.

Genetic Factors

AD has genetic and nongenetic mediators (Wang and Ding 2008; Sleegers et al. 2010). It is categorized by age of onset, early-onset or familial Alzheimer disease (FAD) and late-onset or sporadic Alzheimer disease (SAD). People who have a family history of early-onset AD (i.e., two or more first-degree relatives with an onset before age 65) have a greater risk than people who have no family history. Early-onset familial AD accounts for about 5 percent of all cases. Genetic factors also likely play a role in the susceptibility to later-onset AD, probably accounting for another 5 percent of cases (Rocchi et al. 2003).

Genes on three chromosomes are associated with early-onset AD: APP on chromosome 21, PS1 on chromosome 14, and PS2 on chromosome 1. These genes have helped elucidate the pathogenesis of AD, using cellular and mouse models to demonstrate that a mutation in APP or the presenilins PS1 and PS2 increases the production of amyloid-beta 42, thought to be the primary neurotoxic peptide. The extent to which environmental risk factors are involved is unclear.

The apolipoprotein E (*APOE*) on chromosome 19, has not been shown to be causative but is associated with an increased risk of late-onset AD (Coon et al. 2007). This gene occurs in three forms, the *APOE2, APOE3,* and *APOE4* alleles, and they play a role in the distribution of cholesterol in the brain. The occurrence of the specific alleles is also associated with the risk of AD. Individuals who have two *APOE4* alleles are more likely to develop AD between the ages of 60–70 years. Conversely, the *APOE2* allele seems to confer some resistance or protection (Rocchi et al. 2003).

The largest genome-wide association study (GWAS) identified two new possible genetic risk factors for late-onset AD (Harold et al. 2009; Bertram and Tanzi 2010). The GWAS study pooled more than 16,000 DNA samples from groups in the United States and Europe. The results revealed associated variations in the sequence of two genes—ApoJ/clusterin (CLU) on chromosome 8 and phosphatidylinositol-binding clathrin assembly protein (PICALM) on chromosome 11—with increased risk, and also found an additional 13 gene variants that merit further investigation.

More research is necessary to determine the roles of the CLU and PICALM variants. CLU levels are frequently elevated when brain tissue is injured, and increased levels of CLU are found in the brains and cerebrospinal fluid of patients who have AD. PICALM may play a role in maintaining the health of synaptic connections that are lost in AD, and PICALM may affect the levels of beta-amyloid deposits in the brain.

Inflammatory Processes

Local inflammation may be an important secondary mechanism in AD neurodegenerative changes (Weiner and Frenkel 2006). Amyloid plaques and other changes create an acute inflammatory response, attracting microglial cells, followed by a response in the complement system, in which the microglia begin opsonizing or marking neuritic plaques for phagocytosis. Two of the major byproducts of the complement system, C3a and C5a, are powerful proinflammatory molecules that exacerbate the localized response and begin a complex cascade of inflammation.

The inflammation causes neurocapillary permeability changes leading to plasma leakage into surrounding tissues followed by swelling, which results in brain tissue damage. In healthy individuals, once the extracellular waste is cleared, the inflammatory response ends, and microglia and other immune cells repair the damaged tissues. However, in individuals who have AD, the production of amyloid results in chronic inflammation and ongoing nerve damage (Combs et al. 2000). Elucidating the complex cascade of deleterious inflammatory events may clarify the neurodegenerative effects caused by the immune response.

Microglial cell activation is a prime research target (Blasko et al. 2004; Petrozzi et al. 2007). In the presence of amyloid plaques, microglia begin to differentiate into phagocytic cells that produce cellular markers and cytokines. One specific cell marker, CD40, plays a major role in microglial cell activation and inflammation when it links with a CD40 ligand. As microglia enter the amyloid plaque, which is rich in the CD40 ligand, they undergo mass activation.

Microglia activation results in phagocytosis of the plaques and production of the proinflammatory cytokines, interleukin-1β (IL-1β) interleukin-6 (IL-6), and tumor necrosis factor-α (TNF-α). Phospholipids in the microglial cell membranes are also degraded into arachidonic acid and then processed by the enzymes cyclooxgenase 1 and 2 (COX-1 and COX-2). The result of the COX pathway is the production of lipid-derived prostaglandin, PGE2, and thromboxanes.

As microglia degrade ingested material they produce nitric oxide, and the combined effect of the production of cytokines, prostaglandins, and nitrous oxide is increased vascular permeability and dilation. Thromboxanes enhance the inflammatory effect by causing vasoconstriction and platelet aggregation in adjacent blood vessels. All of these effects contribute to the increasingly neurotoxic inflammatory response in AD.

Neuronal Damage and Death

The neurotoxic processes occurring in Alzheimer disease result in neuronal injury, dysfunction, and death (Kim et al. 2007). Recent studies have described how neuronal excitotoxicity causes them to bind with glutamate, which leads to neuronal death. Glutamate signals cells to transport calcium, which is normally used to trigger the release of neurotransmitters from synaptic vesicles. However, as calcium accumulates within the neuron, calcium-activated proteolytic enzymes, calpains, begin to degrade essential proteins (Richard et al. 1999). When calcium/calmodulin kinase II (CaM-KII) is activated, phosphorylation of various proteins and enzymes occurs, increasing their activity and triggering apoptosis. Increasing cellular concentrations of calcium also increases electron transport within mitochondria, causing oxidative stress that contributes cell death through necrosis.

Treatment

There are currently two strategies to treat and manage AD, and other approaches are being tested or developed in clinical and preclinical trials. Behavioral, psychological, and environmental strategies help individuals and family caregivers cope with the progressive dementia, psychiatric disturbances, behavioral and psychological symptoms, and functional dependency (chapters 10 and 15). Pharmacologic treatments include cognitive-acting drugs, appropriate psychotropic drugs, if needed, and nutritional interventions. A great deal can be done to enhance the physical and mental health of "individuals-turned-patient" throughout the course of the illness.

A number of valuable clinical reports are available. The American Association of Geriatric Psychiatry (www.aagpgpa.org/prof/position _caredmnalz.asp), the American Psychiatric Association (www.psychiatryonline.com/ pracGuide/pracGuideTopic_3.aspx), and the American Academy of Neurology (www.aan .com/professionals/practice/pdfs/gl0012.pdf) have published practice guidelines for the treatment and management of AD and related dementias (Lyketsos et al. 2006). The American Psychiatric Association has also published consensus guidelines for dealing with agitation (www.psychguides.com/gagl.pdf).

Cognitive-Acting Drugs

The FDA has approved five antidementia drugs; four are anticholinesterase inhibitors, and one acts on NMDA receptors. Although many drugs are in various stages of development and several substances may be promising for prevention, there are no cures at this time, and the medications to date are considered neuroprotective.

Cholinesterase Inhibitors

Four antidementia drugs, as of this writing, belong to a class of drugs known as cholinesterase inhibitors: tacrine (Cognex), now off the market; donepezil (Aricept); galantamine (Reminyl); and rivastigmine (Exelon). These agents increase the amount of acetylcholine and prolong its activity by inhibiting the activities of the synaptic enzyme, acetylcholinesterase, which deactivates acetylcholine.

Evidence-based guidelines recommend cholinesterase inhibitors as standard therapy for AD (Fillit et al. 2006; Doody 2008). Cummings (2003) emphasized the importance of research to clarify the utility and effectiveness of these drugs: what drug to choose, when to initiate treatment, how to measure a positive response, when to switch to other cholinesterase inhibitors, how long they can be used effectively, how to minimize side effects, and when to use in dementias other than AD. Because the average cost in the United States ranges from approximately $1,200 to $1,800 a year, cost effectiveness is a continuing concern.

Each cholinesterase inhibitor has different pharmacologic properties and therefore different effects and side effects. Donepezil has a longer half-life and is administered once a day, whereas rivastigmine and galantamine have shorter half-lives and are given twice daily. Donepezil and galantamine are metabolized by hepatic cytochrome P450 enzymes, and rivastigmine is metabolized in the kidneys and excreted in urine.

Tacrine (Cognex) was the first antidementia drug approved by the FDA in 1993, and it reportedly slowed the rate of cognitive losses in about 30 percent of people treated. However, about half also showed elevated values of certain liver enzymes (Gracon et al. 1998). Because of the risk for liver toxicity and a management schedule requiring periodic blood tests, tacrine is rarely prescribed even though it is still available.

Studies using donepezil (Aricept) show that the disease progression is slowed and nursing home placement delayed for periods up to two years or more (Geldmacher et al. 2003). As with other medications in this class, side effects initially involve loss of appetite and gastrointestinal symptoms.

Rivastigmine (Exelon) was released in the United States in 2000, although it had been tested and used previously in Europe and Latin America. It seems to be well tolerated because it is eliminated through the kidneys, and patients show significant improvement in their cognitive abilities compared with those taking a placebo. Rivastigmine appears to enhance overall cerebral metabolism, and it improves the functioning not only of people who have AD but also of those who have vascular dementia, mixed dementia, or Lewy body dementia (P McKeith et al. 2000; Vincent and Lane 2003; Erkinjuntti et al. 2004).

Rivastigmine may be more effective for certain individuals because it inhibits both butylcholinesterase and acetylcholinesterase (Plosker and Keating 2004). Acetylcholinesterase and acetylcholine decrease as AD progresses, whereas butylcholinesterase increases. As a result, rivastigmine is reportedly effective in both later and early stages of the illness. However, the pharmaceutical company making rivastigmine has issued a warning about the increased risk for cerebrovascular accidents in patients who are taking this medication compared to controls over a two-year period.

Galantamine (Reminyl) is a different class of acetylcholinesterase inhibitors that increases the amounts of acetylcholine in the brain in two ways (Loy and Schneider 2006): it inhibits the cholinesterase that breaks down acetylcholine, and it also stimulates other brain receptors to release more acetylcholine. There is evidence that at higher dosages galantamine enhances cognitive functioning, but because initial side effects include nausea and vomiting, it is essential to start with a low dose and slowly increase the dose (Rockwood et al. 2001).

Acetylcholinesterases may affect the course of AD, but the effect is not universal, and approximately half of patients show little or no benefit. At this time, there are no markers to indicate which patients are likely to respond, and the cost of the medications is problematic for families as well as third-party payers. The National Institute for Clinical Excellence (NICE), an arm of the British Medical Research Council, questioned the effectiveness of acetylcholinesterase inhibitors (Loveman et al. 2006), and the British government is reviewing its continuing coverage.

Memantine: Drug Affecting NMDA Receptors

Memantine, a N-methyl-D-aspartate receptor blocker commercially termed Namenda, is a noncompetitive NMDA receptor antagonist that has been used clinically for the treatment of dementia in Germany for more than ten years. The European Union's Committee for Proprietary Medicinal Products approved it for the treatment of moderate to severe AD in 2002 (Wimo et al. 2003). Clinical trials in the United States suggested that it was safe and reduced clinical deterioration (Reisberg et al. 2003), leading to approval by the FDA in 2003.

Memantine regulates the activity of glutamate and may improve cognitive functioning when beta-amyloid toxicity is present (Rogawski and Wenk 2006). Memantine selectively blocks glutamate from binding with NMDA receptors of presynaptic neurons (Danysz et al. 2000). The voltage-gated magnesium (Mg2+) blocked ion channels associated with the NMDA receptor are not depolarized, which normally causes the release of magnesium and the influx of calcium. As a result, excitotoxicity triggered by glutamate in both synaptic neurons is prevented (Molinuevo et al. 2005).

A mild, chronic malfunction of glutamate systems leading to excessive amounts of glutamate, which causes overstimulation of nerve cells, calcium overload, and cell death, has been implicated in many neurodegenerative disorders (Danysz et al. 2000). At least 70 percent of the fast excitatory synapses in the brain use glutamate as a transmitter, and glutamate activates three major classes of receptors: alpha-amino-3-hydroxy-5-methyl-4-isoxazolepropionic acid (AMPA) receptors, N-methyl-d-aspartate (NMDA) receptors, and metabotropic receptors coupled to phospholipase or adenylate cyclase. Memantine is believed to exert a neuroprotective effect by blocking NMDA receptors so they are not overstimulated by excess amounts of glutamate (Danysz and Parsons 2003).

Because of its low potential of interaction, memantine can be effectively combined with acetylcholinesterase inhibitors (McShane et al. 2006), and the combination of memantine and donepezil is reported to have a synergistic effect (Tariot et al. 2004). The most common side effects in clinical trials include hallucinations, confusion, dizziness, headache, and fatigue. While these reactions were typically mild, a few patients experienced other rare effects including anxiety, hypertonia, vomiting, cystitis, and increased libido.

Other Drug Treatments Not Currently Approved by the FDA

Anticholinesterase Inhibitors

Heptylphysostigmine (Eptastigmine) has a longer-term effect in the body than donepezil, and the cognitive and behavioral data have been promising (Braida and Sala 2006). Most patients tolerate the drug reasonably well, although some have shown serious adverse effects. Several acetylcholinesterase inhibitors are being evaluated in clinical trials (Colombres et al. 2004)—Taketa (TAK-147),

huberzine A, and Ganstigmine (CHF 2819). Takeda attaches to the enzyme acetylcholine esterase to block its activity. It increases brain metabolism and stimulates the growth of brain cells that use acetylcholine (Ishihara et al. 2000). Huperzine A has been reported to improve cognitive functioning in China (Wang et al. 2006). Ganstigmine is being studied for a number of neurodegenerative conditions, including AD (Jhee et al. 2003).

Drugs Acting on Muscarinic and Nicotinic Acetylcholine Receptors

Drugs that stimulate muscarinic or M receptors cause the release of extra acetylcholine and increase the production of the harmless beta-amyloid instead of BAP42 found in Alzheimer plaques (Georgi 2005). There are five types of M receptors, but most research has focused on the M1 receptor (Fisher et al. 2003), and at least two compounds are being tested for activity and tolerance: talsaclidine (Wienrich et al. 2001) and CI-1017 (Lockwood et al. 2006). At least two agents are being tested for their impact on nicotinic receptors: SIB-1553A promotes the release of acetylcholine (Rao et al. 2003), and Nefiracetam appears to increase nicotinic activity in the hippocampus (Moriguchi et al. 2007).

Antioxidants

Antioxidant therapies, which include vitamins C and E, ginkgo biloba, and selenium, are being investigated for their role to reduce oxidative damage in AD (Behl and Mooseman 2002). Vitamin E has been reported to slow progressive decline in AD, but the effects are not as compelling in other dementias (Berman and Brodaty 2004). Studies of the effects of ginkgo biloba for dementia have yielded both positive and negative results (Gertz and Kiefer 2004; LS Schneider et al. 2005). The federal government has funded larger-scale studies of ginkgo biloba (DeKosky et al. 2006), and results to date indicate that ginkgo biloba does not reduce the overall incidence rate of dementia or AD in older adults who have normal cognition or mild cognitive impairment (DeKosky et al. 2008).

Estrogen

Data on estrogen replacement therapy and AD have been equivocal until recently. Long-term clinical trials of estrogen and progesterone suggest that estrogen is not protective and may indeed increase the risk of dementia (Shumaker et al. 2003). The Women's Health Initiative Study also reported a higher risk of breast cancer associated with postmenopausal use of estrogen and progesterone, resulting in termination of the clinical trial (Rapp et al. 2003). Several publications from the Women's Health Initiative Memory Study report that hormone therapy decreases cognitive functioning, especially in persons who have lower cognitive functioning at the start of treatment and recommend against the use of estrogen or a combination of estrogen and progesterone to prevent dementia or cognitive deficits (Espeland et al. 2004; Shumaker et al. 2004).

Nonsteroidal Anti-Inflammatory Drugs

Observations that people who had rheumatoid arthritis treated with anti-inflammatory medications were less likely to show AD symptoms led to trials of nonsteroidal anti-inflammatory drugs (NSAIDs) and low doses of prednisone (Townsend and Pratico 2005). It is not clear why steroids or other anti-inflammatory medications might be effective, but it is possible that they mediate local inflammatory responses in the brain that occur during neuronal loss (Klegeris and McGeer 2005). A meta-analysis of observational studies between 1996 and 2002 suggest that NSAIDs are protective against the development of AD (Etminan et al. 2003). Other analyses have corroborated the findings (Szekely et al. 2004). However, the appropriate dose, duration of use, and risk-benefit ratio are unknown.

Future Biological Treatments
Neural Growth Factor

Neural growth factor (NGF) may have potential therapeutic effects for AD (Wiliams et al. 2006). Originally NGF had to be delivered to the exact site by neurosurgical stereotaxic approaches, but now genetically modified cells able to produce NGF can be injected into the brain without implantation (Tuszynski 2007). NGF has been identified for its interactions with the cholinergic basal forebrain (Auld et al. 2002). NGF specifically binds to cell surface receptors TrkA and p75 (NTR), which are unique to these cholinergic neurons, and the decreased NGF, TrkA, and NTR expression is believed to alter the cholinergic system in the pathogenesis of AD (Ginsberg et al. 2006).

Cerebrospinal Fluid Shunts

Eunoe, Inc., developed the COGNIShunt System, which is a cerebrospinal shunt designed to improve CSF clearance without the drainage that occurs with hydrocephalus shunts (Silverberg et al. 2003). Initial studies suggested that the device is well tolerated, and a small sample of patients showed improvements in cognitive functioning (Silverberg et al. 2004). However, a prospective randomized double-blind clinical trial showed no differences, and the trial was terminated because a number of subjects developed central nervous system infections that were treated successfully (Silverberg et al. 2008).

Secretase Inhibitors

Inhibitors of beta- and gamma-secretase enzymes are being studied in hopes of preventing the abnormal deposition of amyloid-beta-42 and the cascading sequence of neurotoxic events (Citron 2004; Pollack and Lewis 2005). The results of a multicenter study of LY450139, a gamma-secretase inhibitor, with a limited number of patients have shown minimal side-effects, changes in the amount of beta-amyloid in plasma and CSF, but no cognitive effects (Fleisher et al. 2008).

Beta Sheet Breakers

A new group of pharmacologically designed peptides are being evaluated for their ability to inhibit the formation of insoluble amyloid fragments (Hetényi et al. 2002). They are called beta-sheet breakers because their mode of action is to inhibit amyloid aggregation by interfering with the conformational change of the 42-amino-acid residue amyloid-beta-peptide chains from α-helices to β-pleated sheets (Rosenblum 2002).

Beta-sheet breakers are similar in structure to amyloid-beta-peptides. They were first created in 1996 by using the C-terminal sequence of the amyloid peptide as a template (Sato et al. 2006). The inhibition stems from the peptide's design, which specifically targets and mimics the region of the amyloid protein that regulates folding. By interfering with beta-sheet formation, the toxic amyloid fragments are dissolved, leading to significant increases in neuronal survival, decreases in inflammatory responses, decreases in amyloid plaque load, and a reduced risk for stroke associated with amyloid aggregation (Sigurdsson et al. 2004). Beta-sheet breakers remain in preclinical development because of their poor penetration of the blood-brain barrier and low metabolic stability (Gozes et al. 2004).

Metal Chelators

Metal chelators target neurotoxic plaque formation and the subsequent oxidative stress that may have potentially therapeutic effects (Huang et al. 2006). These compounds suppress the ability of amyloid-beta-peptides to bind large metal ions such as copper, zinc, and iron; and free amyloid-beta-peptides are dissolved and cleared, preventing their aggregation as plaques (Bush 2003). The suppression of amyloid-beta-peptide reactivity also decreases the production of hydrogen peroxide and the cascade of reactive oxygen species production. One metal chelator, clioquinol, appears promising (Chen et al. 2007).

Ampakines

Ampakines, a new class of drugs developed to modulate neuronal stimulation on the AMPA receptor, function by binding to the AMPA receptors of neurons and altering the amount of sodium that enters via the designated ion channels (Arai and Kessler 2007). By increasing both the strength and length of the depolarization triggered by glutamate, ampakines are believed to increase long-term potentiation as well as other important behavioral and cognitive processes during the glutamate defi-

cient stages of AD. One ampakine, CX-516 or Ampalex, is currently being investigated for its effectiveness and safety in healthy older adults and people who have AD (Wezenberg et al. 2007; Zarate and Manji 2008).

Vaccines

The amyloid cascade hypothesis has stimulated research to develop vaccines to reduce amyloid and consequently cognitive dysfunction. Hardy (2009) suggested that although the amyloid hypothesis has generated some testable predictions, it has not led to successful clinical trials. Schenk and associates first demonstrated that actively immunizing amyloid precursor protein (APP)–trangenic mice with an amyloid-beta-peptide vaccine significantly reduced the production of brain amyloid (Selkoe and Schenk 2003). Other researchers demonstrated that active immunization would protect these transgenic mice from developing memory impairments. Later studies showed that passive immunization using intranasal administration of amyloid-beta-peptide and the passive transfer of anti-amyloid-beta antibodies could also reverse memory deficits, even when administered for brief periods (Maier et al. 2006).

These findings led to a vaccination trial of Betabloc, an amyloid beta peptide, in persons who have AD, but the phase II trial was halted because 6 percent of the participants developed meningoencephalitic symptoms (Okura et al. 2006). Further investigations of anti-amyloid-beta antibody therapy and other forms of vaccination are ongoing to overcome the brain inflammation. Okura and colleagues (2006) developed a nonviral DNA vaccine that contained DNA sections that code for the beta amyloid plaque used in the earlier vaccine. The goal was to elicit more gentle immune reactions rather than the system-wide toxic responses previously observed against amyloid. Early treatment of transgenic mice before amyloid-beta deposition reduced plaque deposition by 16–38 percent, whereas treatment of transgenic mice after amyloid-beta deposition reduced plaque deposits by 50 percent. Neuro-inflammation was not observed in mice even after long-term vaccination. Nonviral DNA vaccines may be a promising approach for safe and effective human trials.

Caffeine

Epidemiological research suggests that high intake of caffeine over decades reduces the risk of AD (Maia and Mendonca 2002). Arendash and colleagues (2007, 2009) studied the long-term protective effects of dietary caffeine intake on cognition and beta amyloid levels in AD transgenic mice. Caffeine, an adenosine receptor antagonist, was added to the drinking water of Swedish mutation (APPsw) transgenic (Tg) mice between 4 and 9 months of age, and behavioral was testing done during the final 6 weeks of treatment. The average daily intake of caffeine per mouse, 1.5 mg, was the human equivalent of 500 mg caffeine, the amount found in five cups (40 oz.) of coffee per day. All the Tg mice given caffeine performed significantly better on multiple cognitive tasks of spatial learning and memory than did Tg control mice, and their cognitive performance was similar to that of nontransgenic controls. Long-term administration of caffeine resulted in lower hippocampal amyloid-beta (Abeta) levels in caffeine-treated Tg mice, and the expression of both Presenilin 1 (PS1) and beta-secretase (BACE) was also reduced, indicating decreased Abeta production as a likely mechanism for caffeine's cognitive protection.

The ability of caffeine to reduce Abeta production was confirmed in SweAPP N2a neuronal cultures, in which concentration-dependent decreases in both Abeta1-40 and Abeta1-42 were observed (Arendash et al. 2009). Although adenosine A(1) or A(2A) receptor densities in the cortex and hippocampus were not altered by caffeine treatment, brain adenosine levels in Tg mice increased back to normal with dietary caffeine, suggesting adenosine's involvement in the cognitive protection provided by caffeine. Thus, moderate daily intake of caffeine may delay or reduce the risk of AD.

Prevention

Although there are suggestions that antihypertensive medications, diets containing omega-3 fatty acids, cognitive engagement, and physical activity may prevent AD, the NIH Consensus Panel on Preventing Alzheimer's Disease and Cognitive Decline that convened in 2010 concluded that "firm conclusions cannot be drawn about the association of modifiable risk factors with cognitive decline or Alzheimer's Disease" (http://consensus.nih.gov/2010/alz.htm).

AD and related brain disorders are complex management challenges as clinicians and families alike learn how patients think and feel when comprehension and communication are difficult or impossible. After reviewing a number of other dementias in chapter 8, chapter 9 describes a range of psychological, behavioral, social, and environmental strategies and tactics to guide the process of communicating, understanding, and interacting with patients.

8

Other Dementias

The nonreversible dementias include vascular cognitive impairment, frontotemporal dementias, dementia with Lewy bodies (DLB), infectious diseases with dementia, tauopathies, nutritional dementias, and others. As research advances improve our knowledge about the etiologies, diagnosis, clinical course, and efficacy of treatment interventions of these disorders, it is imperative for health professionals to maintain state-of-the-art clinical practice. Updated information can be found on several authoritative web resources, including the National Institute of Neurologic Disorders and Stroke (www.ninds.nih.gov), the ADEAR website maintained by the National Institute on Aging (www.nia.nih.gov/Alzheimers/), and eMedicine (www.emedicine.medscape.com).

Consensus clinical criteria for the different types of dementias include the following: NINCDS-ADRDA diagnostic criteria for Alzheimer disease (McKhann et al. 1984), proposed revisions of the NINCDS-ADRDA diagnostic criteria (Dubois et al. 2007), NINDS-AIREN criteria for vascular dementia (Roman et al. 1993), consensus diagnostic criteria for Lewy body dementia (McKeith et al. 1996, 2004), the Manchester-Lund criteria for frontotemporal dementia (Lund and Manchester Groups 1994), and consensus diagnostic criteria for frontotemporal lobar degeneration (Neary et al. 2005). These standards are only guidelines based on expert-based consensus and do not consider procedures to identify coexisting dementias.

Vascular Cognitive Impairment

Cerebrovascular pathology causes a group of dementias referred to as VCI or vascular cognitive impairment (Black and Iadacola 2009). The term *vascular dementia* is used to refer to cases of VCI in which persons have met the traditional criteria for dementia, and *vascular mild cognitive impairment* (vMCI) is used for persons who have mild cognitive deficits believed to be due to vascular pathology (Meyer et al. 2005). VCI includes cerebral autosomal dominant arteriopathy with subcortical infarcts (CADASIL), familial forms of cerebral amyloid angiopathy (CAA), small vessel disease, subcortical pathology, single infarcts, and other cerebrovascular pathology. Although vascular dementias are separable from Alzheimer disease, the two can occur together as a mixed dementia in about 24–28 percent of patients (Kalaria 2002). Current diagnostic criteria do not easily identify mixed dementias, but the coexistence of cerebral infarcts with Alzheimer disease is associated with faster cognitive decline (Sheng et al. 2007).

Diagnosis

Individuals who have vascular dementia present with signs and symptoms similar to those of AD, but vascular dementias have several different risk factors (Gorelick 2004; Alagiakrishnan and Masaki 2009). These include hypertension, atherosclerosis, ischemic heart disease, diabetes, smoking, hypercholesterolemia, and increased homocysteine levels. Vascular dementias typically have an abrupt onset, a patchy quality of cognitive deficits, a stepwise progression, with losses often followed by partial recovery of functioning (www.emedicine.com/med/topic3150.htm).

Several scales are useful to identify the presence of vascular dementia, but the most useful is the Modified Hachinski's Ischemia Scale (Hachinski et al. 1975). Factors considered in these scales include hypertension, cardiovascular problems such as atrial fibrillation and bradycardia, ischemic events, diabetes, blood changes in coagulation and hyperviscosity, arteritis, pulmonary diseases, alcohol and substance abuse, and hyperlipidemia. Although the Hachinski scale is heavily weighted toward stroke, it remains a quick "bedside" screen to differentiate AD and vascular dementia, but not mixed dementias or the other subtypes of vascular cognitive disorders (Moroney et al. 1997).

Diagnostic criteria for vascular dementias have incorporated neuroimaging and cognitive standards. These include the California Alzheimer's Disease Diagnostic and Treatment Centers criteria for probable and possible ischemic vascular dementia (Chui et al. 2000), the ICD-10 criteria for vascular dementias (WHO 2007, www.who.int/classifications/icd/en/), the National Institute of Neurological Disorders and Stroke-Association Internationale pour la Researche et l'Enseignement en Neurosciences (NINDS-AIREN) diagnostic criteria for probable and possible vascular dementia (Roman et al. 1993), and the DSM-IV-TR criteria for dementia of the vascular type (APA 2000). Studies comparing the clinical criteria show significant differences in patient classification depending on the criteria used, and the Hachinski scale has a higher inter-rater reliability than any of these criteria (Pohjasvaara et al. 2000; Lopez et al. 2005).

CT and MRI brain scans show multiple infarcts in the dominant hemisphere and limbic system, multiple lacuner strokes, or periventricular white matter lesions (van Straaten et al. 2004; Nagata et al. 2007). Although neuroimaging findings show significant variability, they are improving our understanding of pathologic changes in different vascular dementias (Vitali et al. 2008).

Vascular dementias are characterized by patchy neuropsychological deficits, usually reflecting the site and severity of cerebrovascular disease in the brain (Graham et al. 2004; Bastos-Leite et al. 2007). People who have vascular dementia usually have better memory functioning than people who have AD but perform more poorly on verbal fluency and executive functioning tests and display more

perseverative behaviors. The presence of damage to the deep white matter layers is usually reflected in slowing and impaired dexterity and executive functioning as well as in dysarthria and other speech impairments.

Types of Vascular Dementia
Binswanger Disease

Binswanger disease, also referred to as subcortical vascular dementia or subacute arteriosclerotic encephalopathy, is a slowly progressive dementia (Román et al. 2002). It is rare, with an age of onset between the fourth and seventh decade. Binswanger disease is characterized by multiple cerebrovascular lesions in the deep layers of the white matter as well as clinical symptoms of memory and other cognitive impairments, language disturbances, reading and writing difficulties, motoric slowing, as well as mood and behavioral changes.

Patients usually have a history of hypertension, seizures, mild strokes, blood abnormalities, large blood vessel disease in the neck, and disease of the heart valves. Prominent features include urinary incontinence, gait disturbances, clumsiness, facial masking, mood swings, lack of impulse control, and aggression. Medical and behavioral symptoms may stabilize or improve for a short period but usually return in most patients. While there is no cure, treatment is focused on symptomatic management of medical conditions (Román 2002, 2003). Although it is believed that early detection and effective treatment of vascular risk factors can prevent or postpone Binswanger disease and other types of vascular dementias, there are no long-term studies supporting this hypothesis.

Cerebral Autosomal Dominant Arteriopathy with Subcortical Infarcts and Leukoencephalopathy.

Cerebral autosomal dominant arteriopathy with subcortical infarcts and leukoencephalopathy (CADASIL), also referred to as hereditary multi-infarct dementia, is the most common form of hereditary stroke disorder (Kalaria et al. 2004). It is caused by pathology in the endothelium of the brain's small blood vessels, leading to hemorrhaging and widespread white matter changes. Brain magnetic resonance imaging shows lacunar infarcts and severe leukoencephalopathy (i.e., demyelinization).

CADASIL is a rare autosomal dominant condition affecting the notch 3 gene on chromosome 19q12, and the age of onset is usually between 30 and 45 years. Although the clinical presentation is similar to Binswanger disease, there is no history of hypertension or other cerebrovascular risk factors. It manifests exclusively with central nervous system symptoms (Taylor and Doody 2008). In about 15 percent of cases, the initial symptoms are severe psychiatric symptoms, which often delays accurate diagnosis (Leyhe et al. 2005). Cognitive impairments show a stepwise progression associated with micro-infarcts, and patients usually have a history of migraines with a visual aura.

A brain MRI should be done in all older patients who present with late-onset severe psychiatric symptoms. CADASIL should be considered as a possible differential diagnosis whenever a marked leukoencephalopathy is detectable (Leyhe et al. 2005). Temporal lobe hyperintensity appears to be a marker for CADASIL, and involvement of the external capsule and corpus callosum may help identify CADASIL. A skin biopsy or genetic testing may be useful but can also be negative (Peters et al. 2005).

Cerebral Amyloid Angiopathy

Cerebral amyloid angiopathy (CAA), also known as congophilic angiopathy, is another rare vascular dementia caused by amyloid deposition in small blood vessels resulting in hemorrhaging (Weller and Nicoll 2003). If the bleeding is significant, symptoms similar to stroke may occur. If the bleeds are small, symptoms (e.g., confusion, seizures, headaches, cognitive impairment) depend on the part of the brain affected and may last for months. There is evidence that CAA is linked to the pathogenesis of AD through cerebrovascular mediation of alpha beta deposition in the brain (Nicoll et al. 2004).

Treatment and Prevention

The American Psychiatric Association has published treatment/management guidelines for the vascular dementias (APA 2007). Prevention of future strokes and continued deterioration are the primary principles for managing vascular dementia (Alagiakrishnan and Masaki 2009). The focus is treating underlying diseases (e.g., hypertension and diabetes), control of major risk factors, and the use of antiplatelet medications (e.g., aspirin, ticlopidine, clopidogrel). Hemorheologic drugs have been shown to increase cognitive functioning. Vascular cognitive impairment can be prevented by appropriate treatment of risk factors in adulthood as well as emerging vascular conditions (e.g., atrial fibrillation, congestive heart failure).

People who have vascular dementias commonly manifest psychological and behavioral symptoms (Aalten et al. 2007), and a mixed dementia manifests substantially increased psychopathology and behavioral disturbances (D Cohen et al. 1993). Patients respond well to behavioral interventions and psychotropic drugs when appropriate. As is the case with all dementias, management of progressive cognitive impairment includes referral to home- and community-based services, financial and legal planning, family support, and interventions to reduce caregiver stress and prevent depression.

Dementia in Parkinson Disease

Parkinson disease, first described as "shaking palsy" by James Parkinson in 1817, is a progressive and disabling illness that is becoming more prevalent as the population ages (Hauser and Pahwa 2009). Parkinson disease is a movement disorder resulting from alterations in dopaminergic neurons, largely in the substantia nigra. The disease may manifest clinically with tremor in arms, hands, and legs, stiffness in the jaws or extremities, slow movement, and unstable posture, coordination, and balance. As a consequence, patients may have difficulty with ADLs. Urinary problems and constipation as well as emotional problems, including depression, emotional lability, and hallucinations, may also occur.

Although people who have Parkinson disease are at heightened risk for dementia, the majority will not develop it (McKeith and Burn 2000). Parkinson disease co-occurs with AD and cerebrovascular disease in 10–30 percent of cases (Aarslund et al. 2005), and depression may accompany Parkinson disease in half of all patients (Weintraub and Stern 2007). When dementia manifests, it is usually slow and progressive, with memory losses, motor slowing, and poor impulse control. However, dementia with Parkinson disease is a complex and controversial diagnosis within the continuum of alphasynucleinopathies, which include Parkinson disease, dementia in Parkinson disease, and Lewy body dementia (Otero 2008).

Risk Factors

Age of onset is one of the best predictors of the occurrence of dementia (Emre 2003). When the age of onset is 50 years or younger, dementia is rare, whereas the risk is higher when Parkinson begins at age 70 or older. The male / female ratio for Parkinson, with or without dementia, is 2:1. Mortality rates appear to be higher in patients who have dementia than in patients who have only Parkinson disease.

The following variables are associated with dementia in these patients (Emre 2003):

· Advanced age at onset of motor symptoms
· Score of 25 or higher on the Parkinson Disease Rating Scale (Martinez-Martin et al. 2004)
· Co-existing depression
· Development of agitation, confusion, mania, or psychosis when patient is treated with L-dopa
· Co-existing cardiovascular disease
· Presence of bradykinesia, postural and gait disturbances

Cognitive Impairment

Patients may show a range of cognitive problems (Elmer 2004). The heterogeneity suggests that the many possible Parkin-son dementia syndromes have different pathophysiologies.

In Parkinson disease with dementia, the results of neuropsychological testing usually show deficits in areas characteristic of frontal-cortical dementia such as the following (Hauser and Pahwa 2009):

· Short- and long-term memory, where cluing may improve performance
· Executive functioning
· Visuospatial impairment
· Language changes such as decreased comprehension of complex grammar and commands and use of shorter phrases

There are at least three general Parkinson dementia syndromes: (1) a mild dementia with features of a subcortical dementia; (2) a more severe dementia with cortical features, yet neuropathologically different than AD; and (3) a severe dementia with changes in the cortex and basal ganglia (Cummings et al. 1998).

Clinical Examination

Clinicians need to be patient during examinations because people who have Parkinson disease, even those who do not have dementia, speak and respond slowly, and they may appear indecisive and anxious. The guidelines for the diagnosis of dementia by the American Psychiatric Association (APA 2000) and the American Academy of Neurology (Suchowersky et al. 2006) describe the diagnostic procedures. There are no special laboratory tests, and imaging does not help establish the diagnosis.

Neuropathological Findings

Parkinson disease is characterized by the loss of dopaminergic neurons of the substantia nigra pars compacta, aminergic brain nuclei, cholinergic neurons, and neurons in the hypothalamus as well as cortical neurons in the cingulated gyrus and entorhinal cortex (Dauer and Przedborski 2003; Hauser and Pahwa 2009). Lewy bodies occur in the cortex, basal forebrain, and the brainstem. Lewy bodies are large, eosinophilic, hyaline inclusion bodies with clear halos, and those occurring in the cortex are smaller and show a less distinct core.

The amount of cell loss in the medial substantia nigra and the hippocampus is associated with the severity of cognitive deficits (Camicioli et al. 2003). The level of cognitive impairment also correlates with Lewy body densities in the entorhinal and anterior cingulated cortex (Kövari et al. 2003). The density of Lewy neurites, not Lewy bodies, in the cornu ammonis 2 field of the hippocampus predicts cognitive impairment (Burn 2006). Lewy neurites are ubiquitin-positive neuronal processes that are dying. Patients who have significant gait disturbances show a faster rate of decline than patients who do not have gait disturbances (Burn 2006).

Treatment

Although no treatments exist for Parkinson disease at this time, medications can ameliorate many symptoms (Hauser et al. 2009). However, appropriate dosing and drug-drug interactions make pharmacotherapy a challenge. Levodopa and carbidopa, which increase dopamine levels in the brain, are the treatment of choice, but long-term use of Levodopa leads to motor deterioration in some patient populations (Fahn et al. 2004). Anticholinergic agents may help control tremor and stiffness but impair cognitive functioning (Katzenschlager et al. 2004). Medications such as bromocriptine, pramipexole, and ropinirol, which are dopamine agonists, may improve symptoms (Lemke et al. 2006; van Hilten et al. 2007). Amantadine may reduce dyskinesia in some patients (Crosby et al. 2003), and rasagiline, a MAO-beta inhibitor, used in conjunction with levodopa has been approved for use in advanced Parkinson disease (Rascol et al. 2005).

Management includes properly diagnosing and treating a broad range of sensory, autonomic, behavioral, and sleep-related symptoms (Pandya et al. 2008). Impaired sense of smell, anxiety, depression, fatigue, and constipation may be due to the Parkinson or medication effects. Orthostatic hypotension, sedation, and temperature regulation can all affect the patient's quality of life. Visual hallucinations, anxiety, depression, apathy, paranoia, and psychosis may occur in 10–30 percent of patients; and patients may manifest a range of sleep disorders, including excessive daytime sleepiness, insomnia, restless legs syndrome, and vivid dreams.

Dementia with Lewy Bodies

In 1913, Frederick Lewy first identified what are now called Lewy bodies in the substantia nigra of patients who have Parkinson disease, but it later became clear that Lewy bodies occurred in other dementias (McKeith 2006). The first international consortium on dementia with Lewy bodies (DLB), held in 1995 (McKeith et al. 1996), had a dramatic impact on clinical practice and research. A second meeting of the international consortium (McKeith et al. 1999) modified the clinical criteria, and in 2003 the consortium met a third time to modify the guidelines again and agree on the first treatment recommendations (McKeith et al. 2005).

DLB was originally believed to be relatively rare, but it now appears to be the second or third most common dementia, accounting for 10–15 percent of autopsied cases (McKeith et al. 2004). DLB and the dementia associated with Parkinson disease (PDD) are clinically defined disorders, and, while there are clinical diagnostic criteria for DLB (McKeith et al. 2005), there are currently no clinical diagnostic criteria for PDD (Emre 2003). Furthermore, neuropathologic studies show a great deal of variability in the density and distribution of Lewy body pathology in DLB and PDD as well as AD and vascular dementias.

The general consensus is that DLB is one entity on a spectrum of Lewy body diseases characterized by the dysregulation and aggregation of alpha-synuclein (McKeith et al. 2006). The clinical features include DLB, Parkinson disease, and autonomic nervous system dysregulation, but it is often difficult to distinguish between DLB and PDD. The 1996 consortium report recommended that DLB should be diagnosed when dementia occurred before or at the same time of the parkinsonism, and the PDD should be diagnosed when the dementia occurred after Parkinson disease had been present for a year or more.

Diagnosis

The diagnostic criteria recommended in the third report of the DLB consortium (McKeith et al. 2005) included central features (i.e., essential for a diagnosis), core features (i.e., two core features indicates probable DLB, and one core feature indicates possible DLB), suggestive features (i.e., features that occur more often than in other dementias), and supportive features (i.e., occur frequently but not proven to be diagnostic). Currently, there are no genotypic or CFS measures associated with a diagnosis of DLB (Galasko 2007).

The central feature of DLB is progressive mental impairment that interferes with functional effectiveness, although the disabilities in DLB are the result not only of cognitive impairment but also of psychiatric, motoric, sleep, and autonomic dysfunction. Deficits in attentional performance, executive functioning, and visuospatial skills are usually prominent. Significant memory deficits may not be present in the early stages, but they usually become apparent with progression of the disorder.

The three core features of DLB are fluctuating cognition with significant alterations in attention and alertness, recurrent detailed visual hallucinations, and spontaneous symptoms of parkinsonism. The assessment of cognitive fluctuations is challenging in clinical practice (Cummings 2004), and it is recommended that caregivers be interviewed thoroughly and that at least one measure of fluctuation be used by trained staff. The Cognitive Assessment of Fluctuation scale (Walker et al. 2000) relies on the judgment of experienced clinicians to assess the frequency and severity of fluctuating confusion over the previous month. The One Day Fluctuation Scale (Walker et al. 2000), a semistructured interview, creates a cut-off score to distinguish DLB from AD and vascular dementias. The Mayo Fluctuations Composite Scale (Ferman et al. 2004) is based on caregiver responses to questions about daytime sleepiness and sleep, periods of staring into space, and episodes of disorganized speech. Visual recurrent hallucinations are common in DLB, and the Neuropsychiatric Inventory (Cummings et al. 1998) is useful to identify their frequency and severity. The intensity of extrapyramidal motor symptoms in DLB is similar to Parkinson disease with or without dementia. The five-item subscale of the Unified Parkinson's Disease Rating Scale (Ballard et al. 1997) identifies symptoms in DLB independent of the severity of dementia: tremor at rest, action tremor, body bradykinesia, and rigidity.

If one or more suggestive features are present in addition to one or more core symptoms, probable DLB is a likely diagnosis. If one or more suggestive features are present, even in the absence of core features, possible DLB can be diagnosed. REM sleep disorder often occurs with vivid, frightening dreams, in which patients often act out but do not remember their dreams. Other sleep disturbances may include excessive daytime drowsiness and sleeping. A positive history of sensitivity to neuroleptics is another suggestive indicator of DLB (Swanberg and Cummings 2002). Finally, dopamine transporter imaging is useful to differentiate DLB from AD (JT O'Brien et al. 2004).

The clinician should interview patients and caregivers about supportive features because they may not consider them to be related to the dementia. Supportive features resulting from autonomic nervous system dysfunction include orthostatic hypotension, repeated falls and syncope, brief unexplained loss of consciousness, urinary incontinence, constipation, sexual dysfunction, and eating and swallowing problems. Other supportive features include auditory and visual hallucinations, depression, delusions, and paranoia. Clinical and imaging studies suggest the following supportive features: intact medial temporal lobe structures on CT and MRI scans, general low uptake on SPECT/PET perfusion scan and reduced occipital activity, abnormal MIBG myocardial scintigraphy, and slow wave EEG activity and sharp transient waves in the temporal lobe.

Exclusion criteria include the presence of cerebrovascular disease supported by focal neurologic signs or white matter lesions seen in imaging, the presence of other physical disorders that could explain the clinical presentation, and when parkinsonism occurs for the first time during severe stages of dementia.

Neuropathology

The neuropathologic hallmarks of DLB are Lewy-related pathology in the brainstem, limbic system, and neocortical areas (McKeith et al. 2005). Lewy bodies are rounded neuronal inclusions in the cytoplasm, and Lewy neurites are diffuse filaments. Both are composed of alpha-synuclein, a protein in the synapses associated with the release of chemicals in the synapse. The cause of the abnormal deposition of alpha-synuclein in Lewy bodies and Lewy neurites is not known.

The third consortium concluded that the likelihood that neuropathologic findings predicted the clinical syndrome of DLB is a direct function of the severity of the Lewy-related pathology and is inversely related to the severity of Alzheimer-type pathology. The group proposed specific neuropathologic research standards to distinguish DLB and AD pathology. The likelihood that the dementia is caused by AD pathology are ascertained according to NIA-Reagan criteria (NIA 1997) which use the CERAD method for evaluating neuritic plaques (Mirra et al. 1991) and a method to stage neurofibrillary degeneration similar to the standards of Braak and Braak (Harding et al. 2000). The likelihood of Lewy-related pathology is assigned, using criteria from the first consortium report (McKeith et al. 1996), and semiquantitative methods are used to grade Lewy body severity from absent to severe. However, the regional pattern of Lewy-related pathology is more significant than counts. The brainstem is affected in almost all cases of DLB, but the severity is variable. The severity of limbic system and neocortex involvement are also variable. The third con-

sortium also recommended an algorithm to assign the pattern of Lewy body pathology in different brain regions.

Frontotemporal Dementia

Frontotemporal dementia (FTD) includes a spectrum of progressive disorders with cognitive decline, personality changes, language impairments, and behavioral abnormalities characterized by clinical and pathological heterogeneity (McKhann et al. 2001; Kertesz et al. 2005). The clinical and neuropathologic features are characteristic of damage to the frontal and/or temporal lobes, and symptoms reflect the anatomic region of the brain affected (Blass and Rabins 2009).

People who have FTD exhibit a broad range of psychopathology, the most striking of which are personality and behavioral changes (Graff-Radford and Woodruff 2007; Blass and Rabins 2009). Disinhibition, socially inappropriate behavior, hyperorality, behavioral and verbal stereotypies, and poor hygiene are prevalent in the early phases of FTD, features that distinguish it from AD. Personality changes may include coldness, passivity, excessive talking, loss of insight, and poor judgment. Patients may show symptoms of mood disturbances including depression, anxiety, apathy, euphoria, and irritability, but psychotic symptoms are rare.

FTD includes a range of clinical and neuropathological variants. Clinical subtypes include the behavioral variants described above, language variants (i.e., semantic dementia, progressive nonfluent aphasia), and motor variants (i.e., corticobasal degeneration, motor neuron disease) (Hodges et al. 2004). Pathological subtypes include cases with tau-immunopositive inclusions (i.e., with or without Pick bodies), cases with ubiquitin immunopositive inclusions, and cases without identifiable histology. There is also a clinical/genetic nosology of FTD linked to chromosome 17.

Pick Disease

The defining features of Pick disease are cortical atrophy affecting the frontal and temporal poles and argyrophilic, round intraneuronal inclusions known as Pick bodies. In 1892, Dr. Arnold Pick published clinical descriptions of patients who presented with symptoms of language impairments, dementia, and shrinkage of the left side of the brain (Kertesz and Kavlach 1996). In 1911, Alzheimer identified swollen structures inside neurons that were atypical of Alzheimer disease, which he called Pick bodies.

Pick disease affects men more than women, and it is estimated that there is one person who has Pick disease for every 100 who have AD (www.ninds.nih.gov/health_and_medical/disorders/Picks_doc.htm). Pick disease usually has an age of onset between 40 and 60 years. The dementia progresses slowly, usually lasting 7–8 years, but the symptoms are different than AD over the course of illness (Duara et al. 1999).

Primary Progressive Aphasia

Primary progressive aphasia (PPA) is characterized by progressive profound language disturbances in the absence of impaired memory and functional status. This disorder is diagnosed when other cognitive abilities and behaviors remain relatively intact, language is the sole impairment for at least the first two years of the disorder, and imaging studies do not show specific lesions accounting for the language deficit (Mesulam 2007). Some patients only manifest language disturbances for a decade or longer, whereas others develop several cognitive impairments after several years. PPA is distinct from progressive dysarthria or phonologic disintegration (i.e., disturbances in word formation) and frontal-lobe dementias with anomia and decreased speech production (Mesulam 2003).

The most common variants of PPA are progressive nonfluent aphasia, semantic dementia, and logopenic progressive aphasia (Amici et al. 2006). Progressive nonfluent aphasia is characterized by labored speech, agrammatism in production (i.e., difficulty forming grammatically correct sentences) and/or comprehension. Patients who have semantic dementia show loss of word and object meaning and surface

dyslexia (i.e., ability to recognize words but not their meaning). Those who have logopenic progressive aphasia have word-finding problems, talk or write with simple but accurate syntax, and have impaired sentence comprehension.

The clinical symptoms reflect neuronal atrophy, decreased blood flow, and decreased glucose metabolism in the language areas of the brain's left hemisphere, known as Broca's and Wernicke's areas and surrounding regions of the frontal, parietal, and temporal cortex (Mesulam 2003). The metabolic functioning of the right hemisphere is unaffected, at least early in the course of the disease.

Neuropathological examinations reveal that about 60 percent of patients have a focal degeneration distinguished by cell loss, gliosis, and mild spongiform changes in upper layers of the cortex, a pattern referred to as dementia lacking distinctive histology (Grossman and Ash 2004). The cerebral cortex may have a few ballooned neurons filled with phosphorylated neurofilament protein, as well as neuronal and glial inclusions containing ubiquitin or the cytoskeletal protein tau. Pick disease occurs in another 20 percent of patients who have PPA.

The epidemiology and risk factors are unknown, and there are no known treatments (Mesalam 2007). Because the symptoms are markedly distinct from AD and other dementias, different aspects of activities of daily living are affected and therefore different interventions are required. Some patients use sign language, laminated cards, voice synthesizers or personal computers to communicate. Speech therapy may lead to effective communication strategies.

Motor Neuron Disease

Most people who have motor neuron disease (MND), also known as amyotrophic lateral sclerosis (ALS), do not manifest dementia, but a small number show frontotemporal dementia (Talbot 2004). Neuropathological characteristics include loss of pyramidal cells in the frontal and temporal lobes, but not the premotor cortex, and deterioration of motor neurons in the hypoglossal nucleus and spinal motor neurons. The average of onset is between 55 and 65 years but may be earlier in cases with a family history. The course of illness in patients who have MND and frontotemporal dementia is more rapid than that observed in patients who have either frontotemporal dementia or MND, and most patients die within three years (Leigh et al. 2003).

Infectious Diseases with Dementia
Spongiform Encephalopathies

Spongiform encephalopathies are a rare group of degenerative conditions in which the brain has a characteristic spongiform appearance (Mariani 2003). They are called transmissible spongiform encephalopathies (TSEs) when there is evidence of animal-to-human or human-to-human transmission (Lasmezas 2003). Prions, abnormally configured proteins without nucleic acids but with the ability to spread under certain circumstances, are believed to be the infectious agents responsible for the transmission of TSEs (Safar et al. 2005; Aguzzi and Heikenwalder 2006).

TSEs include kuru, sporadic Creutzfeldt-Jakob disease (CJD), iatrogenic CJD, familial CJD, variant CJD, and animal spongiform encephalopathies. Kuru, a disease characterized by tremors, blurred vision, gait problems, stupor, and death within a year, was an epidemic in New Guinea, Africa, in the 1950s (Goldfarb 2002). Gajdusek demonstrated that kuru was transmitted as a result of cannibalism, particularly of brain tissue (Gajdusek 1976).

The prevalence of TSEs is one in one million persons, and symptoms include dementia, tremor, and ataxia (Hoch 2009). More than 50 percent of people who have CJD die within six months; very few live two years (Ladogana et al. 2005). Iatrogenic transmission of CJD by contaminated surgical instruments and electrodes in patients receiving corneal transplants, dura mater grafts, or purified hormones is very rare (P Brown et al. 2006). Approximately 200 patients have been affected in the United States since 1960. About 10 percent of cases of CJD are familial, with an autosomal dominant pattern of transmission, and about 100 fami-

lies have been identified (Zerr et al. 2009).

The animal spongiform encephalopathies include scrapie, transmissible mink encephalopathy, and bovine spongiform encephalopathy (BSE) (Gavier-Widen 2005). BSE, also referred to as mad cow disease, was first reported in 1986 in Great Britain, but it has also occurred in other countries (McGarity 2005; Odeshoo 2005). The peak of infected cows occurred in 1993, when more than 1000 cows were being diagnosed every week (Mariani 2003). BSE, which manifests with head tremors, unsteady gait, weight loss, and aggressive behaviors, was traced to cattle feed that contained meat from sheep infected with the scrapie agent, causing a disease in sheep similar to CJD. Few animal cases are being diagnosed at present because of the elimination of millions of infected animals, strict requirements for animal feed, ban on milk products from infected cows, and a ban of beef on the bone. BSE has been transmitted to humans who ate infected beef, with the first case of variant CJD reported in 1995 (Mariani 2003). More detailed information can be found at the United Kingdom CJD Surveillance Unit website (www.cjd.ed.ac.uk).

The differential diagnosis of the variant CJD is a tentative one, and clinical symptoms differ from sporadic CJD (van Everbroeck 2004). Most people who have variant CJD develop psychiatric symptoms first—depression, apathy and withdrawal, anxiety, and insomnia—followed by headaches and loss of consciousness. In later stages, patients may become aggressive and confused, hallucinate, and be in chronic pain. Common features of sporadic CJD include myoclonus (i.e., muscular jerking and twitching of the arms, legs, and body), visual symptoms, ataxia, dysarthria, and psychiatric symptoms.

There are no consensus diagnostic guidelines or documented treatments for CJD. The disease progresses rapidly, making it difficult to diagnose in the early stages. A protein in the cerebrospinal fluid called 14-3-3 was identified as a diagnostic marker for the disease (Huang et al. 2003).

HIV-Associated Dementia

Although the human immunodeficiency virus (HIV) and AIDS are usually associated with younger persons, they are also a major concern in older populations (Linsk 2000). With available treatment, infected individuals are living into their later years, and states with surveillance systems report that 10 percent of new cases of HIV are age 55 or older (Stoff et al. 2004). Risky sexual behaviors, not contaminated blood transfusions, are now the most common antecedents in the older age group.

Older people who have AIDS are frequently seen later in the progression of the disease, and symptoms are often confused with AD because of an unfounded low index of suspicion for this sexually transmitted disease (Illa et al. 2008). The diagnosis of HIV is not made until shortly before death in more than 20 percent of persons age 60 or older.

Central nervous system complications may arise from the HIV virus itself or from opportunistic infections, tumors, or drug-related complications. HIV encephalopathy and the AIDS dementia complex (ADC) are neurologic complications that arise after primary HIV infection (McArthur et al. 2005). HIV encephalopathy is part of the acute HIV syndrome during seroconversion. HIV-associated progressive encephalopathy (HPE) is a syndrome characterized by cognitive, motor, and behavioral problems. ADC, also known as HIV-associated dementia complex (HAD), is characterized by cognitive, motor, and behavioral features, and it usually develops in advanced AIDS when CD4 lymphocyte counts fall below 200 cells/mm. With the advent of highly active antiretroviral therapy (HAART), a less severe condition, minor cognitive motor disorder (MCMD), has become more common than ADC.

HAART has become the cornerstone of care (Brew 2004). The Multicenter AIDS Cohort Study in the United States prospectively followed 2,734 American men with HIV. Before HAART (1990–1992), the incidence of HIV dementia was 21 cases per 1000 person-years; after the availability of HAART (1996–1998), the incidence decreased to 10.5 cases per 1000 person-years (Yamashita et al. 2001). HIV-associated progressive multifocal leuko-encephalopathy (PML) is a significant clinical problem even with the use of HAART (Antinori et al. 2003). It is serious disease affecting as many as 77 percent of patients, and the course is usually rapid decline and death.

Several mechanisms likely mediate the process by which HIV infection leads to ADC (Toborek et al. 2005): (1) HIV neuroinvasion, in which HIV enters the brain by infected monocytes and other infected CD4+ cells; (2) cellular proteins that cause widespread damage with the secretion of chemokines, proinflammatory cytokines, and other neurotoxic factors; (3) HIV proteins that are toxic to neurons or cause damage by activating astrocytes, microglia, and macrophages to release cytokines or other neurotoxic substances; (4) autoimmune disease leading to anti-CNS antibodies and neuronal damage; and (5) changes in the release of neurotransmitters.

ADC and HPE affect many aspects of cognitive, behavioral, and motor functioning. Patients usually present with poor concentration, mental slowness, motor problems, loss of interest in activities, decreased libido, and forgetfulness. The early signs are often subtle, but over time they evolve into a generalized dementia with memory loss, language, and neuropsychological deficits characteristic of subcortical dementia. The early phases reveal psychomotor slowing, memory loss, word-finding difficulties, and the executive functioning deficits that occur with subcortical dementia. As the disease advances, severe psychomotor slowing and language impairments lead to akinetic mutism.

Neurosyphilis

Syphilis is a systemic infectious disease transmitted by sexual contact, and it is caused by the spirochete *Treponema pallidum,* which attacks the parenchyma of the brain (Timmermans and Carr 2004). Despite the widespread availability of antibiotics, the proportion of patients who have syphilis and central nervous system problems, neurosyphilis, has been increasing since the 1980s along with other sexually transmitted diseases (Kerani et al. 2007). Neurosyphilis is usually clinically apparent after a latent period of 10–20 years post primary infection, although the coexistence of HIV/AIDS infection has altered this temporal frame. The nervous system may be affected at any stage of the infection, and psychiatric symptoms may occur at any time (Lair and Naidech 2004). Depression and anxiety are common in the early stages, and as syphilis progresses, psychiatric symptoms may include insomnia, confusion delusions, high bodily concerns, irritability, and periods of euphoria and confabulation (Sanchez and Zisselman 2007).

Chronic meningitis is the pathologic basis of the four forms of neurosyphilis that occur in 15–20 percent of people who have untreated syphilis: asymptomatic syphilis, meningovascular syphilis, progressive paralysis, and tabes dorsalis (Cohen 2005; Marra 2009). Asymptomatic neurosyphilis occurs in 15 percent of persons who have latent syphilis. No clinical symptoms are observed, but patients may show cerebrospinal fluid abnormalities. Patients who have meningovascular syphilis caused by occlusion of small blood vessels manifest cognitive decline, agitation or apathy, and stroke-like symptoms, including hemiplegia, aphasia, and seizures. This form of neurosyphilis usually occurs 4–7 years after infection, and symptoms usually disappear after treatment with penicillin.

Parenchymal neurosyphilis may present as progressive paralysis or tabes dorsalis. Progressive paralysis usually develops 10–15 years after infection, and clinical features include progressive frontal lobe dementia, dysphoria or elation, apathy, psychotic symptoms, personality changes, and significantly impaired psychosocial functioning. Tabes dorsalis results from the destruction of posterior horn cells and tracts, and symptoms include gait disturbances, sharp pains in the legs, bladder problems, delayed pain recognition, pupil abnormalities, and spinal ataxia. Psychiatric symptoms are very rare. Tabes dorsalis usually occurs 10–20 years after infection and progresses slowly if not treated.

A sequence of tests is recommended to detect neurosyphilis (Luger et al. 2000). The first is to test for syphilis using nontremonal screening for blood antibodies (i.e., VDRL, RPR). If positive, the diagnosis of syphilis is confirmed using treponemal tests (e.g., FTA-Abs or MHATP); and to confirm neurosyphilis, VDRL are detected in the cerebrospinal spinal fluid. Cerebrospinal fluid analysis almost always reveals abnormalities (e.g., primary lymphocytosis and increased protein levels). In addition to a lumbar puncture, other tests may include CT or MRI imaging or a cerebral angiogram.

Neurosyphilis can be prevented by early diagnosis and treatment of primary and secondary syphilis (Marra 2009). Consistent follow-up to ensure patient adherence to an antibiotic regimen is necessary to prevent neurosyphilis from developing. When neurosyphilis is diagnosed, it should be treated aggressively with penicillin. Treatment outcome is a function of the type and severity of symptoms present before diagnosis, including HIV-AIDS.

Tauopathies

Tauopathies, dementias in which abnormal tau proteins are found in neurons and glial cells, are associated with a mutation of the tau gene on chromosome 17 in persons who have AD, Parkinsonian disorders, argyrophillic grain disease, progressive supranuclear palsy, and corticobasal degeneration (Rademakers et al. 2004; Iqbal et al. 2005).

Argyrophilic Grain Disease

Argyrophilic grain disease (AGD), also known as Braak disease, is a late-onset dementia characterized by personality changes, emotional lability, and memory problems (Ferrer et al. 2008). Braak and Braak (1987) first described the comma-shaped argyrophilic (i.e., silver-staining) grains in the brain cells of the limbic system (i.e., mediobasal temporal/entorhinal cortex, hippocampus, and amygdala). Because these argyrophilic grains or coiled bodies consist of abnormally phosphorylated tau protein isoforms with four microtubule-binding repeats, AGD is known as a 4-R tauopathy. The cause is as yet unknown, and AGD appears to be sporadic with no evidence of a genetic link.

Although the original studies underscored the lack of Alzheimer changes, a large series of studies have demonstrated the association of AGD with AD as well as Pick disease, progressive supranuclear palsy, corticobasal degeneration, Creutzfeldt-Jakob disease, Parkinson dementia, and Lewy body dementia (Ferrer et al. 2008). As a result, some investigators question whether AGD is a distinct entity (Tolnay and Clavaguera 2004).

Corticobasal Degeneration

Corticobasal degeneration (CBD) is a rare disorder characterized by symmetrical or asymmetrical atrophy in many areas of the cerebral cortex and basal ganglia (Wadia and Lang 2007). The first clinical report was published in 1968, and although early studies suggested that CBD was a distinct entity, the current consensus is that there is significant heterogeneity in the clinical spectrum, the corticobasal syndrome (CBS), and the neuropathology of CBD (Boeve et al. 2003).

The age of onset is usually between the sixth and eighth decade, and although it progresses gradually over 6–8 years, patients ultimately become unable to walk (Wadia and Lang 2007). Symptoms include those similar to Parkinsonism, such as akinesia, rigidity, and impaired balance as well as cognitive and visual-spatial impairments. Other symptoms may include apraxia, language disturbances, myoclonus, and dysphagia (Mahapatra et al. 2004).

A number of diagnostic criteria have been proposed for CBD or CBS, but none have been validated at this time (Mahapatra et al. 2004). They are based on clinical observations and reviews of the literature, and there is considerable overlap between them. Wadia and Lang (2007) identified core and supportive features. Core features include insidious onset and progressive course; cortical dysfunction manifest by at least one focal or asymmetrical

sign of ideomotor apraxia, alien limb, cortical sensory loss, visual or sensory hemineglect, constructional apraxia, myoclonus, and apraxia of speech/nonfluent aphasia; and evidence of basal ganglia dysfunction manifest by focal or asymmetrical appendicular rigidity and/or focal or asymmetrical appendicular dystonia. Supportive features include evidence of focal cognitive impairment with intact learning and memory, and focal or asymmetrical atrophy, especially in the frontoparietal cortex, on imaging studies.

Clinical diagnosis is difficult in early stages until cognitive impairments become prominent. However, accurate diagnosis rests on neuropathological findings (Wadia and Lang 2007): neuronal loss and gliosis in the basal ganglia and all cortical layers, but particularly in the superior frontal and parietal gyri; ballooned neurons that contain the tau protein; loss of myelinated axons in the white matter; neuronal inclusions similar to Pick bodies. Lewy bodies and neurofibrillary tangles are absent. The substantia nigra shows neuronal loss with extraneuronal melanin, gliosis, and neurofibrillary inclusions, called corticobasal bodies.

Although the etiology is unknown, the accumulation of the tau protein suggests a relationship to a mutation in the tau gene. There are no treatments at this time to slow the course of corticobasal degeneration, and patients do not respond to medications used to treat Parkinson-like symptoms. Clonazepam may improve myoclonus. Occupational, physical, and speech therapy as well as assistive devices may be helpful to manage the patient's progressive impaired functioning.

Progressive Supranuclear Palsy

Progressive supranuclear palsy (PSP), also called dementia-nuchal dystonia or Steele-Richardson-Olszewski syndrome, is a rare brain disorder that causes significant persistent difficulties with gait and balance as well as supranuclear gaze palsy and dementia (Golbe 2001; Venmans et al. 2009). PSP is one of the tauopathies with neuropathologic evidence of widespread glial tau inclusions and neurofibrillary tangles in the subcortical gray matter.

The prevalence rate is 5 per 100,000, the incidence rate ranges from 0.3 to 1.1 per 100,000, and it occurs equally in men and women (Vanacore et al. 2001). Patients frequently manifest mood alterations, behavioral and psychological changes, including depression and apathy, as well as progressive mild dementia. This disorder is often difficult to diagnose because the symptoms are similar to more common movement disorders such as Parkinson disease, and certain symptoms may develop late or not at all.

The most distinctive symptom is the inability to focus the eyes correctly, the result of lesions in supranuclear nucleus that coordinate eye movements. As a result, patients may report dizziness, have a stiff or awkward gait, lose their balance when walking, or fall. Other common early symptoms are mild memory impairments and personality changes such as anhedonia, irritability, angry outbursts, emotionally lability, or apathy. As the disorder progresses, almost all patients develop blurred vision and difficulties controlling eye movements (e.g., inability to maintain eye contact, shifting gaze downward, moving eyelids, which causes the automatic closing of the eyes, protracted or intermittent blinking, or difficulties opening the eyes) (Golbe 2001). Some patients will exhibit slurred speech, swallowing difficulties, or hand tremor.

The etiology of this tauopathy is not known, but there are several theories (Kowalski et al. 2004): a viruslike agent, genetic mutations, environmental exposure, or free radical damage. Effective pharmacologic treatments are limited. Slowness, stiffness, and balance problems may respond to antiparkinsonian agents such as levodopa, levodopa combined with anticholinergic agents, or amantadine, but the effect is usually temporary. Antidepressants may improve PSP symptoms, although this is unrelated to their antidepressant effect. Speech problems, visual abnormalities, and swallowing difficulties are not responsive to medications.

There are a number of nonpharmacologic treatments. Many patients profit from weighted walking aids to counteract the tendency to fall backward. Bifocals or prism glasses are frequently prescribed to correct difficulties looking down. Physical therapy can help maintain flexibility and range of motion.

Patients who have this disorder deteriorate progressively over time, but it is not directly life-threatening. However, patients are at risk for serious complications such as choking and pneumonia secondary to swallowing problems, head injury, and fractures caused by falls. Most patients live ten years or more after the initial symptoms with adequate clinical care, and pneumonia is the most common cause of death.

Wernicke-Korsakoff Syndrome

Wernicke-Korsakoff syndrome, typically associated with alcohol abuse, is caused by thiamine deficiency (Xiong and Daubert 2009). The syndrome has two symptom clusters: Wernicke encephalopathy and Korsakoff syndrome. Wernicke encephalopathy involves damage to nerves in the central and autonomic nervous system, which causes ocular abnormalities, ataxia, and acute confusional states. Korsakoff syndrome or Korsakoff psychosis, which involves impaired memory and learning, usually develops when Wernicke symptoms diminish. Chronic heavy alcohol use is the most common antecedent of Wernicke-Korsakoff syndrome, which in turn leads to nutritional deficiencies, but other causes may include persistent emesis, systemic disorders, starvation, and procedures such as chronic dialysis. The prevalence ranges from 1 to 3 percent but is significantly higher in specific populations that have alcohol problems and malnutrition (e.g., homeless persons and psychiatric inpatients). Onset may occur from 30–70 years of age, and men are at a slightly higher risk.

Although thiamine deficiency causes a widespread reduction in cerebral glucose metabolism, clinical symptoms reflect focal damage (Xiong and Daubert 2009). Metabolic alterations in the brain stem, affecting the abducens nuclei and eye movement centers in the pons and midbrain, cause ocular motor abnormalities. However, because ocular cells are not destroyed, rapid and complete improvement usually occurs with thiamine therapy. Ataxia reflects cerebellar damage, especially the superior vermis, and about 40 percent of patients recover completely. Vestibular paresis is observed in the early phases of the disorder, and it usually improves with treatment. Memory impairment is caused by damage in the medial thalamus, connections with the medial temporal lobes, and amygdala. However, this neuronal damage appears to be irreversible, because memory does not always improve with treatment, and only 20 percent of patients show complete recovery.

The way thiamine deficiency leads to damage is not fully understood. Potential mechanisms include changes in cerebral metabolism resulting from decreases in transketolase, pyruvate, and acetylcholine; decreases in synaptic transmission; and impaired DNA synthesis. Differences in clinical signs and symptoms and the observation that not all patients who have thiamine deficiency develop the Wernicke-Korsakoff syndrome suggest that a genetic predisposition may exist in some persons.

Changes in mental status, which occur in 90 percent of patients, may occur concurrently with ophthalmoplegia and ataxia, but they usually follow these signs and symptoms by days to weeks. A patient's mood may vary, manifesting as blunted affect or apathy; and a patient in acute alcohol withdrawal will present with acute delirium tremens. Stupor or coma may occur in more severe cases but not in early stages, and if patients are not treated, the condition will progress to death. A global confusional state, characterized by apathy, distractibility, and indifference to surroundings, commonly occurs in early stages. Spontaneous speech is minimal, and when patients are questioned directly, they are generally disoriented. The timely administration of thiamine usually improves attentiveness and orientation.

Persons who have the Korsakoff amnestic state are alert and, when evaluated, manifest the amnestic features of the Korsakoff psychosis. They display significant anterograde amnesia (i.e., learning) and retrograde amnesia (i.e., impaired recent and remote memory). A patient will be able to repeat a set of numbers or objects but will not be able to recall them. The loss of certain recent and remote memories leads to confabulation.

Wernicke encephalopathy is a clinical emergency (Xiong and Daubert 2009), and intravenous thiamine (50–100 mg) is the treatment of choice to quickly reverse the ophthalmoplegia, improve ataxia and early mental confusion, and prevent the development of the amnestic state. In patients whose disease has gone unrecognized and untreated, the severe and extended thiamine deficiency will have caused permanent deficits (e.g., memory loss, severe ataxia).

Depending on the patient's symptoms and condition, thiamine should be continued daily (50–100 mg) and supplemented by magnesium and potassium, electrolytes that are often low in alcoholics. The B vitamins should also be given to those who are seriously and chronically malnourished. Thiamine should be administered to chronically malnourished patients before giving intravenous glucose, because glucose may deplete thiamine and precipitate Wernicke-Korsakoff syndrome. A balanced diet is an essential component of treatment.

Because chronic alcohol abuse is the most common cause of Wernicke-Korsakoff syndrome, referral to an alcohol recovery program is another core aspect of treatment. Those who have other etiologies should be referred to the appropriate medical consultation. Some patients may require physical therapy for gait abnormalities, which may be permanent, depending on their severity and the timeliness of therapy.

9

Managing the Behavioral and Psychological Symptoms of Dementia

Since Alzheimer first described prominent paranoia, delusions of sexual abuse, hallucinations, and screaming in his famous patient, Auguste D, psychiatric and behavioral disturbances have been a prominent research priority and a challenge for clinical practice (Katona et al. 2007; Lyketsos 2007). The geriatric mental health community has developed recommendations for diagnosing neuropsychiatric symptom in DSM-V to improve the limited attention in DSM-IV-TR (Jeste et al. 2006).

An international consensus conference in 1996 recommended that the term *behavioral and psychological symptoms of dementia* (BPSD) be used to describe disturbances in perception, thought, mood, or behavior that occur in patients (Finkel and Burns 2000). Behavioral symptoms, which are based on direct patient observation, include repetitive questions, restlessness, wandering, agitation, screaming, cursing, hoarding, culturally inappropriate behaviors, physical aggression, sexual aggression, and severe violence. Psychological symptoms, which are based on patient and informant interviews, include symptoms of anxiety, depression, paranoid thinking, hallucinations, and delusions. Detailed information is available in a comprehensive resource published by the International Psychogeriatric Association—The Behavioral and Psychological Symptoms of Dementia Educational Pack, accessible online at www.ipa-online.org/ipaonlinev3/ipaprograms/bpsdarchives/bpsdrev/toc.asp.

The etiology of rapidly emerging behavioral disturbances requires a comprehensive physical and psychiatric examination of the individual, evaluation of changes in the living environment or routines, a review of interactions of the patient with others, and a diurnal record of the problematic behaviors and their onset, severity, and possible precipitating factors. Cohen-Mansfield (2000, 2004) developed a framework to group different causes of behavioral disturbances: (1) the direct effect of brain degeneration causing disinhibition and inappropriate behaviors; (2) the response to an unmet need that patients cannot communicate (e.g., pain, hunger); (3) behaviors that continue because patients are reinforced by the attention they receive; and (4) the inability of patients to adapt to changes in their environment.

BPSD create considerable emotional distress for family members and formal caregivers (Shultz and Martiere 2004). BPSD in patients living at home are likely to lead to increased caregiver depression, frequent hospitalizations, earlier nursing home placement, domestic violence, and homicide or homicide-suicide. The manifestation of these symptoms in long-term care residents may lead to the use of restraints, sedating medications, or psychiatric hospitalization, depending on the facilities ability or propensity to deal with behavioral problems. Sedation and keeping the person in bed can have a cascading effect that may result in decubiti and infections as well as accelerated physical and mental deterioration.

A great deal can be done to manage BPSD to maximize the emotional well-being of patients and caregivers and restore a safe, comfortable living environment (M Snowden et al. 2003; Cohen-Mansfield and Mintzer 2005). Understanding the complex set of events and circumstances at the root of these problems, evaluating the patient thoroughly, and responding with appropriate individualized treatment/management plans are essential to success.

Clinical Presentation of Symptoms

BPSD may occur throughout the course of dementia, and most, if not all persons with dementia, will manifest them (Lyketsos et al. 2002). Depression and anxiety may occur more frequently in mild dementia, whereas severe psychotic-like symptoms and agitation may be more common in people who have moderate or moderately severe dementia (Holtzer et al. 2003). Psychotic symptoms are markedly diminished in advanced stages, probably due to significant neurodegenerative and physical deterioration (Leroi et al. 2003). Agitation and wandering are likely to emerge in most patients, and their prevalence increases over the course of the illness, somewhat correlated with a decline in cognitive functioning (Holtzer et al. 2003; Lai and Arthur 2003). Although BPSD may occur in any of the dementias, specific symptoms and their prevalence may vary according to the type of dementia, as described in chapter 8.

Psychological Symptoms

The most problematic psychological symptoms are delusions, hallucinations, misidentifications, depression, anxiety, and apathy.

Delusions and Hallucinations

Delusions are reported to occur in 10–75 percent of patients, with paranoid or persecutory delusions being the most common (Bassiony et al. 2000; Paulsen et al. 2000). The five most frequent delusions reported using the Behavioral Pathologic Rating Scale for Alzheimer's Disease (BEHAVE-AD; Reisberg et al. 1997) include: (1) people are stealing things; (2) the house is not the patient's home; (3) the spouse or caregiver is someone else; (4) the patient believes that he or she has been abandoned; and (5) the patient believes that his or her spouse has been unfaithful. Verbalizations that people are stealing are the most frequent delusion, manifest in 18–40 percent of patients, followed by expressions of abandonment in 3–18 percent of patients, and infidelity in 1–9 percent of patients. Delusions may also be a risk factor for physical aggression.

Between 12 and 50 percent have hallucinations (Wragg and Jeste 1989). Visual hallucinations are the most common, occurring in up to 30 percent of patients, and they are most common in those who have mild or severe cognitive impairment. As many as 80 percent of people who have Lewy body dementia experience visual hallucinations. Other patients may have hallucinatory experiences that are threatening and become integrated into a full-blown delusional system. About 10 percent of patients have auditory hallucinations, but tactile or olfactory hallucinations are uncommon. Patients who have dementia and have visual or auditory impairment (e.g., visual agnosia or impaired contrast sensitivity to language and sound) are at particularly high risk for hallucinations.

Patients who have significant brain damage, particularly parts of the brain affecting executive functions, often have catastrophic reactions to failure or become violent if angry and frightened (Smith et al. 2004). The risk for aggression and violence increases when these patients are also paranoid. These behaviors may range from verbal assaults to physical assaults, including homicide against family members at home or staff and other residents in long-term care facilities.

A consensus panel of the American Association of Geriatric Psychiatry refers to the symptoms of hallucinations and delusions as psychosis associated with Alzheimer disease, vascular dementias, or other dementias. To qualify for the diagnosis, symptoms must be severe enough to be disruptive and occur after the onset of dementia, with no premorbid history (Jeste and Finkel 2000). The diagnostic criteria include:

- Patient has hallucinations and/or delusions
- Patient meets criteria for diagnosis of Alzheimer disease or another dementia
- No history of psychotic symptoms before the dementia diagnosis
- Psychotic symptom(s) must be present for at least one month and disrupt patient's functioning

- Diagnosis of schizophrenia and other psychotic disorders are excluded
- Psychotic symptoms are not caused by delirium
- All other medical causes of psychotic symptoms are excluded

Misidentifications

Misidentifications are due to disorders of perception interacting with cognitive dysfunction (Harciarek and Kertesz 2008). They are misperceptions of external stimuli, in contrast to hallucinations, which occur in the absence of external stimuli. The four main classes are: (1) seeing people in the home (e.g., phantom boarder syndrome); (2) not recognizing oneself (e.g., mirror reflection); (3) mistakenly identifying others; and (4) believing television images and events are real.

Depression

Major depressive disorders (MDD), reviewed in chapter 10, are reported to occur in 10–20 percent of patients, and another 40–50 percent have symptoms of depression (Wragg and Jeste 1989). About half of patients who have vascular dementias also have MDD, and patients who had a history of MDD before the dementia diagnosis have a high risk of recurring MDD. Fluctuating symptomatology, accompanied by anhedonia, self-rejection, irritability, and anxiety are prominent symptoms of a typical depressive profile in dementia.

Consensus diagnostic criteria for depression in Alzheimer disease (Olin et al. 2002) are reviewed in chapter 7. Depression is most readily recognized early in the course of dementia when individuals are able to describe feelings and are functioning reasonably well. Detection in later stages is more difficult, but there are a number of useful clinical scales relying on observed and reported behaviors (chapter 3). Depressed patients who have dementia may express suicidal ideation or commit suicide and should be evaluated for dangerousness and lethality (chapters 7 and 18). A history of major affective disorder, a prior suicide attempt, or suicide in the family is a significant risk factor. At-risk individuals should be thoroughly evaluated, treated with antidepressant medications, and carefully monitored.

Anxiety

Anxiety may appear as fearfulness, confusion, agitation, or other behavioral problems (Seignourel et al. 2008), but anxiety may also occur independently of problem behaviors (Reisberg et al. 1997). Anxiety can escalate when patients travel or move to new environments, and even small environmental changes may provoke anxiety and agitation. In long-term care facilities, changes such as the unfamiliar face of a new aide or a move to a different room, even in the same facility, can be the stimulus for stress associated with fear and anxiety. Prevention of relocation anxiety can best be done by preparing the patient (e.g., explaining repeatedly that a change will occur, transporting familiar belongings to the new room, and involving family members to support the patient).

Cognitively impaired patients often shadow relatives relentlessly at home because of fears of being alone, and caregivers, in turn, may become upset with the clinging behavior and lack of privacy. When family members leave the home or just use the bathroom (and close the door), patients may become extremely agitated, and caregivers are often conflicted about preventing the patient's upset or leaving home for essential trips. Hiring part-time household help early in the dementia is a helpful tactic to deal with negative patient responses to a family member's absence, but the patient will need time to develop a trusting attachment to others.

The "Godot syndrome" is a common result of anxiety in which patients repeatedly ask questions. The repetitiousness, which results from memory loss coupled with impaired focused thinking, can become burdensome for caregivers. Caregivers often become irritated and angry and criticize the patient, only to recognize what they are doing and feel guilty.

Apathy

Apathy is one of the most prevalent BPSD, occurring in at least 50 percent of patients

(Lyketsos et al. 2002). Apathetic patients present with flat facial expression and affect, speak softly with little vocal inflection, and show little interest in other persons or activities. Symptoms of apathy and depression may be difficult to distinguish, because both conditions may present with lack of interest and energy, psychomotor retardation, lack of motivation, and poor psychological insight. Apathetic patients are usually not dysphoric and do not display the somatic and vegetative symptoms of depressive disorders.

Behavioral Symptoms

The most common and distressing behavioral symptoms for caregivers to cope with are violence and physical aggression, wandering, restlessness, agitation, and sexual disinhibition. Common behavioral symptoms that are more manageable include crying, cursing, repetitive questioning, and shadowing others.

Violence and Physical Aggression

Physical aggression and violence are often used interchangeably to refer to physical, sexual, and other behaviors that have a high potential to cause physical harm, psychological distress, or death. Paveza and colleagues (1992) reported that 16 percent of individuals who have dementia living at home had shown severe violent behaviors in the year following diagnosis. Resident-to-resident violence in nursing home facilities is a serious problem that affects the culture of safety and well-being of residents. Nursing staff at all levels and other employees have been forced to deal with resident violence and aggression, but research is lacking to adequately inform clinical responses and interventions (Institute of Medicine [IOM] 2001b).

Physical aggression is a major management challenge in long-term care settings (Lyketsos et al. 2006; Lyketsos 2007), but it appears that only a small subset perpetrate violent injury and/or death. Cohen (2004) estimated that the prevalence of dementia-perpetrated homicide is 0.22 per 100,000 persons who have dementia, and half occur in long-term care facilities.

The following antecedent factors increase the risk for homicidal behavior in people who have dementia (Cohen 2004): history of previous violence or "other-directed" behaviors, history of alcohol abuse, active paranoia and psychotic symptoms and behaviors, psychotic depression, vascular dementia with behavioral disturbances, history of catastrophic reactions, traits such as low frustration tolerance and aggressivity, and a history of dealing with dangerousness and/or violence (e.g., military/law enforcement/firefighter occupations). Precipitating factors are more difficult to identify, but these are not willful and intentional acts to injure and kill. They are tragic outcomes of a combination of circumstances: the individual's sensory, cognitive, emotional, and physical status; the individual's fearfulness and ability to communicate; impaired executive functioning; the lack of awareness and preparedness of others who interact with the patient; biopsychosocial and environmental stressors; and the availability of firearms, knives, heavy objects, and other lethal means.

Wandering

Wandering refers to meaningless walking, often with identifiable movement patterns (Algase et al. 2007), and it includes several behaviors: repeatedly checking for someone or something, stalking or shadowing, aimless walking, night walking, elopement, and excessive activity. The prevalence rates vary from 10 to 70 percent, depending on the populations and settings studied.

Long-term care residents who begin wandering in the absence of a previous history need to be evaluated for a possible change in medical status (Kallimanis-King et al. 2009). Wandering behaviors, ranging from circumstances in which individuals elope from home or long-term care facilities, get lost, or fall and injure themselves, are dangerous (Nelson and Algase 2007). If not successfully managed, wandering may lead to extended nursing home or home care and untimely death (Aud 2004).

A number of technological interventions have been developed to prevent falls, wandering, and bed-rail entrapment as well as to improve patient handling (Nelson et al. 2004). There also has been significant progress toward developing evidence-based protocols for assessing and managing wandering behaviors in community, residential, and hospital settings (Nelson and Algase 2007).

Agitation

Agitation is operationally defined as inappropriate behavior distinguished by excessive verbal and/or motor activity (Cohen-Mansfield 2002, 2004). Agitated behaviors can be grouped into several subcategories: verbally nonaggressive behaviors (e.g., interruptions and negative comments); verbally aggressive behaviors (e.g., shouting, cursing); and physically nonaggressive behaviors (e.g., pacing and restlessness). Agitation needs to be distinguished from intentional aggression.

The likelihood of agitation increases with the severity of dementia, from 38 percent in mildly impaired individuals to 66 percent in more severely impaired persons, and as many as 80 percent of nursing home residents manifest agitation (Ballard et al. 2001). Hallucinations and paranoid ideation often coexist with agitated behaviors. This is especially likely in Pick disease, other frontal lobe dementias, and Creutzfeldt-Jakob disease. Dementia with Lewy bodies is often associated with visual hallucinations as well as fluctuating attention, but it is not clear to what extent Lewy bodies are associated with agitation and paranoia.

Other sources of agitation occur, particularly in advanced stages of dementia. These include the sundowner syndrome, in which agitation increases significantly at the end of the day and may be associated with circadian rhythm disturbances (Bachman and Rabins 2006). They are more common in the vascular dementias, Lewy body dementias, and supranuclear palsy (Bhatt et al. 2005).

Inappropriate Sexual Behavior

Inappropriate sexual behavior is defined as a sexually related action done at an improper time and/or directed at an inappropriate individual. It is estimated that 7–17 percent of people who have dementia exhibit these behaviors over the course of the disease (Black et al. 2005). People may not remember or may reject their partner, may believe the partner is a stranger or a previous partner, or may even accuse the partner of being a whore. They may not remember having had intercourse or engaging in other sexual activities and demand more sex, sometimes exhibiting anger and aggressive behaviors if they are denied.

Inappropriate sexual behavior in the middle and later stages of dementia occurs more frequently in men than women (Alagiakrishnan et al. 2005; Buhr and White 2006). This behavior may include undressing, exposing genitalia, masturbating in public, making lewd sexual references, and touching or fondling other people. Such sexually aggressive behavior is relatively rare and is the result of sexual disinhibition from brain damage that has impaired the individual's executive functioning as well as the presence of paranoia and psychosis (Guay 2008). Such behavior may lead to legal problems, especially if the victim of the inappropriate action is an unwilling individual who calls law enforcement, or, if the parties are residents of a long-term care facility, the administration of the facility (Kamel and Hajjar 2003).

Cultural Factors

Cultural beliefs and practices influence the reported prevalence and manifestation of BPSD (www.ipa-online.org/ipaonlinev3/ipaprograms/bpsdarchives/bpsdrev/toc.asp). In some cultures, caregivers are likely to deny the presence of BPSD because of perceived stigma or reverence for the older person (Dilworth-Anderson and Gibson 2002).

Patient/family reactions to behavioral and psychological symptoms as well as the choice of management interventions depend on several factors:

- Beliefs about aging and the role of older people
- Beliefs about memory changes with aging
- Religious beliefs and cultural norms
- Size and location of racial/ethnic community
- Availability of family and other caregivers
- Perceived burden

- Availability and accessibility of culturally appropriate health care services

Management

The American Psychiatric Association and American Academy of Neurology have practice guidelines for management based on evidence-based reviews of the literature (Doody et al. 2001; Lyketsos et al. 2006; Rabins et al. 2007). A number of reports from expert consensus groups and panels contain practice parameters for non-pharmacologic management, and there are many excellent review articles (Teri et al. 2002; Livingston et al. 2005; Alexopoulos et al. 2007).

The recommended strategic framework for managing behavioral and psychological symptoms includes:

- Identify the problem behavior(s) or symptom(s).
- Prioritize the problems and work with one at a time.
- Gather detailed information about the frequency of occurrence, severity, temporal course, location(s) where problem behaviors occur, and presence of other persons.
- Clarify factors that trigger the behavioral disturbance.
- Identify the consequences of the behavior for the patient, family, and others around the patient if in a day care or long-term care environment.
- Develop a specific care plan tailored to the patient and caregiver(s). Engage family members to set management goals and involve the patient within the boundaries of their abilities. If possible, generate several approaches to deal with the situation and choose the one most likely to work best.
- Work with family members or formal staff caregivers to anticipate problems when the care plan is implemented and generate possible solutions. Prepare caregivers for the time required, because change is not immediate.
- Find ways to praise patients and caregivers for their efforts.

- Evaluate the patient's behavior and care plan frequently and modify as needed.
- Identify standards to evaluate whether the plan is working.

A physical examination is necessary to rule out sources of pain and discomfort that may result from a change in physical status, circulatory problems with pain in the extremities, infections, stool impaction, decubiti, dental caries or rotting teeth, fractured bones, or even tightly fitting clothes and shoes. A drug review is necessary to examine the possible impact of new medications, side effects, and drug-nutrient interactions that may cause discomfort. Visual changes, including cataracts and glaucoma, and hearing loss can provoke paranoia and agitation from persons who cannot understand or express their reactions and needs. Many environmental factors can overstimulate patients and provoke agitation, including loud noises, television, warm or cold ambient temperature, erratic illumination, being with too many people, being exposed to another resident who is wandering or disrupts nighttime sleep, behavioral problems of other residents, relocation to another room or residential setting, or any significant environmental changes.

Working with caregivers who interact with patients on a daily basis is a critical component of effective management and prevention of problem behaviors. It is essential to obtain a history of the patient's premorbid personality, lifestyle, daily routines, and preferences. Patients who have dementia are people who have needs and desires and who need to feel comfortable, safe, and secure in the context of a disease that interferes with virtually every aspect of their lives. The simple irritations of having an assigned roommate who snores; of being too hot or too cold; of having a stranger, sometimes of the opposite sex or another race, assist with toileting or bathing, can be upsetting and lead to behavioral disturbances if the emotional impact of these circumstances is not understood and addressed.

Family caregiver partnerships and interventions are discussed in chapter 15. Unless family caregivers are educated about what happens over the course of dementia, inappropriate demands, unrealistic expectations, getting angry, and blaming the patient for failures can rapidly toxify a household, causing more anger and frustration, agitation and other problem behaviors, and an unpleasant environment for everyone. These situations are also associated with the risk of patient-caregiver and caregiver-patient abuse.

Psychological and behavioral interventions require education of family caregivers to reinforce positive behaviors in the patient and ignore others, to provide a structured daily routine, to maintain a level of environmental stimulation appropriate to the patient's abilities, to deal honestly with patients' questions within the limitations of the dementia, and to provide opportunities for physical exercise and social interactions within a structured daily routine.

Strategies for effective management to minimize and/or prevent agitation include:

• Structuring the environment to make the patient feel safe
• Implementing stimulating, but not overstimulating, daytime activities
• Involving patients in active physical activities rather than passive activities
• Avoiding or minimizing daytime napping
• Implementing early evening activities that engage but do not overstimulate patients
• Providing light stimulation in the late afternoon for sundowners
• Establishing bedtimes consistent with patient's history
• Minimizing noise
• Maintaining the consistency of lighting in the environment
• Avoiding having people wait for meals, particularly in noisy restaurants or cafeterias
• Providing assistance for those who cannot feed themselves, ideally in separate quiet areas
• Providing finger food and liquids frequently throughout the day
• Providing bedtime snacks that promote sleep
• Considering the value of pets

Maximizing comfort, pleasure, and activity is the key to enhancing the quality of life and minimizing BPSD for people who have dementia. The goal is to attempt to fit the pattern of care to the patient's history and current functioning rather than to force behavioral changes in order to accommodate caregivers or institutional rules. The alternative is to try to develop an effective compromise.

Managing Sexually Aggressive Behavior

Inappropriate sexual behaviors are similar to other BPSD. Their occurrence is caused by several factors: the direct effect of brain degeneration; the response to unmet needs such as physical discomfort caused by hunger, thirst, loud noises, drug effects, or pain that the patient cannot communicate; constipation, fecal incontinence, or irregular bowel movements; the inability to adapt to the environment; and a history of sexual behaviors (e.g., sex offender).

In contrast to other behavioral disturbances, inappropriate sexual behaviors are a delicate issue for most people, and discussions to identify how to manage them create situations that may be embarrassing for caregivers. However, not to help caregivers overcome resistant feelings and deal with these issues will lead to continued sexual disturbances and increasing frustration and embarrassment as well as anger, resentment, and sometimes abuse of the patient.

Psychological, behavioral, and environmental interventions are often effective in minimizing or extinguishing the inappropriate behavior (Alagiakrishnan et al. 2005; Light and Holroyd 2006). Medications should never be the only treatment strategy. However, medications such as the atypical antipsychotics have been used as the first-line treatment to reduce symptoms for serious aggressive outbursts, exhibitionism, and sexual touching, especially in severely impaired, nonverbal, and volatile patients.

Institutions often have significant problems with inappropriate sexual behavior. Other residents, family members, administration, and line staff frequently react strongly and assertively to such behaviors. Protecting other residents is a valid primary concern, but this is best done by developing a strategy to manage untoward behaviors while protecting others from harm (Kamel and Hajjar 2004). Residents who are not cognitively impaired but have romantic inclinations should be allowed to have personal intimacy. Staff members need to be mindful that age and residential status per se do not preclude the development of a supportive affectionate bond with others.

Caregivers need practical guidance and support to develop a plan to manage sexually inappropriate behaviors in a calm responsive manner. When more harmless behaviors occur at home (e.g., taking off clothes), bring a robe and help the person put it on. Because disrobing often occurs when a person is uncomfortable because of problems such as tight clothes or itchy skin, experiment with ways to change the undressing behavior (e.g., dress the person in comfortable workout clothes and tennis shoes or let the person choose his or her favorite clothes). Caregivers should be encouraged to take the patient for a physical evaluation to identify medical sources of discomfort.

Masturbation is a particularly unnerving behavior for many caregivers. If the person is masturbating when others are present, he or she should be guided calmly to the bedroom or other private place, covered with a robe, and distracted with another activity. When inappropriate sexual behaviors occur in a public place, caregivers should inform others that the person has dementia and does not understand that their behaviors are inappropriate and then guide the person to the nearest private area and distract him or her. Ways to prevent inappropriate public masturbation include being attentive to regular toileting; monitoring problems such as urinary tract infections, vaginitis, and impaction; showing affection throughout the day and night by appropriate touch; and keeping the person actively involved in activities.

Caregivers need preparation for knowing when it is appropriate for a spouse to consider whether they are able or want to continue to have sexual relations with their partner. Clinicians need to interview the partner directly and thoughtfully about issues such as whether sex is still comfortable, whether the needs of both partners are being met, and whether sexually aggressive behaviors are increasing, placing the caregiver at risk for injury. There are many options, ranging from separate sleeping arrangements at home to placement in an assisted living residence or nursing home.

Pharmacological Management

Although nonpharmacolgical interventions are the first-line treatment after a thorough assessment of the causes of behavioral disturbances, there may also be a role for medications (Martinon-Torres et al. 2004). Pharmacological treatment is appropriate when symptoms are severe, psychotic in nature, and seriously adversely affect the patient's and family's ability to function and when there is no evidence for delirium or medical and environmental triggers that can be ameliorated. Before making the decision to administer medication, the clinician should consider several issues:

- Have behavioral, psychological, and environmental management strategies been tried, and do they need supplementation with medications?
- Is the behavior or the underlying etiology responsive to medication?
- What class of medication should be considered?
- What side effects as well as medication and nutrient-medication interactions should be anticipated?
- How long should the medication be used?
- What medications is the patient taking?

The current synthesis of research regarding pharmacologic agents for BPSD indicates that efficacy is limited and adverse side effects are common (Sink et al. 2005). When pharmacological approaches are indicated for agitation, Trazadone appears to be the consensus treatment. Haloperidol may be effective to stabilize aggressive patients, but it is not effective for agitation or other BPSD (Lonergan et al. 2002). However, adverse events such as extrapyramidal symptoms and somnolence are common, outweighing the possible benefits. Low doses of the atypical antipsychotics, risperidone and olanzapine, may be effective for agitation. Depression can be effectively treated, but it is often missed if patients are not able to communicate verbally. Antidepressants may be effective for treating depression in dementia but do not ameliorate other psychiatric and behavioral disturbances.

The FDA has required black box warnings regarding the increased risk for cerebrovascular events with atypical antipsychotics, and the clinician should carefully consider the use of these medications in the context of the patient's overall health status. There have also been concerns about weight gain that occurs in patients taking atypical antipsychotic drugs. This weight gain may predispose patients for a metabolic syndrome and increase the risk of type II diabetes.

These issues require that clinicians proceed with caution, and it is prudent to discuss the risks and benefits of potentially beneficial medications with the patient, if possible, as well as with appropriate caregivers. Asking the patient and/or caregivers questions is a helpful strategy to assess their comprehension of the potential risks and to ensure that they are fully informed. The discussion should be documented in the patient's chart along with a plan to monitor the patient and withdraw the medication when it is no longer needed.

10

Mood Disorders

The mood disorders of later life—depression and bipolar disorder—are characterized by considerable variability in clinical symptoms and diagnostic specificity, brain changes, and response to treatment. If these disorders are not diagnosed and treated, they can be associated with reduced functional effectiveness, excess disability, unnecessary suffering, an impoverished quality of life, increased rate of suicide, increased use of medical care, and increased strain on caregivers (Liebowitz 1996; Charney et al. 2003; Evans et al. 2005).

There is only modest agreement about strategies to disaggregate depressive disorders into component subtypes (Blazer 2009). An extensive literature suggests the existence of a spectrum of geriatric depressive disorders ranging from subsyndromal to major unipolar and bipolar depression (Alexopoulos and Kelly 2009). Depressive symptoms in older people are not accurately reflected by the criteria described in DSM-IV-TR (Blazer 2009), and it remains to be seen whether DSM-V will accurately reflect geriatric diagnostic criteria.

Types of Mood Disorders

DSM-IV-TR classifies mood disorders as follows:

- Major Depressive Disorder (Single Episode or Recurrent)
- Dysthymic Disorder of early onset (before age 21) or later onset
- Depressive Disorder not otherwise specified
- Bipolar Disorders I and II
- Bipolar Disorder not otherwise specified
- Adjustment Disorder with Depressed Mood and/or Anxiety
- Psychotic Depression

- Mood Disorder secondary to a medical disorder or substance abuse

There is also an entity, not a diagnostic category, called Depressive Disorder, which is a syndrome lasting more than 2 weeks, but not directly due to a medical condition or a reaction to grief. This disorder varies in severity, and symptoms may be influenced by factors ranging from medical co-morbidities to cultural expectations and practices. The symptom cluster includes sadness, anhedonia, anorexia and weight loss, sleep problems, motor agitation or retardation, loss of energy and motivation, guilt, cognitive loss, and thoughts of death.

Older patients may manifest atypical symptoms characterized by lack of sadness and/or symptoms of anxiety, panic, and/or masked depression with somatization (Blazer and Steffans 2009). Clinicians may sometimes empathize with the patient's circumstances, believing that these symptoms are reasonable reactions, and thus overlook the need for a clinical diagnosis and treatment.

Epidemiology

Depressive symptoms are the most common mental health problems in older people. Twenty-five percent of older people living in the community report mild symptoms, and Major Depressive Disorders (MDDs) occur in 1–9 percent, a rate similar to that in younger populations (Pirkis et al. 2009). Nonmajor forms of depression, also known as minor depression, affect at least 50 percent of residents in long-term care facilities and as many as 25 percent of patients in primary care settings (Teresi et al. 2001; Snowden et al. 2003). Minor depression is defined by a distinctive cluster of symptoms, including depressed mood, psychomotor retardation, poor concentration, constipation, and poor perception of health (Rapaport et al. 2005). This profile is associated with cognitive deficits and physical illness and does not correspond to any particular DSM category.

Subsyndromal depressive spectrum disorder refers to another nonmajor clinically significant depression (Lyness et al. 2006). It is defined by the presence of two or more depressive symptoms occurring together for most or all of the time for at least 2 weeks and associated with social dysfunction in people who do not meet the diagnostic criteria for minor depression, major depression, or dysthymic disorder.

The prevalence of bipolar affective disorder ranges from 0.1 to 0.4 percent in the United States, but 10–20 percent of older patients who have mood disorder have bipolar disorder (Sajatovic et al. 2005a). Late-onset bipolar disorder is rare, but the recurrence of remitted disease is common, and the prevalence is expected to grow with increasing life expectancy (Sajatovic and Blow 2007).

Appropriate Responses to Loss versus Clinical Depression

Grief and sadness are normal reactions to death, changes in health, and stressful circumstances. In the short term, individuals experience a reactive depression, losing interest in pleasurable activities and experiencing emotional pain, insomnia, fatigue, boredom, and restlessness. Most people eventually find ways to deal with their losses with the support of their psychosocial network and using adaptive coping strategies. Some people, however, do not recover and are unable to cope with the routine demands of daily life.

When symptoms persist over 4 to 6 weeks or become more severe, the clinician's index of suspicion for clinical depression should be high. The acronym SIG E CAPS provides a heuristic framework for evaluation (Abraham and Shirley 2006):

S: Sleep disturbances
I: Lack of *I*nterest or pleasure in almost all activities
G: Inappropriate *G*uilt / feelings of worthlessness / hopelessness
E: Lack of *E*nergy
C: Concentration difficulties and indecisiveness
A: Lack of *A*ppetite
P: *P*sychomotor agitation or retardation
S: Suicidal ideation, plans, or attempts

With the exception of suicide, many of these symptoms commonly occur with frailty and / or illness. However, it is not normal for them to persist, worsen, and threaten an individual's welfare. Not discriminating appropriate emotional reactions to significant losses and clinical depression can be one of the more significant factors responsible for the underdiagnosis and suboptimal treatment of depression in primary care.

Bereavement professionals disagree about distinctions between normal, abnormal, and complicated grief reactions (Bonanno and Kaltman 2001). Some symptoms and behaviors help determine whether patients are experiencing normal prolonged grief reactions to loss or are clinically depressed. Intense yearnings are a core feature of extended grief reactions but not of severe depression (Maciejewski et al. 2007). Other indications of complicated grief include the existence of the following characteristics more than a year after a loss: intense intrusive thoughts and emotional pangs, feeling alone and empty, avoiding tasks that evoke memories of the deceased, persistent sleep disturbances, and excessive loss of interest in activities (Horowitz et al. 2003).

Supportive or socialization therapy, psychoeducation, Internet-based cognitive-behavioral interventions, and monitoring symptoms can be beneficial (Shear et al. 2001; Zhang et al. 2006; Wagner and Maercker 2007). Allowing patients to work through the grieving process is preferable, and monitoring those who have severe or complicated grief is essential. Treating depression does not block the grieving process, but not treating it increases the likelihood of complicated grief reactions.

Diagnosis

Diagnosis rests on physical, neurologic, and psychiatric examinations, including a review of medications and psychosocial stressors (Sajatovik and Blow 2007; Ellison et al. 2008; Blazer and Steffens 2009). Accurate diagnosis depends on taking time to have conversations with the person and informants, when available. Sensitive biological markers for depression and bipolar disorder do not exist at this time. A variety of rating scales reviewed in chapter 3 are useful screening tests to assess the severity of symptoms but do not replace a careful interview.

Many physical illnesses cause or coexist with depressive symptoms (Lyness et al. 2006), including AD and related dementias, endocrine disorders, neoplastic diseases, chronic infections, and collagen diseases. Other psychiatric disorders may also co-occur with depression, such as alcohol abuse/misuse, anxiety, and personality disorders (Devanand 2002).

Prescription medications may cause depression (Alexopoulos et al. 2001; Savoy 2004): cardiovascular drugs, such as beta blockers, reserpine, clonidine, digitalis, and alphamethyldopa; hormones, such as corticotrophin and glucucorticoids; anticancer agents, such as cycloserine; psychotropic medications, such as benzodiazepines; anti-inflammatory drugs, such as nonsteroidal anti-inflammatory agents and sulfonamides; and other medications, such as L-dopa, cimetidine, and ranitidine.

The clinician needs to consider a number of age-specific issues in the diagnosis. Because anhedonia is often more pronounced than sadness per se, clinicians should ask questions about sources of personal pleasure. Anorexia, weakness, fatigue, and weight loss are typical, especially in very old, severely ill patients, and if the clinician misinterprets these symptoms as physical illness, individuals may be at risk for deterioration and death. Homebound older persons living alone may be especially difficult to diagnose because of their frailty, limited mobility, weakness and fatigue, and social isolation. Older patients are often preoccupied with somatic symptoms and pain, which frequently exacerbates depression, and although they are often not aware of or do not communicate emotional distress, they frequently ruminate about problems and are more melancholic than younger adults. Sometimes the diagnosis of depression can be made only after a successful response to a trial of antidepressants.

Major Depressive Disorder

Major depressive disorder (MDD) can be a single episode or a recurrent condition, and it is characterized by somatic or vegetative symptoms, behavioral changes, and psychological reactions. It is a painful and incapacitating illness in which life feels overwhelming and miserable. William Styron, the Pulitzer prize-winning author, described his depression as feeling "condemned" to a life in which "the entire body and spirit of a person is in a state of shipwreck" (Styron 1990).

The following characteristics increase the risk for a MDD (Cole and Dendukuri 2003): a previous episode of MDD, intense psychosocial stressors, acutely disabling conditions, chronic co-morbidities, dependency on alcohol and drugs, a family history of depressive disorders, female gender, and functional impairments and disabilities interfering with independence.

To be diagnosed with *MMD* using DSM-IV-TR criteria, a person must have at least five of the following symptoms present nearly every day:

1. Depressed mood most of the day
2. Loss of interest or pleasure in usual activities, nearly every day for at least two weeks
3. Loss of appetite with associated weight loss or overeating with sudden weight gain (a monthly gain or loss of more than 5% of body weight)
4. Insomnia or sleeping a lot
5. Agitated behaviors
6. Loss of energy or fatigue
7. Feelings of worthlessness or excessive guilt
8. Decreased ability to concentrate and make decisions
9. Ongoing thoughts of death, suicidal ideation or actions

To be diagnosed with *minor depression,* a person must have had two to five of these symptoms for at least 2 weeks duration. Patients often have fewer vegetative symptoms and more subjective symptoms (e.g., worry, irritability, lethargy).

MMDs may include psychotic symptoms, and psychotic depression is more prevalent in later life than middle adulthood (Blazer 2009). Some individuals have mood-appropriate, nonbizarre delusions, such as refusing help because of beliefs of being a burden (delusions of guilt) or being convinced they have cancer or a terminal illness (somatic delusions). Other people may exhibit more troublesome delusions, such as feeling their spouse is planning to end a long-lived marriage (delusions of inadequacy), paranoia, or potentially dangerous hallucinations. Older persons are less likely to express guilt and self-deprecation than younger adults.

Depression may co-occur with AD, but the features and course differ from the DSM-IV-TR criteria for MMD. Provisional criteria for the diagnosis of depression in AD, developed by an NIMH workgroup (Olin et al. 2002), requires the presence of at least three symptoms of MDD for at least two weeks. Two symptoms were also added to the list of nine for MDD—irritability and social withdrawal/isolation—but none of the eleven symptoms has to be present "nearly every day." Decreased cognitive ability was eliminated because of the nature of dementia.

The NIMH criteria identify a higher proportion of people with AD who are depressed relative to DSM-IV-TR and other criteria (Teng et al. 2008). However, the two symptoms added—social isolation and irritability—do not predict depression. Symptoms most associated with a diagnosis of depression were psychomotor changes, fatigue, and guilt/worthlessness. Ongoing studies, including the Depression in Alzheimer's Disease Study-2 (Martin et al. 2006; Rosenberg and Lyketsos 2006) will continue to evaluate the precision and usefulness of diagnostic criteria.

Depression affects 50 to 70 percent of patients who have probable AD, and the prevalence decreases with increasing cognitive impairment (Zubenko et al. 2003). Depression in this instance is characterized by concentration difficulties, indecisiveness, and limited dysphoria (Alexopoulos 2004). There are gender differences, with men having more coexisting agitation and more severe symptomatology overall (Cohen et al. 1993).

Bipolar Disorders

Less is known about geriatric bipolar disorders than about depressive disorders (Charney et al. 2003; Depp and Jeste 2004; Sajatovic and Blow 2007). Bipolar disorder is gender neutral, and the age of onset varies considerably from childhood to age 50, with most cases first coming to clinical attention between ages 15 to 24. Although some patients who have recurrent depressive episodes have the first manic episode after age 50, this is relatively uncommon and suggests the likely influences of medical disorders (Sajatovic et al. 2005a). The hallmark of bipolar disorders or manic-depressive disorders is the occurrence of mania in the person's history. Bipolar disorders are characterized by mood swings of both depressive and manic behavior, and although mood shifts are usually gradual, they can occur rapidly or be separated by years. Using DSM-IV-TR criteria, bipolar disorders include type 1, with mania and usually recurrent depression, and type 2, recurrent major depression with hypomania. Type 1 is known as classic manic-depression, with episodes of major depression alternating with episodes of mania, whereas type 2 is a milder disorder consisting of depression alternating with less extreme manic behavior (hypomania). The latter does not manifest with psychotic symptoms or cause severe impairment in personal, social, and work activities. Cyclothymia, another form of bipolar illness, is characterized by oscillating mood swings of lesser intensity, but it rarely has its onset in later life.

A history of at least one episode of mania is required for the diagnosis. There are two types of mania, euphoric and dysphoric, and patients who have bipolar disorder can manifest both types. Euphoric patients are on a high, in love with themselves and the world, seem full of energy, need minimal sleep, exhibit pressured speech (i.e., rapid outpouring at words often with loose association), and are grandiose. Dysphoric patients experience a different kind of high. They talk fast and have grandiose thoughts but they are also agitated, angry, destructive, and often paranoid. Younger patients who have mania are more likely to present with euphoria and grandiosity, whereas older patients are more likely to present with depressed mood and manic symptoms, such as pressured speech and poor sleep patterns (Almeida and Fenner 2002).

Some patients may have had previous episodes of depression as well as subsequent cycles of mania and depression. To be diagnosed with a manic episode using DSM-IV-TR criteria, patients must have a period of persistently elevated, expansive, or irritable mood lasting at least one week, and three or more of the following symptoms in the same period:

1. Inappropriate grandiosity or inflated self-esteem
2. Significantly decreased need for sleep
3. Unusually talkative with pressured speech
4. Rapidly racing thoughts
5. Very distractible
6. Increased agitation and goal-directed activities
7. Excessive time spent in pleasurable activities without awareness of negative consequences

Older patients presenting with bipolar disorder in the manic phase can be a challenging differential diagnosis, because they frequently show confusion, disorientation, memory problems, and agitation. Disorders considered in the differential would include agitated depression, dementia, schizophrenia, delirium, and medication side effects.

Bipolar disorders are a chronic condition with no currently known cure, but they can usually be managed effectively. They typically cause substantial social problems that affect marriage, work, and family; and patients need to be protected from the possible negative consequences of poor judgment and excessive

activity. Over time, even in periods of remission, the chronicity and unpredictability of symptoms can lead to legal, marital, and job problems as well as medical complications and suicide.

Bipolar disorders are costly financially and socially, making them a challenging public mental health issue (Kleinman et al. 2003; Simon 2003). Older adults who have bipolar disorder use four times the services of those who have MDD (Bartels et al. 2000). The course is episodic but highly variable, and it often coexists with substance abuse and anxiety disorders. Morbidity and mortality risks are high, and a significant proportion of people die from complications of risky behavior, heart attack, or suicide (Conwell 2001; Depp and Jeste 2004).

Cyclothymic Disorder

Cyclothymic disorder, which is rare in older adults, is a chronic bipolar disorder consisting of short periods of mild depression and hypomania that may last a few days or several weeks. The onset is separated by short periods of normal mood. Individuals who have cyclothymia are never totally free of symptoms of either depression or hypomania for more than a few months at a time. Although cyclothymic disorder is not as severe as MDD and bipolar disorder, it affects all aspects of the patient's life.

Adjustment Disorders with Depressed Mood

Adjustment disorders with depressed mood are a persistent over-reaction to an acute or chronic stressor lasting more than six months and impairing the individual's cognitive, emotional, social, or occupational functioning. There are several adjustment disorders, which are classified by the predominant symptoms of depression, anxiety, mixed symptoms, or unspecified symptoms.

Dysthymic Disorders

Dysthymia is characterized by chronic mild depressive symptoms of at least two years duration. It may coexist with MDD and has been called a double depression (Hybels et al. 2008). The somatization shown by older patients and the feelings associated with limitations in activities all help mask the condition, and it is often misinterpreted as a normal consequence of the infirmities of older adults.

Dysthymic disorder usually begins in childhood or adolescence. To be diagnosed with a dysthymic disorder using DSM-IV-TR criteria, the patient must have a depressed mood most of the day, more days than not, for at least two years and have at least two of the following symptoms:

1. Poor appetite or overeating
2. Insomnia or sleeping too much
3. Low energy and fatigue
4. Poor self-esteem
5. Difficulty with concentration or decision-making
6. Feelings of hopelessness

Although dysthymia is less severe than a MMD, the consequences can be just as significant: increased morbidity, emotional anguish, severely impaired functioning, and risk for suicide. Some people have described living with dysthymia as seeing the world through dark glasses: they are able to function and get on with life, but they are not happy.

Dysthymia in older people may have a different etiology, a later age of onset, and less severe psychiatric morbidity than younger adults (Hybels et al. 2008). It is often a reaction to health status, major stressors, and perceived functional decline.

Depression with Psychotic Features

The prevalence of psychotic depression is about 4 percent in depressed older persons living in the community, and it occurs in 20–45 percent of hospitalized depressed older patients (Blazer 2009). Psychotic depression appears to be associated with cognitive impairment, especially in patients who have vascular dementia. Delusions and hallucinations, either congruent depression-related guilt feelings, or incongruent thought intrusions, or paranoia, characterize the psychotic features. Psychiatric symptoms impair reality testing.

Etiology

Depression

Depression and Medical Illness

Any review of the biological causes of depression must begin with medical conditions, because depression is frequently a co-morbid condition with almost all medical illnesses in older adults (Evans et al. 2005). Depression may also occur when individuals are trying to change health behaviors: smoking cessation or compliance with dietary, exercise, or medication regimens. The conclusion of several comprehensive reviews of the literature on depression and medical disorders is that depression is more than the secondary consequences of these medical conditions (Blazer 2009).

The relationship between depression and heart disease has been studied more thoroughly than other co-morbidities (Lichtman et al. 2008; Nemeroff 2008). In addition to the high prevalence rate of depression in patients who have coronary artery disease, people who have co-morbid depression after a myocardial infarction are more likely to have poorer outcomes, including death rates, than cardiac patients who do not have depression (Barth et al. 2004). Long-term survival is inversely associated with the severity of depression. This same relationship has also been observed in patients after coronary artery bypass graft surgery as well as in patients who have isolated systolic hypertension.

Several theories have been proposed for the shared mechanisms linking depression with cardiovascular disease, including platelet activation, catecholamine release, and proinflamatory cytokines (Joynt et al. 2004). Evidence that platelet activation is increased in older depressed adults is one possible mechanism placing them at heightened risk for ischemic heart disease, including early mortality (Chen 2009). Decreased appetite and poor nutrition may lead to a low body mass index, frailty, and failure to thrive (Blazer 2009). Depressed older adults have higher cytokine interleukin 6 levels, indicative of increased anti-inflammatory activity. Free fatty acid composition has been related to depression in community-residing older people, and it is an independent factor unrelated to inflammatory reactions (Tiemeier et al. 2003).

Biological Etiologies

The present consensus about the etiology of depression can be described as a gene-environment interaction model for complex diseases that is similar to cancer and diabetes, with a focus on impaired vascular circulation, three monoamine neurotransmitter systems—serotonin, norepinephrine, and dopamine—as well as stress and hormones associated with the hypothalamic-pituitary-adrenal axis (Nemeroff and Owens 2009).

Alexopoulos (2004) proposed the vascular depression hypothesis, suggesting that cerebrovascular disease not only is a risk factor for a geriatric depressive syndrome but also may precipitate or perpetuate depression in older adults who have dementia. This hypothesis is supported by several factors: the co-occurrence of depression with hypertension, diabetes, coronary artery disease, and stroke; the high frequency of silent stroke and white matter hyperintensities in geriatric depression; and the association of depression with brain lesions affecting the basal ganglia and prefrontal cortex (Alexopoulos 2006; Santos et al. 2009). The results of imaging studies revealing white matter hyperintensities and neuropathological correlates of small strokes in older depressed patients suggest that cerebral circulatory compromise is a primary rather than secondary cause of geriatric depression.

Geriatric depression is associated with several metabolic and structural changes in the brain (Alexopoulos 2004; Nemeroff 2008). The findings of functional imaging studies suggest that depression is associated with abnormal metabolism, usually increased, in limbic regions, including the amygdala, pregenual and subgenual anterior cingulate cortex, and posterior orbitofrontal cortex as well as the posterior cingulate and medial cerebellum. In contrast, reduced blood flow is seen in the lateral and dorsolateral prefrontal cortex, dorsal anterior cingulate, and caudate nucleus. Reduced bilateral activation of the dorsal anterior cingulate and the hippocampus has been observed in severely depressed older patients (de Asis et al. 2001). Decreased prefrontal activation and increased caudate activation has also been observed (Alexopoulos et al. 2008).

There is reduced activity of serotonergic neurons, reduced numbers of serotonin transporter (SERT) binding sites (i.e., the binding site for SSRIs) in the midbrain and amygdala, reduced presynaptic serotonergic receptor density in the midbrain, and reduced postsynaptic serotonergic receptor density in the mesiotemporal cortex (Muller and Schwartz 2007; Gerretson and Pollack 2008). These findings suggest that there is a net reduction in the number and/or functioning of the presynaptic serotonergic nerve terminals and a reduction in postsynaptic serotonergic signal transduction.

The importance of serotonergic circuits is underscored by the consistent finding that persons who have the s allele of the promoter region of the SERT gene (SLC 6A4) are at heightened risk for depression associated with early life abuse or neglect (Vergne and Nemeroff 2006; Nemeroff and Owens 2009). The effect is dose-dependent in terms of the s allele as well as the frequency and severity of abuse. Those most vulnerable to depression have the s/s genotype, the least vulnerable have the l/l genotype, and those with the s/l genotype have intermediate risk. Furthermore, imaging studies show that individuals who have s/s and s/l genotypes have reduced SERT binding sites compared to l/l individuals.

Neurochemical and neuroendocrine studies have demonstrated the importance of the norepinephrine circuit in depression, including treatment-resistant depression (Robinson 2007). Norepinephrine reuptake inhibitors (e.g., desipramine, nortriptyline) are effective antidepressant medications. Low levels of norepinephrine metabolites are present in the urine and cerebrospinal fluid of depressed patients. Postmortem examination of the cortex of people who have been depressed and committed suicide shows an increased density of beta-adrenergic receptors. Finally, significant life stress, which increases the activity of norepinephrine brain circuits, is associated with the development of depression.

Dopamine also plays a significant role in depression (Dunlop and Nemeroff 2007; Robinson 2007). The dopamine hypothesis of depression is consistent with the inability to experience pleasure, one of the most important diagnostic symptoms of depression, and it is well documented that anhedonia is mediated by the dopaminergic circuit. Postmortem and imaging studies have shown reduced dopamine transporter binding sites and increased postsynaptic dopamine D2/D3 receptor density, evidence of reduced availability of synaptic dopamine in depression. Together, these results suggest that medications that increase the neurotransmission of dopamine (e.g., monoamine oxidase inhibitors, dopamine receptor agonists) or triple (serotonin, norepinephrine, and dopamine) reuptake inhibitors under development are effective treatments for depression.

Several well-known findings support a significant role for hyperactivity of the hypothalamic-pituitary-axis (HPA) in the etiology of depression: high levels of cortisol and other HPA hormones observed in depressed and suicidal persons, the high prevalence of severe depression and anxiety in patients who have Cushing disease, and the increased production of glucocorticoids in healthy persons under stress (Gillespi and Nemeroff 2005).

Psychosocial Factors

Psychosocial variables play a significant role in the etiology of depression. The results of a major study of more than 22,000 persons aged 50–104 from ten countries revealed that physical health as well as measures of absolute and relative social and economic deprivation predicted the occurrence of depression (Ladin et al. 2009). Using a stress-diathesis model for depression, depression-inducing stress involves a mixture of social, psychological, and biological factors that are likely to vary in their impact on individuals and be mediated by genetic vulnerability, developmental history, personality and cognitive variables, coping styles, culture, and environmental influences.

Genetic Contributions

The genetic and genetic-environmental interactions in the spectrum of depressive disorders are difficult to summarize (Smith et al. 2007; Blazer 2009). Genetic studies have indicated that Met 66 allele carriers are twice as likely to have geriatric depression compared to carriers of the Val 66 allele homozygote (Taylor et al. 2007). Lavretsky et al. (2008) found that dopamine transporter genotypes but not serotonin transporter genotypes were associated with impaired executive functioning and methylphenidate response, while Steffens et al. (2007) showed that Apo lipoprotein Ee4, lower MMSI, and older age were correlated with the volume of grey matter lesions in geriatric depression. Finally, candidate genes have been associated with psychosocial as well as biological triggers for depression, and this research may elucidate the etiology of late- and early-onset depression (Smith et al. 2007).

Bipolar Disorders

The precise etiology and pathogenesis of bipolar disorders are unknown, but twin, family, and adoption studies suggest a prominent genetic component, with first-degree relatives of patients who have bipolar disorder at a sevenfold higher risk than the general population (Barnett and Smoller 2009; Craddock and Sklar 2009). The results of a European genome-wide association study of bipolar disorder suggest that bipolar disorder involves multiple genes, each with modest effects (Baum et al. 2008). In studies of the Old Order Amish in Pennsylvania, researchers developed a genetic tree with data dating back to eighteenth-century England demonstrating strong genetic influences on bipolar illness (Shaw et al. 2005). Genome-wide linkage analyses provided evidence that regions on chromosomes 6, 13, and 15 have susceptibility loci for bipolar affective disorder, suggesting that bipolar affective disorder in the Old Order Amish is inherited as a complex trait. Molecular genetic and imaging studies suggest that cell death in parts of the frontal cortex and hippocampus are implicated (Lyoo et al.

2004). There is also evidence that individuals susceptible to bipolar disorder experience an increasing number of neuronal insults from excessive and chronic stress-related glucocorticoid stimulation (van Rossum et al. 2006).

Treatment

Treatments are effective when evidence-based guidelines are used (Colenda et al. 2003). However, despite advances in pharmacotherapy and psychotherapies, currently about 20 percent of older persons do not respond to treatment, and another 20–30 percent respond partially (Fava 2003; Mulsant et al. 2004). Although NIMH cites treatment response rates of 80 percent for people who have major depression, the results of the National Comorbidity Survey Replication showed that only 42 percent of patients responded adequately to treatment (Kessler et al. 2003). Older adults who have double depression have the same treatment response as older adults who have MDD alone (Hybels et al. 2008).

The American Psychiatric Association's evidence-based guidelines are not specifically focused on older persons, but they emphasize the impact of co-morbid conditions and drug effects in this age group (Fochtmann and Gelenberg 2005). The Expert Consensus Panel Treatment Guidelines on Late-Life Depression (Alexopoulos et al. 2001; Charney et al. 2003) are based on expert consensus, not evidence-based practice. The Canadian Coalition for Seniors' Mental Health has published national practice Guidelines for the assessment and treatment of depression (Buchanan et al. 2006). There are also several expert recommendations for the treatment of depression in Alzheimer disease (Olin et al. 2002; Lyketsos and Lee 2004).

Many studies show the effectiveness of coupling primary care and specialty psychiatric care in the treatment of late-life depression (Skultety and Rodriegues 2008). Screening patients in primary care with appropriate referral to specialists improves outcomes, including decreased depressive symptomatology, stabilization of medical conditions, and improved

psychosocial support for patients and family members (Arean and Ayalon 2005; Bogner et al. 2005; Knight and Houseman 2008). The success of PROSPECT (Prevention of Suicide in Primary Care Elderly: Collaborative Trial) has demonstrated that depression, hopelessness, and suicidal ideation can be identified and treated successfully in the primary care setting through the use of depression mental health managers (Mulsant et al. 2004; Alexopoulos et al. 2005a; www.nrepp.samhsa.gov/programfulldetails.asp?PROGRAM_ID=113). The largest geriatric depression treatment study to date is IMPACT (Improving Mood-Promoting Access to Collaborative Treatment; http://impact-uw.org/about/implement.html). The results indicated that about half of all older patients who have major depression have a 50 percent reduction in symptoms (Unutzer et al. 2002; Bruce et al. 2004; Hunkler et al. 2006). The UPBEAT (Unified Psychogeriatric Biopsychosocial Evaluation and Treatment) program of the Veterans Administration had low patient compliance with protocols, and although the protocol led to improvement, treatment outcomes were minimal for other psychiatric morbidity (Oslin et al. 2004).

The Sequenced Treatment Alternatives to Relieve Depression (STAR*D), the largest study of treatment-resistant depression in the United States to date (www.edc.pitt.edu/stard/public/), focused on identifying what to do after a failed treatment response and created an empirical basis for practice guidelines. The objectives were to determine what subsequent treatment strategies to adopt, in what order, and in combination(s) that were acceptable to patients, to provide the best clinical results with the least side effects. A secondary objective was to identify costs and cost offsets in primary care and specialty care settings.

STAR*D included four levels of treatment choices (Rush et al. 2004). Level 1 was treatment with citalopram, and persons who got well continued on the medication for a year. Those who did not get better went to level 2, where they had two choices: (1) switch treatments and be randomized to sertraline, bupropion, venlafaxine-ZR, or cognitive behavioral therapy; or (2) add treatment and be randomized to bupropion, buspirone, or cognitive-behavioral therapy. Those who did not get better went to level 3, where they had two choices: (1) switch treatments and be randomized to mirtazapine or nortriptyline; or (2) add treatment and be randomized to lithium or tri-iodothyronine. Those who did not get well went to level 4, where they were taken off all medications and randomized to tranylcypromine or venlafaxine and mirtazapine.

Results indicated that patients can get well after trying several treatment strategies, but the odds of recovery diminished as additional treatment strategies were needed (Rush et al. 2006). About half of the participants were symptom-free after the first two treatment levels, after which remission rates decreased. Over the course of all four levels, about 70 percent of those who did not withdraw from the study became symptom-free. Two significant indicators of successful treatment outcomes emerged. Individuals who became symptom-free had a better chance of staying well over the follow-up period, compared to those who experienced only symptom improvement. Individuals who required several treatment levels to become symptom-free had more severe depressive symptoms and more co-morbidities at the beginning of the study, and they were more likely to relapse during a one-year follow-up phase. These results underscore both the need for a better understanding of how different people respond to different treatments and the challenges in finding effective short- and long-term treatments.

Pharmacological Management

When choosing pharmacologic therapies for older patients, clinicians need to consider potential adverse side effects, drug and drug-nutrient interactions, and patient limitations (Small 2010). The general indications for pharmacological intervention include:

- Presence of moderate to severe depression
- Presence of suicidal thoughts and behaviors
- Existence of symptoms for two or more years

- Ineffective psychotherapy or lack of trained psychotherapists
- Significantly impaired social/work functioning
- Presence of depression with psychotic symptoms
- Prior positive response to an antidepressant
- Patient requests medication.
- Patient has responded well in the acute and continuation phases of drug therapy, and maintenance therapy is planned.

There are several excellent resources for drug efficacy and prescription information (Savoy 2004), guidelines for geriatric medication management and combined medication/psychological treatment (Nierenberg et al. 2007; Adams et al. 2008; Chew-Graham et al. 2008), consensus guidelines (Alexopoulos et al. 2001), and evidence-based pharmacologic interventions for geriatric depression (Shanmugham et al. 2005).

As of this writing, the FDA has approved 10 types of antidepressants and 36 different brands. The principal groups are selective serotonin reuptake inhibitors (SSRIs), tricyclic antidepressants (TCAs), monoamine oxidase inhibitors (MAOIs), and newer compounds that include serotonin norepinephrine reuptake inhibitors (SNRIs), noradrenergic specific serotonergic antidepressants (NASSAs), norepinephrine reuptake inhibitors (NRIs), norepinephrine and dopamine reuptake inhibitors (NDRIs), selective serotonin reuptake enhancers (SSREs), melatonergic agonists, and augmenter drugs.

No single antidepressant is significantly more effective than another, and no single drug results in success for all patients. Side effects vary, and clinicians should become familiar with drugs in each classification in order to be prepared to switch or supplement medications when patients do not respond or have adverse side effects. Combining two or even three medications may also be helpful. Drug selection depends on many factors:

- Type and severity of depression
- Pharmacokinetics
- Side effect profile

- Simplicity of dosing
- Need for monitoring
- Overdose safety
- Prior response to drug
- Presence of dementia
- Coexisting medical illnesses and current medications
- Degree to which a drug could interfere with a patient's lifestyle
- Cost

Some antidepressant drugs, SSRIs and SNRIs in particular, may take 6 weeks or more before patients notice significant improvement, and patients need support from clinicians and family members in the acute treatment phase. Treatment response is usually stepwise, with cycles of improvement and decline. The temporary return of symptoms is common and does not predict outcome. The addition of newer antipsychotic medications may also contribute to symptom relief, although not without the risks attendant to the atypical antipsychotics described in chapter 12 (i.e., strokes and increased vascular morbidity).

Increased activity and improved sleep are usually the first responses to treatment, and mood is among the last symptoms to improve. Side effects need to be closely monitored and medications changed when side effects are intrusive. Suicidal ideation needs to be carefully monitored, because severely depressed patients are at higher risk for suicide early in treatment when they have more energy but still have a depressed mood and feelings of hopelessness. Hospitalization, or at least close 24-hour monitoring, may be clinically indicated.

The results of the PROSPECT and STAR*D studies emphasize the importance of careful patient monitoring. Early response (i.e., 4–6 weeks) is a positive indicator, but patients who have heightened anxiety, are socially isolated, have low socioeconomic status or low educational attainment, are male, and do not have an early response, should be considered as candidates for augmentation or medication change.

Selective Serotonin Reuptake Inhibitors

Selective serotonin reuptake inhibitors (SSRIs) are usually prescribed as the first-line treatment for depression (Taylor et al. 2006). Five SSRIs have been approved for use in the United States: fluoxetine (Prozac), sertraline (Zoloft), paroxetine (Paxil), citalopram (Celexa), and escitalopram oxalate (Lexapro). They are equally effective and have a greater benefit/risk ratio than TCAs and MAOIs (Kaspar and Heiden 2004).

SSRIs are safe if a patient overdoses, because there is no systemic or cardiac toxicity. About half of patients taking SSRIs do not have side effects, and those who do can usually tolerate them. The most common side effects are gastrointestinal, such as nausea, diarrhea, and dry mouth, but these tend to fade within a few weeks. Central nervous system symptoms such as anxiety, agitation, and insomnia as well as sedation, neuromotor side-effects, or bradycardia may also occur.

Sexual dysfunction, ejaculatory problems in men and anorgasmia in women, may also occur. It is important to inquire about these symptoms because patients may be too embarrassed to disclose them or may stop taking their medications because of sexual dysfunction. These symptoms are usually treatable or may be managed by adjusting the dose or prescription of medications to enhance sexual arousal.

Serotonin-norepinephrine reuptake inhibitors (SNRIs) act on the two neurotransmitters identified as playing a role in mood disorders, anxiety and obsessive-compulsive disorder, and neuropathic pain (Vossen et al. 2009; Seo et al. 2010). Like the SSRIs, SNRIs reportedly enhance neural regrowth via other influences on NMDA receptors. A long and growing group of SNRIs are currently available, including Venlafaxine, Desvenlafaxine, Sibutramine, Nefazedone, Duloxetine, Desipramine, Milnacipram and Bicifadine. The side effects vary but include sedation, anxiety, and a withdrawal syndrome if discontinued abruptly.

Tricyclic Antidepressants

Before the approval of SSRIs, TCAs were the standard treatment for depression (Saltzman 2004). Common TCAs include desipramine(Norpramin), amitriptyline (Elavil), nortriptyline, clomipramine (Anafranil), and doxepin(Sinequan). These drugs appear to be as effective as the SSRIs, but they have a quinadinelike effect, have the potential for cardiotoxicity, and can be lethal in an overdose. Side effects may include anticholinergic effects such as dry mouth, blurred vision, sweating, urinary retention, and tachycardia; orthostatic hypotension; sedation, weight gain, and sexual dysfunction. TCAs are less expensive than the SSRIs, but their side effects and toxicity make them less desirable for people of all ages.

Monoamine Oxidase Inhibitors

MAOIs are usually used only after other drugs have not worked (Saltzman 2004). Common MAOIs include Nardil (phenelzine), Parnate (tranylcypromine), and Marplan (isocarboxazid). MAOIs are comparable in efficacy with other antidepressants, but they have significant untoward side effects if patients eat foods that have tyramine, including but not limited to cheese, yogurt, smoked foods, soy sauce, bananas, caffeine, and chocolate.

Other medications that alter norepinephrine levels can also be dangerous when used with MAOIs, causing a dangerous rise in blood pressure with the risk of stroke. Drugs to avoid include antihistamines, decongestants, any cold medications, codeine, narcotic pain relievers, and some forms of anesthesia. Side effects may include orthostatic hypotension, weight gain, and sexual dysfunction.

Other Antidepressant Drugs

There are many other effective antidepressants (Savoy 2004). These include atypical noradrenalin and dopamine reuptake inhibitors, bupropion and buproprion SR (Wellbutrin); serotonin reuptake and 5HT2 receptor inhibitors, trazodone (Desyrel) and nefazodone (Serzone); serotonin and noradrenaline reuptake inhibitors, venlafaxine (Effexor); duloxetine (Cymbalta), a potent serotonin and norepinephrine inhibitor with less potent dopaminergic effects; and the noradrenergic and specific serontonergic antidepressant, mirtazapine (Remeron).

Drug Treatment for Very Old Patients

Data are scarce regarding the use, efficacy, and side-effects of antidepressants in persons age 85 or older, especially those who have severe depression, dementia, or multiple co-morbidities (Roose et al. 2004). Medications may have limited effectiveness for very old people living in the community because of poor compliance due to the lack of home health care or family, and therefore psychosocial support is an important adjunct to drug therapy.

Drug Treatment for Patients who Have Alzheimer Disease or Other Dementia

Depression can be successfully managed, but the efficacy of antidepressants is reduced in patients who have dementia and major depression, particularly in the oldest-old (S Thompson et al. 2007). Cognitively impaired patients who respond to treatment show less improvement than patients who only have MDD. All classes of antidepressants may be effective, but SSRIs are the preferred first line of treatment followed by SNRIs. However, efficacy data are limited across drug classes.

Phases of Treatment

Pharmacologic treatment has three phases—acute, continuation, and maintenance. Most drugs require 8 to 16 weeks to achieve the optimal therapeutic effect. Patients should be monitored carefully to ensure compliance, and where indicated, to prevent suicide, particularly early in treatment when the patient may sleep and act more purposefully but psychological improvement such as feelings of hopelessness and guilt have not yet occurred. If suicidality is an issue, close observation, even possible hospitalization, may be indicated (chapter 17). Psychotherapeutic approaches and ongoing support, in combination with medication, will enhance the prospects for recovery.

Weight Gain

Antidepressant medications have been promoted as weight-reduction aids, perhaps on the assumption that some anxious patients habitually eat to reduce stress and insecurity. However, many medications, SSRIs in particular, have the opposite effect. Weight gain as an undesirable consequence of pharmacologic treatment with some antidepressants and atypical antipsychotics is a significant issue in choosing medication and assessing the balance between clinical benefit and longer-term problems (Ness-Abramof and Apovian 2005).

Several factors contribute to increased weight in addition to drugs: metabolic slowing from hormonal changes, secondary sedative effects that reduce caloric need, and food cravings. The antihistamine sedative effect of some antidepressants, particularly TCAs and NASSAs, may cause increased appetites. Antidepressant medication may also have a positive response on the immune system, and a monitored exercise regime coupled with an appropriate diet (i.e., low fat, low protein, and controlled carbohydrate snacks and dinners) may enhance treatment outcome.

Psychotherapy

Four evidence-based types of psychotherapy, which are time-limited and manual-based, are effective in treating geriatric depression alone or in conjunction with pharmacotherapy: Cognitive-Behavioral Therapy, Interpersonal Therapy, Problem-Solving Therapy, and Brief Psychodynamic Therapy (Mackin and Arean 2005). Although none of these psychotherapies is empirically more effective than the other, different people may derive more benefit from one or another. Psychotherapy is as effective as antidepressants in mild to moderately severe depression, but the improvement is slower than drugs in the beginning of treatment (Thompson et al. 2001).

Most studies demonstrate the value of joint pharmacotherapy and psychotherapy over the use of either modality alone (Alexopoulos et al. 2001; Charney et al. 2003; Moutier et al. 2003; Pinquart et al. 2006). Psychotherapy

is appropriately used alone when patients are not severely depressed, do not want to take antidepressants, are not at risk for self harm or neglect, or have stressful psychosocial circumstances. It is used jointly with medication when patients have not responded to one or more antidepressants. Medications alone or in combination with psychotherapy are recommended for the treatment of severe depression, although cognitive behavioral therapy may be as effective as drugs (Hollon et al. 2005). Major depression with psychotic or melancholic features is best treated with medication or electroconvulsive therapy rather than psychotherapy alone.

Cognitive-Behavioral Therapy

Cognitive-behavioral therapy (CBT) integrates two types of therapy: cognitive and behavioral (Beck and Alford 2009; www.beckinstitute.org). Cognitive therapy focuses on thoughts, beliefs, and attributions, and patients learn to recognize and change maladaptive thinking. In behavioral therapy, individuals learn how to change behaviors. There are several approaches to CBT, including rational emotive behavioral therapy, rational behavior therapy, rational living therapy, cognitive therapy, and dialectic behavior therapy.

These approaches are all based on a cognitive model of emotional responses (i.e., that an individual's thoughts cause depressive feelings and behaviors, not other people or circumstances). CBT targets maladaptive thinking and behavior and teaches the patient rational self-counseling skills to change how they think, feel, and react. It is based on the theory that most emotional and behavioral responses are learned, and the goal is to teach individuals to unlearn unwanted reactions and learn new ways of reacting.

Many studies have demonstrated CBT's efficacy in the treatment of depression and other disorders in all age groups (Butler et al. 2006). Therapy usually occurs weekly over a 3- to 6-month period. It is highly structured, and the therapist's objective is to learn the patient's goals and achieve them. Successful therapy requires a collaborative relationship, but the therapeutic alliance is not the focus of therapy. The therapist's role is to listen actively, ask questions, teach, and encourage, and the patient's responsibility is to talk, learn, practice, and implement what is learned. The CBT approach is based on an educational model. There are specific goals for each therapy session, the patient is taught specific concepts and techniques, and homework is assigned.

CBT is effective with older people (Pinquart et al. 2006; Wilson et al. 2008), and evidence-based practice guidelines exist for using CBT with older outpatients (Snowden et al. 2008). The intervention consists of up to twenty 50- to 60-minute sessions using a standardized manual, and it includes strategies to facilitate learning (e.g., repeated presentation of information using different modalities, slower presentation rates, and modeling behaviors). Where appropriate, patients are taught to monitor and increase pleasant events in their daily lives.

Interpersonal Therapy

Interpersonal therapy (IPT) is based on the premise that depression has many causes, but it is always expressed in the context of interpersonal relationships (Klerman et al. 1984; Weissman 2006). IPT deals with three component processes: symptom formation, social and interpersonal relations, and personality. Symptom formation and interpersonal relationships are the intervention targets but not personality issues. However, knowledge about individuals' personality and the role personality plays in the expression of depression and cognitive impairment are important in formulating interventions.

Patients learn to resolve interpersonal difficulties, such as conflicts, dealing with grief, role changes, health problems, and functional impairments. Therapists help patients test the reality of their perceptions, understand their affect, and learn to change maladaptive feelings and behaviors. IPT usually occurs weekly for about twenty sessions and focuses on one or two issues most related to the depression. The first sessions are devoted to identifying the most salient interpersonal difficulties, with the remaining sessions devoted to improving interpersonal and communication skills and self-concept. Ongoing maintenance of IPT improves the quality of life in geriatric mood disorders.

IPT is effective alone or in combination with medications (Dombrovski and Mulsant 2007; Wilkinson 2007; Hinrichsen 2008). Hinrichsen and Clougherty (2006) wrote a manual for the use of IPT with depressed older adults, and Miller and associates (2009) modified IPT for older adults who have cognitive impairment (IPT-CI).

The major change in IPT for older depressed adults who have cognitive impairment is the partnership of caregivers and identified patients in a process that provides psychoeducation for both, opportunities for problem solving separately and together, and opportunities for mediating disputes. Caregivers not only are directly involved in the therapeutic process but also are encouraged to use their knowledge and skills between sessions to help patients use intact abilities to deal with changed roles, develop new roles appropriate for their cognitive abilities, and adjust to increased dependency.

The International Society for Interpersonal Therapy (ISIPT) is a valuable resource for articles, manuals, and forms for documenting progress (www.interpersonalpsychotherapy .org).

Problem-Solving Therapy

Problem-solving therapy (PST) is highly structured, focused on the present, and actively involves individuals to develop solutions for current problems (Mynors-Wallis 2000; Gellis and Kenaley 2008). The PST model has two components: problem orientation and problem-solving style (Nezu and D'Zurilla 2006). Problem orientation refers to how individuals perceive problems, make attributions about the causes of problems, and perceive the degree of control to deal with problems. The second component focuses on how to identify problems solving styles.

PST is effective in treating depression in older adults (Mynors-Wallis et al. 2000;

Charney et al. 2003; Arean 2009; Gellis and Kenaley 2008; Gellis and Bruce 2010), and it is effective in older depressed patients who have impaired executive functioning, a group usually unresponsive to medication (Alexopoulos et al. 2003). Its effectiveness in the treatment of depressed, cognitively impaired older people is being evaluated in a clinical trial supported by the NIMH scheduled for completion in 2011 (http://clinicaltrials.gov/ct2/show/NCT00601055).

Brief Psychodynamic Therapy

Brief psychodynamic therapy (BPT), developed from psychoanalytic theory, focuses on techniques to help patients in a short period of time, not years of psychoanalysis (Leichsenring and Leibing 2007). The goal is to effect changes in experiences that cause an individual's symptoms. The causes of emotional distress are often conflicts about which the individual is unaware, and the goal of therapy is to clarify the conflict responsible for the patient's symptoms.

Messer (2004) identified six characteristics and practice techniques essential for effective BPT:

• Patient has relatively mature interpersonal relationships
• A clear clinical foci on intrapsychic conflicts, maladaptive interpersonal relationships, or negative feelings about the self
• A mutually agreed upon time limit to achieve change
• Goal setting to use time wisely
• Active questioning, interpretation, and confrontation, if necessary
• Emphasis on issues of separation, loss, and limitations in life during the termination phase

A small literature suggests that BPT is useful in older adults as a sole therapy or in combination with pharmacologic treatment (Mackin and Arean 2005; Scogin et al. 2005).

Psychotherapy in Primary Care Settings

An emerging literature shows the effectiveness of psychotherapy for depressed older people in primary care (Bartels et al. 2002a,b; Unutzer et al. 2003; Bruce et al. 2004; Gum et al. 2006; Arean et al. 2008; Skultety and Rodriguez 2008). About 10–12 percent of older primary care patients have MDD or dysthymia, but few have access to treatment. Most depressed older adults prefer to receive treatment in the primary care setting, and most have a preference for psychotherapy, which is often not available in primary care.

Effective primary care approaches have included adapting short-term psychotherapies to be administered in this setting, use of geriatric evaluation management teams, and developing integrated systems that identify depression in the primary care setting and refer patients to appropriate treatment settings (Arean et al. 2008). Examples of integrated care models include, but are not limited to, the Gospel Oak Study in London (Blanchard et al. 1994a); the Prevention of Suicide in Primary Care Elderly Collaborative Trial (PROSPECT; Bruce et al. 2004), a multiple-site trial in New York City, Philadelphia, and Pittsburg; Improving Mood-Promoting Access to Collaborative Treatment (IMPACT: Unutzer et al. 2002), a multiple-site study at 18 primary care sites across the United States; and a multiple-site intervention to treat minor depression and dysthymia in primary care (Williams et al. 2000). The integrated care model is also effective in reducing mortality in older depressed persons (Gallo et al. 2004, 2007).

Electroconvulsive Therapy

Electroconvulsive therapy (ECT) is a safe and effective treatment for MDD in older adults (Dombrovsky and Mulsant 2006; Rudisch and McDonald 2006), but to date a well-designed randomized controlled trial to test its efficacy against antidepressants remains to be done (Stek 2003). More research is also needed to evaluate the long-term efficacy of ECT, increased risks for morbidity and mortality, as well as cost-effectiveness. Finally, the exact mechanism of action during and after seizures is not well understood (Grover et al. 2005; Sanchez et al. 2009).

ECT can be extremely effective when

patients have a psychotic depression, have not responded to antidepressant drugs, or have treatment-resistant mania (Kelly and Zisselman 2000; Baghai and Moller 2008). ECT works rapidly and can be lifesaving, particularly for suicidal patients and those who are severely medically ill. It can be administered in a hospital or on an outpatient basis, and treatment requires informed consent.

The American Psychiatric Association's Task Force on the Practice of Electroconvulsive Therapy describes practice guidelines and procedures (APA 2001). Patients should be given anesthesia and be closely monitored medically. Most people tolerate ECT well, and about 80 percent recover from depression with six to eight treatments. Maintenance ECT significantly reduces the likelihood of relapse, but if maintenance ECT is not possible, antidepressants should be used even if the patient did not respond to them initially.

Guidelines have been established to limit the number and frequency of treatments, and this has done much to minimize the side effects of confusion and memory loss. Depending on patient characteristics and co-morbidities, many patients who have AD or related dementia may be treated successfully with ECT (Rao and Lysetkos 2000). However, some patients are at risk for more confusion and delirium and therefore may be poor candidates for ECT (Tielkes et al. 2008).

Newer Therapeutic Approaches
Transcranial Magnetic Stimulation

Transcranial magnetic stimulation (TMS) is a relatively new noninvasive technology that influences brain physiology (Busko 2007; Alexopoulos and Kelly 2009). During TMS, capacitors are rapidly discharged into an electrical coil to produce a magnetic field pulse. When this coil is placed near the head, the magnetic field enters the brain and induces an electrical field, which depolarizes neurons and causes biological effects. Evidence for a possible antidepressant effect was noted during studies on Parkinson disease, and since 2002, a number of studies have demonstrated an antidepressant effect when TMS is administered to the left prefrontal cortex (Loo and Mitchell 2005). TMS shows promise and is being tested in clinical trials. However, it is not as effective as ECT and may cause seizures in older patients (Gershon et al. 2003).

Vagal Nerve Stimulation

Vagus or vagal nerve stimulation is a brain stimulation procedure designed to treat depression when standard treatments have not worked (Sackeim et al. 2007; Alexopoulos and Kelly 2009). A pulse generator is surgically implanted in the chest, and a wire is threaded under the skin to connect the pulse generator to the left vagus nerve in the neck. The pulse generator sends out electrical signals along the vagus nerve to the brain. The FDA approved this technique in 2005 for persons age 18 or older who have a severe or recurrent depression, have had a long-term depression of two years or longer, or are treatment-resistant (Shuchman 2007).

Treatments for Bipolar Disorder

Management of bipolar disorder in later life is often difficult because patients often have severe symptomatology and substantial medical co-morbidities, and those who are treated frequently do not respond well and have recurring episodes and a high mortality rate (Young et al. 2005; Gildengers et al. 2008). Unfortunately, treatment efficacy research is almost nonexistent (Sajatovic 2002).

Three types of drugs are commonly used to treat bipolar disorders: mood stabilizers, antidepressants, and antipsychotics (Hirschfeld et al. 2003; Young et al. 2005). Mood stabilizers are the primary treatment for most people (Young 2005). Lithium, marketed as Eskalith, Lithane, Lithobid, Lithonate, and Lithotabs, is the oldest and most common mood stabilizer for long-term prophylactic treatment, and it is the international gold standard for comparison with other treatments. A combination of lithium and divalproex may be effective in patients resistant to treatment with lithium alone. This combination may help some older patients, but the other medications, including the newer anticonvulsants, atypical antipsychotics, and antidepressants, have not been well studied for efficacy (Young el al. 2005).

Expert Consensus Guidelines recommend lithium and divalproex as first choices for treatment (Yatham et al. 2005; Young 2005). APA practice guidelines recommend that first-line therapy for patients who have bipolar disorder and are severely ill include lithium or divalproex and an atypical antipsychotic, whereas first-line treatment for less ill patients includes one of the three agents alone (APA 2001). Second-line treatments currently include anticonvulsants, such as lamotrigine and carbamazepine, but these are also widely used as a first-line treatment. Many older patients who have type 1 or type 2 bipolar disorder tolerate lithium well, but others do not (Depp and Jeste 2004; Sajatovic et al. 2005a,b). Lithium has a controversial history (Baldessarini et al. 2002). Some patients have side effects such as nausea, fatigue, diarrhea, weight gain, tremors, or frequent urination. Long-term data on the prophylactic use of drugs other than lithium, including the newer mood stabilizers, are limited, and no agent provides full protection from recurrences of bipolar illness. Long-term use of lithium is the only treatment consistently associated with lower rates of suicide attempts and suicide (Cipriani et al. 2005; Freeman and Freeman 2006).

Because toxicity is a serious potential side effect of lithium, careful management is necessary (Sajatovic et al. 2005a,b). Neurotoxicity as reflected in falls, polydipsia, polyurea, and cardiac conduction abnormalities has been reported. The literature is unclear regarding the serum plasma lithium concentration appropriate for older people. Ranges of 0.5 mEq/l–0.8 mEq/l have proven effective in some studies whereas 0.8 mEq/l–1.2 mEq/l have been reported in others. Patients taking diuretics or anti-inflammatory medications and patients who have cardiac insufficiency or decreased renal clearance, which are common in older persons, need careful monitoring. Diet, hydration, and other medications may also influence plasma levels.

Lamotrigine appears to be an effective and relatively safe medication, but with a serious side effect (Aziz et al. 2006; Sajatovic et al. 2007). Lamotrigine-related rashes may in relatively rare instances lead to Stevens-Johnson syndrome, a severe condition that may require hospitalization because of its effect on the mucosa and rashes involving the mouth, anus, and other parts of the body (Mockenhaupt et al. 2008). Less than 1 percent of patients develop a serious rash, but those patients who do, particularly early in treatment, should be taken off the drug.

Some patients require two or three drugs to stabilize their mood (Young et al. 2004). Antidepressants may be prescribed for persons who manifest significant depression. Antipsychotic medications may be prescribed for patients who have psychotic features to calm them in an acute manic phase while waiting for the mood stabilizer to take effect. The major older antipsychotic drugs include Thorazine (chlorpromazine), Mellaril (thioridazine), Trilafon (perphenazine), Stelazine (trifluoperazine), Clozaril (clopazine), and Haldol (haloperidol). The newer so-called atypical antipsychotics include Risperdal (risperidone), Zyprexa (olanzapine), Abilify (aripiprazole), Geodon (ziprasidone), Seroquel (quetiapine), and Invega (paliperidone). The older antipsychotics are now used less frequently because of their side-effect profile.

As with all drugs, these medications need to be monitored for side effects, which may include slowed speech and thinking, sleepiness, restlessness, confusion, stiffness, or parkinsonlike movements. Long-term effects (e.g., tardive dyskinesias) are also an important potential issue for geriatric patients. Tapering antipsychotics for patients who have psychiatric symptoms during the maintenance phase is controversial and is a matter of clinical judgment, but using a minimal effective dose is a sound practice.

Although mood-stabilizing and antidepressant drug therapy is the primary pharmacologic treatment for bipolar depression, psychosocial treatment is effective to increase compliance with drug regimens, decrease hospitalizations and relapses, improve quality of life, and help patients cope with stress (Miklowitz and Otto 2006).

Treatment goals, according to guidelines, are focused on stabilizing an episode with the objective of remission of symptoms. However, the nature of the disease often makes a complete recovery with return to premorbid functioning impossible. Long-term studies show that patients are symptomatic 50 percent of the time, and while most can recover from an acute episode, less than 40 percent fully recover functioning. Thus, patients can recover from acute episodes but still not be well (Perlis et al. 2006).

Family Involvement

Mood disorders affect the entire family, making family and friends feel angry, frustrated, and guilty (Soares and Young 2007). These negative reactions usually occur when family members do not understand that a relative is depressed. They also occur when the depressed person denies having a problem and other family members become frustrated with the deepening depression and the helplessness of not being able to overcome the resistance to seeing a professional. More than half of depressed adults report that their family members do not understand them. A vicious cycle can evolve when the negative emotional reactions of family members aggravate the sadness or mania, hopelessness, and low self-esteem of the depressed person.

Family members often express frustration and resentment because they receive so little information about mood disorder and medications. Education about the complexities of depressive and bipolar illness is essential for successful treatment. Family members need to know the symptoms and what precipitates episodes, and also to understand the patient's vulnerability to future episodes.

Family-focused psychoeducational treatment (FFT), which consists of 21 sessions over a 9-month period, increases the resiliency of bipolar patients (Rea et al. 2003; Miklowitz and Otto 2006). FFT includes education about bipolar illness, self-management, communication training, and problem-solving skills training. In addition to reducing the severity of symptoms, conflict, and re-hospitalization, FFT increases positive verbal and nonverbal interactions among the patient and family members.

It is common for adults who have mood disorder to resist or refuse help. They frequently deny having problems, and feelings of fatigue, helplessness, and hopelessness paralyze the person from taking action. Some resist asking for help because they feel worthless and guilty about causing trouble for others. And if clinicians are uncomfortable or embarrassed dealing with mood disorders, this will reinforce the denial or make the patient dig in his or her heels to resist help.

Family members need to be the clinician's partner in treatment, but this risks breaching patient confidentiality without their consent. Family members need to be patient and persistent, and clinicians need to assure the patient and family members that living with and caring for someone who has a mood disorder is stressful and difficult. Ideally, consent should be obtained when patients are not symptomatic, but even in the absence of a patient's permission to share information, family members can be helped to cope with the stress of their family life by referral to self-help groups and education about mood disorders without sharing personal diagnostic information.

Principles of Managing Mood Disorders

1. Maintain a high index of suspicion for mood disorders. Many older patients do not have obvious symptoms matching the DSM-IV-TR diagnostic criteria.

2. Be attentive to gender differences in symptom presentation.

3. When patients are mildly to moderately depressed, consider psychotherapies before using antidepressants as the first step in treatment.

4. Use SSRIs or SNRIs as the first drug treatment. Start older patients on a low drug dose, monitor side effects, increase dose gradually, and be available and supportive until posi-

tive effects are noted. Educate the patient and family about the time involved.

5. Monitor patients carefully, especially during the early stages of treatment. In severe depression, suicide risk may increase early with antidepressant medication because the patient's energy and activity level improve before mood improves. Monitor suicidality throughout treatment.

6. Educate family members and prepare them for the difficulties everyone will face until the patient is feeling better. Be aware of cultural differences in the patient's expression of affect and caregivers' expectations.

7. Most patients require long-term management to prevent relapse.

11

Anxiety Disorders

Anxiety disorders are among the most prevalent psychiatric conditions across all age groups (Saltzman 2004; Somers et al. 2006; Lyketsos 2007), but relatively little research has been done on anxiety disorders in older people (Cassidy and Rector 2008; Hesley and Vanim 2008). Estimates of the prevalence of anxiety disorders in community-residing older persons range from 1 to 19 percent, but the prevalence is probably higher in populations that have dementia, depression, or other medical conditions (Somers et al. 2006; Flint 2007). Generalized anxiety disorder (GAD) is the most common anxiety disorder in older adults, with prevalence rates reported from 1 to 14 percent, followed by phobic disorders, with prevalence rates from 0.7 to 7.0 percent (Flint 2007; Pinquart and Duberstein 2007). Ford and associates (2007) reported findings from the National Survey of American Life (NSAL; Jackson et al. 2004) that among older black Americans, post-traumatic stress disorder (PTSD) is the most prevalent anxiety disorder and the most prevalent of any psychiatric disorders in their sample.

Anxiety is a natural emotional reaction to situations that create fear, from waiting for surgery to hearing a fire alarm, and it usually evokes a response to become more alert and take action. In more severe forms, anxiety disorders are incapacitating, and they are often not detected because the somatic symptoms, cognitive distortions, and heightened physiological arousal can be similar to those in medically ill older adults. The following case illustrates some of the challenges of recognizing anxiety disorder in older persons.

EM, a 79-year-old World War II veteran, had been in excellent health until he fell on the tennis court and broke his hip. Although he recovered successfully from surgery, he was afraid to play tennis again. He also withdrew from his two other passions: golf and fishing. EM was aware of his behavior and complained to his wife and friends that he felt nervous and keyed up all the time. He worried about everything and everyone—his wife, his three sons, and their families. EM would phone his wife, DM, five times or more on the two days she worked at a local art gallery. When his son, who lived more than a thousand miles away, called each week, EM would obsess over every word throughout the day and lie awake worrying about what his son was not telling him.

DM was distressed because her husband's symptoms were similar to those he had ten years ago when a drunk driver hit him on the way home from work. Only now, EM was much worse, even though nothing serious had occurred. He refused to see a psychiatrist and was driving DM "crazy" with his constant worrying, insomnia, and health complaints. EM spent hours in the bathroom and complained of nausea and constipation as well as headaches, weakness, difficulty swallowing, and vague muscle aches. He was anxious and fearful every night, had trouble falling asleep, and when he would wake up to urinate, he would usually pace around the house, unable to sleep, waking his wife. EM no longer met his friends for daily morning walks at the mall because he reported feeling light-headed and was afraid of falling. He also stopped reading, one of his favorite hobbies, complaining that he could not concentrate or remember anything. EM was convinced that he was in the early stages of dementia, and he became angry with his wife for not being more concerned about his health.

One night EM awoke with chest pains and was taken to the emergency room. The staff found nothing wrong and released him in the morning, advising him to see his doctor. At a follow-up visit with his primary care physician, DM insisted that her husband talk about his problems. He was hesitant, but DM indicated that she would tell the doctor if he did not do so himself.

After being referred to a geriatric psychiatrist, EM was diagnosed with generalized anxiety disorder. His doctor thought that it dated back to a car accident and was exacerbated by his fall and surgery, although EM had probably been anxious throughout his adult life. Successful treatment with psychotherapy and medications liberated EM from the paralysis of his illness, and he became a vital, active individual again, fully engaged with his wife, family, and friends.

Differential Diagnosis

Anxiety disorders usually occur for the first time between ages 18 and 45, and the prevalence is higher in women than in men (Yates 2009). These conditions rarely begin de novo in later life, and most older adults who have anxiety disorder have had one or more episodes earlier in life. With the exception of phobias, the late-onset of significant anxiety symptoms are usually associated with a new or exacerbated medical condition, major depression with secondary symptoms of anxiety, cognitive impairment, substance abuse, or major trauma.

DSM-IV-TR classifies the following major anxiety disorders: Generalized Anxiety Disorder (GAD), Panic Disorder, Phobic Disorders, Obsessive Compulsive Disorder (OCD), Post-Traumatic Stress Disorder (PTSD), Anxiety Disorders Secondary to Medical Conditions, and Anxiety Disorders, Not Otherwise Specified. Most anxiety disorders have common characteristics, but significant features distinguish the different anxiety disorders.

Co-morbidity among anxiety disorders is common in all age groups. It occurs in most cases of GAD (Nutt et al. 2006), and in other anxiety disorders two or more diagnosable conditions usually coexist (Kroenke et al. 2007). Symptomatic anxiety frequently occurs

with major depression and physical disorders in older adults, and if not diagnosed and treated appropriately, outcomes may include diminished quality of life, impaired functional effectiveness, and increased risk of mortality (Mulsant et al. 2003).

Generalized Anxiety Disorder

The core characteristic of generalized anxiety disorder (GAD) is excessive, unrealistic, and uncontrollable worries about many life circumstances. The DSM-IV-TR criteria include:

1. Excessive anxiety or worry occurs most days for at least six months about a number of events or activities.
2. The person finds it difficult to control the worry.
3. Worries are associated with three or more of the following six symptoms (with at least some symptoms present for more days than not for the past six months):

· Restlessness or feeling keyed up or on edge
· Easily fatigued
· Difficulty concentrating or mind going blank
· Irritability
· Muscle tension
· Sleep disturbance

In contrast to younger patients, older individuals who have GAD do not usually avoid situations as a result of their disorder (Flint 2007). When the impairment is mild, persons usually function appropriately in social activities, whereas in severe cases, GAD interferes with daily functioning and may affect physical health. GAD frequently occurs together with alcohol and substance abuse, depression, or another anxiety disorder.

GAD is distinguished by its long duration and impairments in functional effectiveness. Acute anxiety, usually caused by a recent stressor, may last for hours or weeks, and although acute stressors are usually not associated with GAD, stress may exacerbate the severity. The evaluation process for individuals who present with symptoms of excessive worry and somatic complaints should include:

- Clarification of symptoms
- Assessment of medical disorders, medications, and functional status
- Assessment of the possibility of substance misuse and prescription drug abuse (e.g., benzodiazepines)
- Evaluation of psychosocial supports
- Review of recent or chronic life stressors
- Evaluation of symptoms of MDD and panic attacks

Panic Disorder

The lifetime prevalence of panic disorder ranges from 1.6 to 2.2 percent, and it usually occurs for the first time in adolescence or young adulthood and diminishes in later life (Madaan 2008). Panic disorder rarely occurs for the first time in older people, but the symptoms are less severe when it does occur (Sheikh et al. 2004). Older patients report fewer panic symptoms, less anxiety and arousal, and lower levels of depression, and those older patients who have late-onset panic disorder report less emotional and physical distress during panic attacks.

Panic disorder is characterized by the occurrence of unexpected recurring panic attacks, which are discrete episodes of intense fear or terror coupled with autonomic over-arousal. DSM-IV-TR criteria require the presence of at least four of the following symptoms for at least one month:

- Chest pain or discomfort
- Choking
- Dizziness, unsteadiness, or faintness
- Fear of dying
- Fear of losing control
- Feelings of unreality, strangeness, or detachment from the environment
- Flushes or chills
- Nausea, stomachache, or diarrhea
- Numbness or tingling sensations
- Palpitations or accelerated heart rate
- Shortness of breath or sense of being smothered
- Sweating
- Trembling or shaking

Clinicians need to distinguish panic disorder from other conditions accompanied by panic symptoms, including phobias and post-traumatic stress disorder; substance abuse, including caffeine or stimulants; withdrawal from alcohol and sedative-hypnotics; or other medical conditions.

Panic attacks can occur at any time, including during sleep, and individuals cannot predict when they will happen. They usually last about ten minutes, but some symptoms may last longer. Several types of panic attacks may occur. The most common is the unexpected attack with no obvious trigger. Individuals may also experience situation-specific panic attacks, which are more likely to occur in certain circumstances, or situational-bound attacks, which occur almost immediately on exposure to a situational trigger.

Patients with panic disorder have a 50–60 percent lifetime prevalence of major depression (Cairney et al. 2008). The onset of depression precedes the onset of panic disorder in a third of patients, while the onset of depression coincides with or follows the onset of panic disorder in the remaining two-thirds. Panic disorders also frequently occur with alcoholism and drug abuse, and individuals may go years before the condition is correctly diagnosed.

Panic attacks lead to an avoidance of the situation in which the attack first occurred (e.g., driving a car), and the lives of some individuals can become so restricted that they become housebound. When individuals are immobilized, as occurs in about one-third of cases, the condition is called agoraphobia. Panic disorders may occur with or without agoraphobia, and agoraphobia may also occur without a history of panic disorder (McCabe et al. 2006). The prevalence of agoraphobia in older populations has been reported to range from 0.6–7.8 percent. It occurs more frequently in women, those who are widowed or divorced, and older adults who have chronic medical conditions.

Phobic Disorders

Phobias are characterized by intense, persistent, and unrealistic anxiety and fear in response to specific situations, and individuals who have phobic disorders either avoid situations that will trigger their fears or endure them but with significant distress. Patients are aware that they have a problem and know that their anxiety is unwarranted

Social Phobias

Social phobias, also known as social anxiety disorders, are characterized by an overwhelming fear of public circumstances. Individuals have intense, persistent fears and beliefs that they are being watched and judged by others. Social phobia has a lifetime prevalence rate of 13.3 percent and a one-year prevalence rate of 7.9 percent in community samples, making it the third most prevalent psychiatric disorder, following substance abuse and depression (Cairney et al. 2007). In community samples, fears of public speaking or performing are the most prevalent phobias, whereas in clinical samples, generalized fears of social interactions predominate. Onset of social phobia typically occurs between 11 and 19 years of age. Although onset after age 25 is rare, it is not uncommon for an existing social phobia to remain unprovoked for years until some situation triggers the syndrome. Slightly more women than men have social phobias.

The DSM-IV-TR criteria include:

• A persistent, marked fear of one or more circumstances where individuals believe their actions will be embarrassing
• Recognition that the fear is excessive or unreasonable
• The feared social or performance situations are avoided or endured with intense anxiety or distress
• Avoidance or distress in the feared social or performance situation(s) interferes significantly with the person's normal routines, social activities, or relationships

Social phobias may be restricted to one sphere of life or, in the most severe form, may affect people anytime they are with others. Common social phobias include fear of public speaking, choking on food while eating with others, being unable to urinate in a public restroom, trembling in front of other people, and not being able to answer questions at work or social gatherings.

Specific Phobias

Specific phobias or simple phobias are a persistent fear of something or someone that poses little or no threat, and they are less troubling than other anxiety disorders (Noyes et al. 2003). Specific phobias are characterized by elevated, irrational fear in response to a specific situation, such as heights, flying, or objects. Exposure precipitates immediate distress, leading to withdrawal from the object or situation and avoidance of further contact. Simple phobias are more common in women and most frequently manifest for the first time in early life. However, phobias can develop de novo in older persons, especially after seeing or experiencing traumatic or violent events.

Some targeted phobias have minimal impact, while others interfere significantly with functioning. For example, persons who have a fear of snakes and live in urban environments may have no trouble avoiding them, in contrast to persons who are afraid of closed places and may not be able to avoid elevators or living on high floors. Some specific phobias, such as fear of large animals, the dark, or strangers, begin early in life, but they may also disappear as the person gets older. Other phobias, such as fear of rodents or insects, storms, water, heights, flying, or enclosed places, typically develop later in life.

Obsessive-Compulsive Disorder

Recurring obsessive or compulsive thoughts and behaviors that cause significant emotional distress characterize obsessive-compulsive disorder (OCD) (APA 2007). Obsessions are senseless, intrusive thoughts and images that individuals cannot suppress, and compulsions are repetitive, purposeful acts or rituals done in response to an obsession. OCD occurs equally in men and women and affects 0.6 to 2.3 percent of the population during any 12-month period, although the prevalence varies in different parts of the world (Crino et al. 2005). OCD is chronic and usually persists for life.

There are few differences in clinical features between younger and older persons. More than 95 percent of people with OCD feel compelled to perform rituals that may include washing or cleaning to be rid of contamination, hoarding to prevent loss, and avoiding persons who might become objects of aggression. Most rituals can be observed, but others, such as repetitive counting or making statements intended to diminish danger, cannot be observed. Obsessions are not always accompanied by compulsions.

Most people are aware that their obsessive thoughts do not reflect actual risks and that their compulsive behaviors are ineffective. OCD, therefore, differs from psychotic disorders, in which people lose contact with reality and justify their behaviors by creating a delusional system where their strange, irrational behaviors make reasonable sense. OCD also differs from obsessive-compulsive personality disorder, in which specific personality traits are defined, such as being a perfectionist. Because people with OCD are aware that their compulsive behaviors are excessive and are afraid of being stigmatized, they often perform their rituals secretly.

Post-Traumatic Stress Disorder

Post-traumatic stress disorder (PTSD) occurs following exposure to an extreme or violent event involving the threat of death or injury (Keane et al. 2006; Gore and Lucas 2009). This could involve a direct personal experience or being a witness to the event. The traumatic event is re-experienced over time, involving flashbacks, recurrent dreams, numbed feelings, autonomic arousal, and avoidance of certain situations. Sleep disturbances are common, and depression is often a co-morbid condition. Traumatic stressors may include military combat, rape, physical abuse or assault, the experience of torture, or natural and man-made disasters. Many older veterans, especially World War II and Korean War veterans, were never diagnosed with PTSD because it was not labeled as such until after the Vietnam War (Clancy et al. 2006). Psychological trauma other than war may also occur later in life, but the incidence of late-onset cases is probably low. The National Center for PTSD maintains an informative website (www.ptsd.va.gov).

Although PTSD is incapacitating, causing severe emotional distress and increased use of health care compared to other anxiety disorders, it is often not diagnosed (Grinage 2003). The events of September 11, 2001, however, raised professional and public awareness of this disorder (Dedert et al. 2009). The lifetime prevalence of PTSD in the United States is about 8-9 percent, and it is twice as common in women as compared to men (Kessler et al. 2005). Approximately 25-30 percent of persons who experience significant trauma develop PTSD, and the number of traumatic experiences is associated with the severity of PTSD and co-morbidities (Sledjeski et al. 2007). Symptoms that do not meet the full criteria for PTSD are common in the general population and may be common in groups at high risk of PTSD, especially veterans (Sayer et al. 2009). For example, although the lifetime prevalence of PTSD in veterans is around 30 percent, a much higher percentage of Vietnam veterans had clinically significant symptoms of PTSD (Schnurr et al. 2003).

The DSM-IV-TR criteria for PTSD are:

1. Persistent re-experiencing of an event occurs in at least one of the following:

- Recurrent and intrusive recollections
- Recurrent distressing dreams/nightmares
- Flashbacks of traumatic event

• Intense psychological distress with internal or external cues to the trauma
• Physiological reactivity on exposure to trauma cues

2. Persistent avoidance of stimuli of trauma and numbing/avoidance behavior demonstrated by at least 3 of the following:

• Avoidance of thoughts or conversation related to the trauma
• Avoidance of activities, places, or people related to the trauma
• Amnesia for important trauma-related events
• Decreased participation in significant activities
• Feeling detached or estranged from others
• Restricted affect
• Foreshortened sense of the future

3. Persistent symptoms of increased arousal demonstrated by 2 or more of the following:

• Difficulty staying or falling asleep
• Irritability or anger outbursts
• Difficulty concentrating
• Hypervigilance
• Exaggerated startle response

Symptoms must last for at least one month and radically disrupt normal activities. Individuals who manifest an anxiety syndrome lasting less than one month after a traumatic event have a condition called "acute stress disorder." The diagnosis requires three or more dissociative symptoms in addition to the unrelenting symptoms associated with PTSD (Benedek et al. 2009). Symptoms lasting less than three months are indicative of an acute condition. Frequently the manifestation of PTSD is delayed, with patients experiencing symptoms six months or more after the traumatic event (APA 2009).

The diagnosis of PTSD may be complicated for many reasons (Hyer and Sacks 2008). Patients may not be aware of the link between their symptoms and the occurrence of a traumatic event. Individuals may not want to reveal the trauma experienced, or the symptoms may be masked by depressive disorders, alcohol and drug abuse, or other co-morbid

conditions. Clinicians need to be straightforward, empathic, and nonjudgmental when interviewing a patient (e.g., "Have you ever been attacked or threatened?" or "Have you ever been in a bad accident or natural disaster?" or "Have you ever witnessed a frightening event?").

Anxiety Disorder Secondary to Medical Conditions

Crippling anxiety can also be a reaction to medical problems. Older persons may have exaggerated beliefs about a symptom (e.g., a headache is a symptom of a tumor, heartburn signals a heart problem). In anxious individuals, however, the obsession with a symptom is the dominant theme in their complaints, and they will frequently see multiple physicians. Isolation and depression will compound the anxiety. Substance-Induced Anxiety Disorder may present with marked anxiety, panic attacks, compulsions, and obsessions associated with use or withdrawal from alcohol and other drugs.

Anxiety Disorder, Not Otherwise Specified

The diagnosis of anxiety disorder, not otherwise specified, refers to disorders that do not meet DSM-IV-TR criteria for anxiety disorder but may include a mixed anxiety-depressive disorder or anxiety associated with early-onset AD and related disorders.

Diagnosis

Many older persons have medical co-morbidities with physical symptoms similar to the physical symptoms of anxiety disorders, and depending on individual circumstances, their fears may be realistic. Agitation and other behavioral disturbances in persons who have mild cognitive impairment may be difficult to separate from anxiety.

There are several indirect approaches to help individuals talk about anxiety. One should inquire about anything that is stressful or causing them to worry more than usual, including future concerns and ask whether they have a hard time putting thoughts or ideas out of their mind. When people report specific physical symptoms, it is important to try to identify how and when the symptoms began. Because agoraphobia is often of late onset and related to illness and traumas, one should probe for information about the time of onset or exacerbation of health problems as well as the occurrence of frightening events. Older people may not volunteer information about stressors that provoke strong anxiety reactions such as fears about safety when robberies have occurred in their community. Fear of driving or shopping or any social activity may occur as a result of a car accident or being assaulted in the mall.

Diagnosis of late-life anxiety is complicated for several reasons (Flint 2007). Older persons often present with purely physical symptoms, and because they usually have several chronic medical conditions and are taking multiple medications, an exacerbation of physical symptoms caused by anxiety may lead clinicians to only focus on physical problems. Men, in particular, tend to ignore or deny psychiatric symptoms, not wanting to appear weak and unable to deal with their emotions. As a consequence, they may be unwilling to disclose their fears.

It is not unusual for patients to be anxious about diseases that have affected other members of the family. The deaths of friends and family members, economic insecurity, family problems, health changes, and other life events may be valid causes of anxiety and emotional distress. The clinical challenge is to recognize when the anxiety is incapacitating, particularly when it is manifest in morbid ruminations about health, loss of memory, or dying that are not consistent with the patient's actual medical status.

Anxiety may be a prodromal sign of health changes, because it is intimately associated with the autonomic nervous system. Minor cognitive impairment, early dementia, delirium, drug side effects, or numerous medical conditions may all affect autonomic nervous system activity, resulting in somatic changes, fear, and incapacitating anxiety. Clinicians should regard anxiety as a serious condition and rule out possible underlying physical and psychiatric etiologies. When somatic symptoms are prominent and the role of anxiety is ignored, the results include frequent physician visits, emergency room visits, and hospitalizations.

Etiology

Anxiety disorders are likely caused by a combination of biopsychosocial factors (Young et al. 2009). There is no direct evidence of a gene(s) for any of the anxiety disorders, but family and twin studies indicate that there are certain genetic commonalities between anxiety disorders, depression, and alcohol and drug abuse (Hettema et al. 2001), and linkage studies also suggest genetic influences in panic disorders (Hamilton et al. 2002, 2004).

Stress is a causal influence in all anxiety disorders, but PTSD has the most clearly defined etiology (Keane et al. 2006). The interrelationships among stress, biologic, and genetic factors are elusive. For example, extreme traumatic experiences may lead to PTSD in the absence of a genetic history or preexisting brain damage, whereas patients who have a positive family history or brain damage may develop an anxiety disorder when exposed to the slightest anxiety-provoking situation. There is significant variability across patients with regard to the impact of the severity and duration of stressful circumstances. Graded stress affects personality development and effective coping styles over the lifespan (Washington 2009), and success in mediating these critical milestones is positive and has an immunizing effect (Edge et al. 2009). Overwhelming stress and the inability to cope accompanied by feelings of powerlessness, however, have a sensitizing effect and are likely to make persons who have this history more vulnerable to anxiety when confronted with fearful or even ambiguous situations (Elzinga et al. 2008; Luecke et al. 2009).

Medical conditions influence the occurrence of anxiety disorders (Culpepper 2009). The metabolic or autonomic disturbances caused by an illness could produce the syndrome of anxiety (for example, hyperthyroidism can produce panic-like attacks). The symptoms of a medical illness such as the sensation of an abnormal heartbeat in arrhythmia could also trigger anxiety. Sometimes medical illness and an anxiety disorder simply coexist.

Abnormalities in the serotonergic, adrenergic, and GABA systems have been implicated in the pathophysiology of panic disorders (Leonard 2006). Panic disorder has also been associated with altered functioning in what has been called a "fear network" in the brain, involving the amygdala, hippocampus, and brainstem centers (Gorman et al. 2004; Kent and Rauch 2004). The amygdala mediates environmental stimulation, and, in vulnerable individuals, may trigger an emotional response by interpreting new information about ongoing events in the context of old memories of threatening situations. This is likely mediated by the hippocampus, which plays an important role in learning and memory. Activated brainstem centers and responses in the hypothalamic-pituitary axis (HPA) cause the somatic and visceral symptoms.

The physiological stress response and its relationship to anxiety, depression, and other medical problems are the subject of a massive scientific literature. A report of the Institute of Medicine (Elliott and Eisdorfer 1982) conceptualized the stress response as an X-Y-Z process with X as the stressor, Y as the immediate response, and Z as a longer-term response. The X variable is any stimulation of the organism, from the molecular to the catastrophic, that serves to alter the balance, or threatens to alter the balance, between the organism and the environment. The Y variable represents a reaction that can range from unconscious physiologic changes to recognition of changes and reactive behaviors. The Z variable or response is the longer-term result of the X-Y sequence, especially when X-Y sequences are repeated and overwhelm the individual's biological and/or psychological ability to adapt. Thus, a single event may lead to an overwhelming reaction that the individual experiences repeatedly,

leading to associated autonomic symptoms such as PTSD. Certain occupations associated with repeated episodes of significant stressful stimuli (e.g., air traffic controllers) may over time lead to the increased probability of certain illnesses such as hypertension.

These X-Y-Z variables are mediated by a host of biopsychosocial factors, the type and intensity of which can alter the phenomenology of the X response and therefore the Y response. Experience with X can diminish or exacerbate a response, for example the reaction to the complex demands of family caregiving, which predictably leads to a variety of Ys that may be deleterious to health, leading to depression and immune suppression. If the context is changed so that the individual experiencing the X complex also has a strong social support system, a history of using religion as a coping style, or any experience that leads to a helpful explanatory system that gives support, the X-Y-Z complex will have a different outcome.

The physiologic stress response, in its simplest terms, involves the central nervous system, mediated by the pituitary influence on the hypothalamus, altering the autonomic nervous system (Kudielka and Kirschbaum 2007). The HPA is considered to be the core of the stress response with its alteration of catecholamines and glucocorticoid steroids (Herman et al. 2005). A number of physiologic feedback loops mediate the elevation of these chemicals, which in turn alters the muscular, gastrointestinal, pulmonary, cardiovascular, cerebrovascular, and central nervous system responses to prepare for action (i.e., the flight or fight response). The HPA response is designed to mediate danger, but its persistence significantly affects the central nervous system and other organ systems, increasing the risks of health problems (Motzer and Hertig 2004).

Treatment

The majority of patients who have anxiety disorders can be treated successfully with behavioral and pharmacological therapies (Pinquart and Duberstein 2007; Benitez et al. 2008).

Medications are generally the first treatment choice because they often have a greater treatment effect, but this decision needs to be made in the context of the individual's medical status and preferences. Treatment is sometimes complicated when older people have more than one anxiety disorder, depression, or substance abuse. In some cases, anxiety may be alleviated by successful treatment of the depressive disorder or substance abuse disorder.

Nonpharmacologic Treatment

Nonpharmacological treatments should be the initial approach to patients who have mild symptoms of anxiety, and they can be effective, alone or in combination with medications, for all anxiety disorders. Unfortunately, psychotherapeutic outcome research in all age groups is in its infancy (Bartels et al. 2004; Wetherell et al. 2005; Ayers et al. 2007). Nonpharmacologic treatments include psychotherapies (e.g., behavioral therapy and cognitive behavioral therapy, discussed in chapter 10) as well as relaxation techniques, such as breathing exercises, and biofeedback.

The goal of behavioral therapy is to modify and control undesirable behaviors. Patients learn to cope with difficult situations, often through controlled exposure in the case of phobias, and develop a sense of control over the stimuli that initiate their anxiety response (Schneider et al. 2005). The objective of cognitive behavioral therapy is to alter unproductive or harmful thought patterns so that the person learns to examine feelings and separate realistic from unrealistic thoughts. Cognitive therapy helps patients reframe subjective cognitive distortions by viewing worries more realistically and then formulating effective plans to manage their anxiety (Hofmann and Smits 2008). It restores mastery and a sense of empowerment. Patients are trained to record specific worries as well as explicit evidence that validates or refutes the extent of their concerns, thereby helping them devise an effective strategy. Patients are also taught that "worrying about worry" sustains or increases their anxiety and that avoiding circumstances causing anxiety or procrastination are not effective coping strate-

gies. Although cognitive behavioral therapy is efficacious to reduce anxiety in older adults, little is known about the mechanism by which it reduces anxiety sensitivity (Hendriks et al. 2008; Hofmann and Smits 2008; Stanley et al. 2009).

Given the limited research at this time, there is no evidence that cognitive-behavioral therapy is more effective than behavior therapy and psychodynamic psychotherapy for most forms of anxiety. Supportive psychotherapy can be helpful with older patients who are socially isolated, frail, and chronically ill. Several patient characteristics are associated with poor response to psychotherapies: patients who have coexisting personality disorders, persons living under the influence of chronic biopsychosocial stressors, and patients who may be depressed and do not expect to feel better (Ayers et al. 2007; Pinquart and Duberstein 2007). A combination of psychotherapy and pharmacotherapy is frequently necessary in these circumstances.

Group psychotherapies can be helpful, but patient composition and the issue of open groups (i.e., people can enter or leave at any time) and closed groups are important clinical considerations (Wetherell et al. 2005). Different psychotherapeutic approaches to the group emphasize that "one size" does not fit all patients, and the needs of patients, rather than the orientation of the therapist takes precedence in all clinical encounters.

When available, but only with the patient's consent, clinicians should include family caregivers in treatment. Family informants may offer a different viewpoint about the patient's problem, because hypervigilant patients often misinterpret information and circumstances because of their fears. Family members may also facilitate creating a therapeutic environment to help the patient develop problem-solving skills by participating in structured social activities and actively minimizing periods of isolation in which the patient may obsess about problems.

Medications

Clinicians should consider prescribing medication when anxiety significantly impairs a patient's daily functioning (Wetherell et al. 2005; Hesley and Vanin 2008). The choice of an anxiolytic drug should be based on the suitability of the drug, the possibility of drug-drug interactions, and the likelihood of dependency in individuals who are vulnerable to addiction. Older patients usually have an adequate, but not dramatic, response to anxiolytic drugs. They may experience some relief, but symptoms may persist, including tension and agitation. Sedation, cognitive impairment, and increased risk of falls and injury are also major concerns.

Benzodiazepines have been the most commonly prescribed antianxiety medications, but they should be avoided in older adults because of their adverse effects (Benitez et al. 2008; Berger et al. 2009; Uchida et al. 2009). Benzodiazepines differ in terms of potency, pharmacokinetics, and lipid solubility. Those with a short half-life (e.g., lorazepam) need to be used carefully, and longer-acting drugs (e.g., diazepam, chlordiazepoxide) as well as very short-acting benzodiazepines, such as triazolam, should generally not be used. Alprazolam should also not be used, because it is highly addictive and tapering a person off the drug is a slow, painful process.

In those rare circumstances when benzodiazepines are prescribed for geriatric patients, the dosage should be lower than that used for younger patients and prescribed on a fixed dosage schedule for a limited time period, 4–6 weeks (Bogunovic and Greenfield 2004). Other strategies should be implemented to reduce the need for medication, and clinicians should advise older patients that the benzodiazepine will be stopped or tapered after a defined period. These medications are difficult to discontinue for psychological and physical reasons after being used continuously for an extended time. It is important, therefore, to discontinue the drug or at least to reduce the dose. Results are best if the drug is discontinued over 3 to 4 weeks during which the dose is gradually tapered every few days.

Clinicians should closely follow patients for harmful side effects (Bogunovic and Greenfield 2004). Benzodiazepines may cause sedation, impair coordination, and have other side effects (e.g., ataxia, slurred speech, poor concentration, memory loss, sleep disturbances, falls, and depressive symptoms). If adverse effects occur, the clinician should reduce the dose or stop the drug even if a patient must be hospitalized during the withdrawal period. A few patients may have a paradoxical reaction (i.e., increased agitation and anxiety), and some may experience a rebound effect (i.e., increased anxiety before the next dose is taken) with short-acting benzodiazepines. In these circumstances, the clinician should consider prescribing medications with longer half-life.

The use of benzodiazepines may play a role in the risk for suicide and homicide-suicide. The results of postmortem studies of older men who committed suicide and/or homicide-suicide showed that, with rare exceptions, they were not being treated with antidepressants, but more than 30 percent were taking benzodiazepines (Malphurs et al. 2005). This may be the consequence of treatment for the manifest anxiety without an evaluation of the underlying depression.

Obsessive-compulsive disorder and posttraumatic stress disorder are more effectively treated by antidepressants, especially the SSRIs (Pinquart and Duberstein 2007).

Most antidepressants have antianxiety and antipanic effects in addition to their antidepressant action, and many have antiobsessional effects. SSRIs have antiobsessional effects, and practice guidelines recommend SSRIs for treatment of anxiety disorders because of their favorable tolerability and safety profiles (Sheikh and Cassiday 2000; Pinquart and Duberstein 2007).

Buspirone is useful for treatment of generalized anxiety disorder and is frequently used as an adjunct to SSRIs. Buspirone is a selective 5-HT_{1A} partial agonist that takes about 4–6 weeks to have therapeutic effect. It is not habit forming and has a safety profile comparable to that of the SSRIs. It does not block panic attacks, and it is not efficacious as a primary treatment of OCD or PTSD.

Principles of Managing Anxiety Disorders

1. Recognize the importance of disabling anxiety and screen for its presence.

2. Differentiate anxiety disorders from anxiety as a symptom of other medical disorders.

3. Treat anxiety disorders in terms of their severity. Mild to moderate anxiety is often successfully treated with an appropriate psychotherapeutic approach. More severe, disabling anxiety usually requires medication management in conjunction with psychotherapy.

4. Educate family and keep them involved.

5. Follow-up care is important to monitor how patients are responding or not responding.

6. Monitor adverse effects of medications.

12

Schizophrenia in Later Life

Over the past decade, less than 1 percent of all published research on schizophrenia has dealt with older persons (Cohen et al. 2008). This is disconcerting, given projections that the number of persons aged 55 or older who have schizophrenia in the United States will double from 500,000 to 1 million people over the next 20 years (Broadway and Mintzer 2007). The costs of health care are higher for older persons who have schizophrenia than for younger patients (Folsom et al. 2002, 2006).

Approximately 85 percent of older persons who have schizophrenia live in the community, usually alone or in assisted living facilities, in homeless shelters, or on the street. Another 13 percent live in nursing homes, 1 percent live in state or county hospitals, and 0.5 percent live in veterans or general hospitals (Cohen et al. 2003, 2008). Cognitive deficits, communication deficits, and functional impairments interfere with the ability to work or maintain productive roles and relationships.

Classification

About 25 percent of older people who have schizophrenia developed the disorder in later life, and 75 percent had the first schizophrenic episode during adolescence or early adulthood. Research on late-onset schizophrenia is limited, partly because until 1994 the American Psychiatric Association's *Diagnostic and Statistical Manual of Mental Disorders* did not acknowledge that schizophrenia could be diagnosed in people who first presented with symptoms after age 45. However, both DSM-IV-TR and ICD-10 have no age restriction for schizophrenia.

The International Late-Onset Schizophrenia Group convened in 1998, and they reached consensus about two later-life subtypes: late-onset schizophrenia with onset between ages 40 and 60, and very-late-onset schizophrenia with onset after age 60 (Howard et al. 2000). The prevalence rate of late-onset schizophrenia is 0.6 percent, whereas the prevalence for very-late-onset is 1.0 percent. The debate continues as to whether late-onset and very-late-onset are distinct pathologic entities (Boyce and Walker 2008).

Late-onset schizophrenia may be neurobiologically distinct from early-onset schizophrenia (Palmer et al. 2003; Moran and Lawler 2005; Boyce and Walker 2008), but patients who have early- and late-onset disorder are similar in several ways: the prevalence of positive symptoms (i.e., paranoid delusions and auditory hallucinations), family history of schizophrenia, cognitive impairment (i.e., learning and abstraction deficits but not delayed recall impairment), nonspecific brain-imaging abnormalities (e.g., mild ventricular enlargement and white matter hyperintensities), chronicity of illness, and higher mortality from suicide and other causes (Jeste and Nasrallah 2003; Sato et al. 2004).

Late-onset schizophrenia, however, is characterized by less-severe negative symptoms (i.e., social withdrawal, emotional blunting, poverty of speech) as well as less-severe learning deficits and the need for lower doses of antipsychotic medications (Jeste et al. 2003, 2005). Partition delusions (i.e., belief that people, objects, and radiation pass through walls) occurs more frequently in late-onset than early-onset schizophrenia. A much higher proportion of women than men manifest late-onset and very-late-onset schizophrenia, and this gender difference suggests that hormonal changes after menopause may play a role.

Diagnosis

Acute psychotic episodes that occur in the context of late-onset schizophrenia, schizoaffective disorder, bipolar disorder, major depressive disorder with psychotic symptoms, delusional disorder, delirium, and a psychotic disorder secondary to medical illness are remarkably similar. They cannot be easily differentiated from each other based on their immediate presentation (Kyomen and Whitfield 2009). Psychosis in later life also requires careful evaluation to exclude organic pathology. The manifestation of very-late-onset schizophrenia differs from the psychosis associated with dementia in both neuropsychological and brain imaging findings. About half of patients who have AD manifest psychotic symptoms, but delusions are simpler (e.g., theft, inability to recognize a family member) and less bizarre (e.g., alien invasion) than the symptoms of schizophrenia (Jeste and Finkel 2000).

Clinicians should carefully evaluate individuals who manifest a new-onset psychotic disorder at any age. The evaluation should include:

• A comprehensive personal and family medical history, including family informants, if possible
• Questions about cultural expectations and practices
• Review of current medications, medication history, and medications used by other family members who may have a similar condition
• The patient's history of medication compliance and medication preferences
• Physical, psychiatric, and neurological examinations, including neuroimaging
• Cognitive screening
• Functional status
• Psychosocial supports

For a diagnosis of late-life schizophrenia, individuals need to meet the DSM-IV-TR criteria for schizophrenia, including duration of the symptom syndrome for at least 6 months, and be age 45 or older. Symptoms include what are referred to as positive symptoms (e.g., delusions, hallucinations, disorganized speech, and disorganized or catatonic behavior) as well as what are identified as negative symptoms (e.g., flattened affect, alogia, avolition, and cognitive impairment). Symptoms must lead to significant social or occupational dysfunction, must not be accompanied by prominent mood symptoms, and must not be exclusively associated with alcohol or other substance abuse.

There are a number of differences between early-onset and late-onset schizophrenia. Patients who have late-onset schizophrenia usually have bizarre delusions, often persecutory, and many patients manifest delusions of being physically and mentally influenced by outside forces. The prevalence of persecutory delusions may be as high as 4 percent, and grandiose, erotic, and physical delusions are observed frequently (Ostling and Skoog 2002). Auditory hallucinations are the second most common psychotic symptom. Thought broadcasting and two voices arguing with each other (e.g., God and Satan) are less common, but they may occur. Patients may also have depressive symptoms. However, loose associations and inappropriate affect are less common than in early-onset schizophrenia.

The following case illustrates a classic example of late-onset schizophrenia:

MA, a 65-year-old divorced female, was involuntarily committed to a psychiatric hospital after a neighbor called the police because she was standing on her front porch partially dressed and holding a kitchen knife. She told the police that she was afraid of hurting herself. In the hospital MA reported talking to Jesus and the Virgin Mary, both of whom were concerned that Satan was inside her. MA also said that when she watched prayer shows on the television, she heard the preachers telling her that she was a vile and evil person. Sometimes she would hear other voices telling her that she should kill herself because she was such a bad person.

MA did not have a previous history of psychiatric problems. She had been a volunteer at the public library after retiring from her position as director of nursing in a nursing home. However, she stopped volunteering and had become more

isolated from her family and friends several months before the hospitalization. MA's family and friends had observed changes in her personality over a 12-month period. She had become withdrawn and disinterested in activities that had previously given her pleasure. MA's sister, who lived a few miles away, reported that she had been talking about hearing voices for several months. The voices spoke to her when she was alone, telling her that she must die because Satan lived inside her body.

After ruling out a number of conditions, including dementia, the psychiatrist diagnosed MA with late-onset schizophrenia and successfully treated her with medication and social support.

MA represents a prototype patient for a diagnosis of late-life schizophrenia: (1) a person who has functioned well throughout most of adult life, albeit sometimes with suspiciousness or schizoid personality characteristics; (2) a person who first manifests persecutory delusions and auditory hallucinations after age 40; and (3) a person who shows improvement in positive symptoms with low doses of antipsychotic medications.

There are significant differences between older and younger persons who have schizophrenia. Illicit drug use and some antipsychotic drug side effects (e.g., acute dystonia) are less common in older patients. However, medical co-morbidities and other drug side effects (e.g., extrapyramidal symptoms, tardive dyskinesia, and cardiovascular symptoms) are more common in older patients. Family and psychosocial support are central to treatment and management in all age groups, but most older persons do not have an involved family member, lack financial resources, and are stigmatized as both old and having a mental illness.

Risk Factors

Family History

As with early-onset schizophrenia, family history is the most common risk factor for late-onset schizophrenia (Howard et al. 2000; Jeste et al. 2005). Familial risk of late-onset

schizophrenia is lower than that observed for early-onset cases but greater than that for the general population. It is not known whether the age of onset is genetically determined, partly because many patients at risk for late-onset schizophrenia do not live long enough to manifest symptoms.

Premorbid Personality Disorder

Individuals diagnosed with late-onset schizophrenia have often been reported to have a premorbid history of reclusiveness and paranoia (Cohen 2003). However, in contrast to persons who have early-onset schizophrenia, who are usually not employed, those who have late-onset disorder have usually been successful achievers in the workplace.

Social Isolation

Although social isolation is common in the older population, it is especially widespread in the patient population with late-onset schizophrenia (Howes et al. 2004). However, it is not clear whether social isolation reflects the influence of premorbid personality factors or of the illness itself or is a risk factor for schizophrenia.

Neuropsychological Abnormalities

People who have late-onset schizophrenia have a pattern of cognitive impairments similar to that observed in people who have early-onset schizophrenia but different from that reported in people who have psychosis associated with dementia (Howard 2001; Barch 2009). The results of imaging studies show focal changes (i.e., reduced volume of the left temporal lobe) and an increased ventricular-to-brain ratio in early-onset schizophrenia.

Female Gender

Late-onset schizophrenia is more common in women than in men, with female-to-male ratios ranging from 2:1 to 22:1 (Cohen 2003). Although women have a greater life expectancy than men, the increased gender ratio is significant. Several investigators have implicated the influence of menopause, especially changes in estrogen levels, on brain-related changes increasing the risk of late-onset schizophrenia in women (Hafner 2003).

Treatment

The treatment of older patients who have late-onset schizophrenia is challenging for many reasons (Sable and Jeste 2002; Cohen 2003; Tune and Salzman 2003; Sokal et al. 2004; Schultz et al. 2005). These patients usually have co-morbid medical conditions and are taking multiple medications. Age-related pharmacokinetic changes also place older patients at increased risk for drug interactions and adverse effects of antipsychotic medications (Uchida et al. 2008). Finally, older persons may be reluctant or unwilling to discuss treatment, and they may refuse to discuss care because of lack of insight, characteristic of the illness (Palmer and Jeste 2006).

Management of Acute Episodes

Principles for clinical management of acute episodes include:

- Being empathic and optimistic in discussions
- Being culturally sensitive
- Speaking clearly
- Emphasizing confidentiality of care
- Conducting a comprehensive assessment of the patient
- Providing written information to supplement information provided during the visit
- Working in partnership with family caregivers and other service providers
- Developing a care plan for the physical, emotional, and social needs of the patient
- Asking the patient for informed consent before beginning treatment
- Communicating the treatment plan with the primary physician
- Including physical as well as social activities in the treatment plan

Pharmacological Treatment

Poor adherence to medication is a serious problem because patients lack insight into their illness, including the importance of medications, often because of the absence of a primary caregiver. This results in relapses, multiple emergency room visits and hospital admissions, as well as a reduced quality of life. Poor adherence and the increased medical contacts are the primary reason the costs of caring for older individuals who have schizophrenia and other psychotic disorders are so high, approximately $50 billion annually (Cohen et al. 2008).

In contrast to the large literature of randomized, controlled drug trials in early-onset schizophrenia, open drug trials and case studies rather than empirical outcome studies have been published about late-onset schizophrenia. Atypical antipsychotic medications, first approved by the FDA in 1989, are currently the first-ranked medications used to improve the acute symptoms of both early-onset and late-onset schizophrenia. Compared to the conventional antipsychotic medications, they reduce the risk of relapse, are associated with higher rates of adherence and compliance, have better safety profiles, and minimize extrapyramidal side effects (Sable and Jeste 2002; Tune and Saltzman 2003; Lieberman et al. 2005). Medications should be dosed at levels significantly below those used for young adults, using a starting dosage of 50 percent of recommended dosage to 25 percent with progressive increments as indicated clinically.

Clinicians must carefully monitor older persons taking atypical antipsychotics for side effects, including sedation, weight gain, hyperglycemia, diabetes, hyperlipidemia, orthostatic hypertension, and cardiac conduction problems (Neil et al. 2003). Although extrapyramidal side effects are less frequent with atypical medications compared to conventional antipsychotics, patients should still be monitored for their occurrence. Elevated prolactin, hyperlipidemia, hyperglycemia, obesity, and cerebrovascular accidents are also potential and serious side effects, underscoring the importance of being cautious when prescribing atypical antipsychotics in vulnerable patients.

Because antipychotics interfere with the glucose transport system through dopaminergic and serotinergic mechanisms, psychotic patients who have risk factors for type II diabetes (e.g., obesity, smoking, a sedentary lifestyle, and a poor diet) need to be followed carefully. When older patients have type II diabetes as well as a psychotic disorder, pharmacologic treatment coupled with lifestyle management can be a challenge.

There is an FDA black box warning that atypical antipsychotics have an increased risk for strokes (Rosack 2005). As is the case with all psychotic patients, clinicians should discuss and consider the risks and benefits of these medications with the patient's medical decision maker. In some circumstances, a nonmedication approach with nursing and/or social work support in a protective, nurturing environment may be more appropriate.

Older men and women incur different risks with the use of atypical antipsychotics (Seeman 2006). Because dopamine inhibits the release of prolactin, dopamine blockade by antipsychotics may increase prolactin levels, leading to decreased libido and decreased bone density in older women. Other effects of elevated prolactin may include breast enlargement and menstrual irregularity, including galactorrhea in younger patients, but data are lacking for women who have late-onset disease. Erectile dysfunction, including ejaculatory problems and decreased spermatogenesis seen in younger patients, has not been studied in men who have late-onset disease.

Conventional first-generation antipsychotic drugs, such as haloperidol and chlorpromazine, are used with patients who do not adhere to the medication schedule and are not able to tolerate or respond to the atypical antipsychotic drugs (Cohen 2003). Clinicians need to follow patients closely, because the conventional antipsychotics may have serious negative side effects, including decreased tolerance, anticholinergic toxicity, and a number of extrapyramidal disorders, including parkinsonism and tardive dyskinesia.

Many state Medicaid programs have restricted access to atypical antipsychotic medications, which are significantly more expensive than the typical antipsychotic medications, because of escalating health care costs (Polinski et al. 2007). The likely impact if these policies continue will be a much-reduced quality of life, increased nonadherence to drug regimens, and increased use and costs of medical care.

Nonmedication Approaches

Nonmedication approaches are necessary for the effective management and treatment of late-life schizophrenia (Berry and Barrowclough 2009). These include:

- Evaluation for visual and hearing impairment and appropriate aides
- Identification of group support systems to reduce social isolation
- Case management for medication adherence, medical appointments, and supportive communication
- Social skills training
- Cognitive-behavioral therapy in conjunction with social skills training
- Cognitive rehabilitation to manage delusions and hallucinations
- Skill training for personal care and instrumental activities of daily living
- Involvement of family members in educational programs and support services

The development and evaluation of psychotherapeutic interventions for older patients who have schizophrenia has been limited. Cognitive-behavioral therapy and cognitive-behavioral therapy coupled with social skills training have been shown to reduce psychiatric symptoms (Arean and Cook 2002; Granholm et al. 2005). Psychosocial interventions to improve personal care and activities of daily living have improved daily functioning and compliance with medication (Patterson et al. 2003), and work rehabilitation has been effective with middle-aged or older individuals who have schizophrenia (Twamley et al. 2005). Clinical trials of the therapeutic effects of cognitive-behavioral training are ongoing (www .clinicaltrials.gov/ct2/show/NCT00832845).

If these interventions significantly enhance the independence and social functioning of older patients, they may prevent excess disability and premature institutionalization and reduce the burden on families and caregivers. Because the quality of life and lifestyle of people who have schizophrenia can be so compromised, an integrated strategy of medication management, psychosocial rehabilitation, and educational supports is the optimal clinical approach. Monitoring the patient's lifestyle, weight, and blood values is a necessary part of the conservative treatment strategy to help but do no harm.

Management of Poor Response or Resistance to Treatment

When patients do not respond well to treatment, clinicians should make sure that an adequate dose of an antipsychotic has been used for a sufficient time to obtain a clinical response. If patients have not responded despite an adequate trial of treatment, clinicians should evaluate and treat other possible causes for the symptoms, including alcohol or drug abuse, medical illnesses, and poor adherence. It may also be useful to expand psychological and psychosocial interventions for six months or more.

Goals of Treatment

The overall goals of treatment for older persons who have schizophrenia are:

- Diminish or eliminate psychosis
- Focus on symptom management and solution of everyday living problems
- Maintain good overall health
- Support adherence to medications
- Maintain decent housing
- Maintain a lifestyle free of alcohol and other substances
- Minimize contacts with law enforcement
- Find and/or maintain significant activities
- Define and support achievement of meaningful personal goals

Other Late-Life Psychotic Disorders

Abnormal Suspiciousness

Older adults who display abnormal suspiciousness frequently have medical disorders and are seen by primary care physicians, not mental health professionals (Ostling and Skoog 2002). These patients may complain about external forces controlling their lives or attempting to hurt them (e.g., beliefs that strangers have tried to get into their home or poison them). These beliefs may also be specifically targeted toward family members or neighbors (e.g., beliefs that their children have deserted them or have plotted to control their assets). The abnormal suspiciousness usually is a psychological reflection that individuals feel that they have lost control of events or circumstances coupled with feelings of isolation, poor social judgment, and sensory impairments.

Intense suspiciousness may occur in some patients who have dementia, especially residents of long-term care facilities, who are frequently distrustful of family and staff members (Schogt 2007). Their accusations are usually disorganized and poorly defined (e.g., possessions missing or staff acting in threatening ways), and they reflect the patient's cognitive impairment and difficulties integrating what is happening around them in the institution. However, elder abuse can be a real possibility, so resident complaints should be investigated (chapter 18).

Transient Paranoid Reactions

Transient paranoid reactions are most likely to occur in older women who live alone. Such patients are adamant that others are trying to hurt them, are plotting against them, or have manipulated them sexually, yet there is no evidence for these circumstances to have occurred. Being socially isolated from others and having sensory impairments may contribute to these distortions. Over time, the content and focus of the hallucinations and delusional thinking usually change from concerns about external threats and what is happening outside the home (e.g., concerns about noises) to incidents inside the home (e.g., reports of the home being broken into, physical assault, sexual molestation, or interactions with aliens). Careful psychiatric, medical, and environmental evaluation of patients and the potential basis for their behavior is warranted. These disorders respond well to minimal doses of atypical antipsychotic medications and supportive care.

Psychotic Disorders Due to Physical or Systemic Disorders

Some psychotic disorders are due to drug intoxication, physical illness, and postoperative psychosis (e.g., psychosis occurring among patients in intensive care units). Visual hallucinations occur more often (as in delirium), yet the psychosis may be organized and elaborate (unlike delirium). These disorders are usually transient and resolve with treatment of the underlying cause or spontaneously. In the midst of the disorder, however, acute management is necessary.

Principles of Managing Schizophrenia

Paranoia and other signs and symptoms of schizophrenia require a comprehensive work-up. The relationship between the symptomatology and other psychiatric conditions as well as medical, postsurgical, and environmental factors requires a rapid comprehensive examination and continued monitoring of the patient to prevent isolation, to maximize treatment adherence, and to minimize untoward consequences to the patient's family.

1. People who have late-onset schizophrenia have distinctive clinical characteristics compared to those with early-onset schizophrenia.

2. The differential diagnosis of psychosis appearing in later life may include many psychiatric disorders, including early- versus late-onset schizophrenia, schizoaffective disorder, bipolar disorder, depressive disorder, delusional disorder, dementia, delirium, and psychotic states due to medical conditions.

3. Atypical antipsychotic medications are the current standard of care for pharmacological management, and the clinician should monitor side effects closely.

4. Psychological therapies, psychosocial interventions that enhance activities of daily living skills, and medication management can reduce the need for hospitalization and institutionalization.

13

Alcohol Abuse, Substance Abuse, and Medication Mismanagement

Alcohol and drug misuse or abuse often go undetected by clinicians who mistake these symptoms for dementia, depression, or other medical conditions (Levin and Kruger 2000; O'Connell et al. 2003). Because of the mistaken belief that alcohol and drug problems are not prevalent in later life, clinicians often miss substance abuse in older adults, which may involve alcohol, prescription medications, over-the-counter (OTC) medications, tobacco, or illicit drugs (Dar 2006). Primary care office visits are often brief, limiting clinicians' time to learn about patients' lifestyles, and even when clinicians suspect substance abuse, they may believe that older people cannot change these bad habits, when the opposite is true.

Older persons frequently deny misusing or abusing substances and are not inclined to seek professional help (Levin and Kruger 2000). Family members may be ashamed of the substance abuse problem and not want to address it, preferring instead to raise the secondary symptoms as a problem without reference to the pattern of addictive behavior.

Failure to diagnose and manage substance abuse can result in serious medical and psychosocial consequences, including the confounding of medication management, other illnesses, intentional or unintentional injury, impaired quality of life, domestic violence, and long-term family difficulties (Gfroerer et al. 2003). Alcohol abuse is responsible for exacerbating a number of conditions, including cardiovascular diseases, immune disorders, gastrointestinal and liver disease, malnutrition, and severe mental health problems (JS Stevenson 2005). The U.S. Substance Abuse and Mental Health Services Administration maintains a comprehensive Older Americans Substance Abuse and Mental Health Technical

Assistance Center website (www.samhsa.gov/ OlderAdultsTAC/index.aspx). Other information sites include the National Institute on Alcohol Abuse and Alcoholism (www.niaaa .nih.gov) and the Hartford Institute for Geriatric Nursing (http://consultgerirn.org/topics/ substance_abuse/want_to_know_more). The Substance Abuse and Mental Health Services Administration (SAMHSA) has also published a comprehensive series of technical reports (SAMHSA 2002, www.oas.samhsa.gov/aging/ toc.htm).

Prevalence

Alcohol and drug misuse and abuse are common in the older population, but the extent, forms, and outcome of abuse and dependence are elusive. Estimates of the prevalence of heavy drinking or alcohol abuse range from 2 to 20 percent (Menninger 2002; Simoni-Wastila and Yang 2006). Many studies of the use of prescription and OTC drugs indicate that older adults consume 25–30 percent of all prescription drugs, use more OTC and prescription drugs than any other age group, and are more likely to consume psychotropic drugs with a potential for misuse, abuse, and addiction (Compton et al. 2007). There is some evidence that the baby boom generation is more likely than earlier generations to have been exposed to drug and alcohol use and may drink or consume drugs at greater rates in later life (Compton et al. 2007).

The proportion of older adults of all racial backgrounds who misuse alcohol, prescription drugs, and/or other substances is growing and will do so in the future (Szapocznik et al. 2007; Johnson and Sung 2009; Paech and Weston 2009). The 2002/2003 SAMHSA

143

National Survey on Drug Use and Health esti-mated that of the 34 percent of adults age 65 or older who drank alcohol in the past month, 7.8 percent reported binge drinking and 1.8 percent reported heavy alcohol use (SAMHSA 2003). An estimated 1.8 percent of adults age 50 or older reported using illicit drugs in the past month, with marijuana the most com-monly used (1.1%) followed by nonmedical use of prescription drugs (0.7%) and cocaine (0.2%). The number of older adults needing treatment for substance abuse is estimated to more than double, from 1.7 million persons in 2000 to 4.4 million persons, in 2020 (Gfroerer et al. 2003).

The prevalence of at-risk and binge drinking reported by older adults is increasing, accord-ing to secondary data analyses of the 2005 and 2006 National Survey of Drug Use and Health (Blazer and Wu 2009). A total of 13 percent of older men and 8 percent of older women reported at-risk alcohol use, and more than 14 percent of men and 3 percent of women reported binge drinking. Binge drinking in older men was associated with higher income and being separated, divorced, or widowed. Among both older men and older women, binge drinking was associated with the use of tobacco and illicit drugs.

In the United States as well as in many other countries, persons age 65 or older con-sume more prescribed and OTC medications than any other age group (Brekke et al. 2006; Repetto 2006; Faggiani et al. 2007). The same age-related physiological changes (e.g., slowed metabolic and clearance mechanisms, changing body composition) that influence the effects of alcohol increase the body's vulnerability to drugs of all kinds, and when adverse effects occur, they last longer. Furthermore, the fre-quent use of multiple drugs places older adults at increased risk for drug-drug and drug-alcohol interactions. At least 83 percent of older adults are estimated to take at least one prescription drug, and 30 percent take eight or more prescription drugs daily. It is common for patients to have multiple specialist physi-cians who may not communicate with one another about prescriptions. Thus the risks for

drug interactions are inevitably increased in those who are most vulnerable and for whom adverse reactions would be the most harmful. Finally, drug misuse may be unintentional if older patients do not understand the instruc-tions for drug treatment, have financial limi-tations influencing whether they can afford medications, purchase inferior medications from subquality sources to save money, or take outdated medications initially prescribed for others.

Older men are more likely to abuse alcohol, whereas older women are more likely to abuse prescription drugs, particularly benzodiaz-epines and OTC drugs. The Surgeon General's Report on Mental Health (1999) predicted that alcohol and drug abuse would increase because the baby boom cohort has a higher level of alcohol consumption and a growing rate of medication abuse than prior generations. Esti-mates are that the current group of approxi-mately 1.7 million older substance abusers will increase to 4.4 million by 2020 (SAMHSA 2004).

Misuse and Abuse of Alcohol
Older Persons and Sensitivity to Alcohol

Age-related biological changes (e.g., decreased body water, enhanced sensitivity to alcohol, and decreased gastric enzymes) make older persons more vulnerable to the adverse effects of alcohol consumption. Total body water and lean body mass decrease with advancing age, and because alcohol is water-soluble, for a specific amount of alcohol, the concentra-tion in the blood is greater in older persons than in younger ones. Age-related decreases in the gastric alcohol dehydrogenase enzyme slow alcohol metabolism, causing the blood alcohol level to remain high for a longer period of time. Thus, a small amount of alcohol can cause intoxication and may lead to increased sensitivity and decreased tolerance. Individuals who have longstanding drinking patterns may become more severely intoxicated as they age.

Excessive, persistent consumption of alcohol can increase the risk for or exacerbate existing health conditions in older persons, including cardiovascular disease, strokes, cirrhosis and other liver diseases, decreased bone density, decreased immunity, malnutrition, gastrointestinal bleeding, insomnia, oral diseases, and psychiatric disorders (Friedlander and Norman 2006; Moos et al. 2009). Individuals who have AD or other dementias frequently have decreased tolerance for alcohol, and the early stages of dementia may be mistaken for alcohol problems. Chronic alcoholism, with its consequent nutritional deficiencies, can also cause Wernicke-Korsakoff dementia (chapter 9).

Levels of Alcohol Consumption

Recommendations about alcohol use should be individualized, depending on risks and potential benefits. Clinicians should screen all patients in routine examinations for excess consumption, problem drinking, or adverse consequences. Because older adults have an increased sensitivity to alcohol and medications and are at risk for drug-alcohol interactions, recommended levels for social use of alcohol are lower for persons 65 or older than for younger people. The Physician's Guide for Helping Patients with Alcohol Problems (www.niaaa.nih.gov) is a valuable resource.

Abstinence is recommended for individuals who have a history of alcoholism, drug abuse, and chronic diseases such as diabetes and congestive heart failure as well as when alcohol use is contraindicated with certain medications. Several studies indicate that moderate levels of alcohol consumption (i.e., one or two regular drinks a day) is associated with lower morbidity, disability, and mortality from coronary heart disease than that among both heavy alcohol users and abstainers across diverse geographical locations and racial groups (Atkinson 2002; Di Castelnuovo et al. 2006; Chen and Hardy 2009). However, some studies show that moderate alcohol intake does not have the same protective value for black males as for white males (Fuchs et al. 2004).

Modest consumption of alcohol has also been shown to improve HDL levels in women (De Oliveira e Silva et al. 2000), but it has been linked to breast cancer in postmenopausal women (Suzuki et al. 2005). Continued

research is important to clarify the health benefits and risks of small to moderate amounts of alcohol and the differential effects of various alcoholic beverages in populations with varying health status (Paganini-Hill et al. 2007; Karlamangla et al. 2009).

The National Institute on Alcohol Abuse and Alcoholism (NIAAA 2005) recommended no more than one standard drink per day for persons age 65 or older, and the TIP Consensus Panel also recommended a maximum of two standard drinks at celebrations but lower limits for women. A standard drink refers to one can (12 oz.) of beer or ale, a single shot (1.5 oz.) of hard liquor, a glass (5 oz.) of wine, or a small glass (4 oz.) of an aperitif, brandy, sherry, or liqueur.

Diagnosis of Alcohol Abuse

DSM-IV-TR criteria for alcohol abuse specify a pattern of alcohol use causing significant impairment or distress, with three or more of the following present at any time in the same 12-month period: (1) need for significantly increased amounts of alcohol or diminished effect with continued use of the same amount of alcohol; (2) presence of the characteristic withdrawal syndrome or alcohol/medications being used to relieve or avoid withdrawal; (3) alcohol used in larger amounts or over a longer period than intended; (4) unsuccessful efforts to control alcohol intake; (5) significant efforts to obtain alcohol or recover from intoxication; (6) withdrawal from social, occupational, or leisure activities because of alcohol use; and (7) continued drinking despite knowledge of serious medical risks.

The DSM-IV-TR criteria do not adequately define alcohol use in the older population. Many older adults do not experience the legal or social consequences more commonly seen in younger persons. The criterion for continued alcohol use despite physical and psychological problems frequently does not apply, because many older people do not understand or accept that the persistent or recurrent problems are related to their drinking. The consumption tolerance threshold is lower in older adults because of increased sensitivity to and bodily distribution of alcohol. Lack of tolerance is not necessarily diagnostic because older adults who have late-onset alcoholism do not develop physiological dependence, nor do they do exhibit signs of withdrawal.

A framework that addresses at-risk drinking and problem drinking is more useful for characterizing drinking patterns in older persons than the DSM-IV-TR (Crome and Bloor 2006). At-risk drinkers are consuming alcohol at a level that has significantly increased the likelihood of negative medical, psychological, or social consequences. At-risk drinking is an important target for interventions because it has been shown to lead to injuries from falls, depression, suicide, cognitive impairment, liver disease, cardiovascular disease, and sleep problems (Thomas and Rockwood 2001; Bartels et al. 2002b; Seitz and Stickel 2007; Lopes et al. 2010). Problem drinking indicates more dangerous levels of alcohol use in which the person is usually unable to control drinking, persists in drinking despite medical problems and/or injuries, drinks out of boredom, and spends time alone drinking rather than maintaining usual social activities.

Types of Problem Drinking

Early-Onset versus Late-Onset Problem Drinking

Early-onset drinkers usually have longstanding alcohol-related problems beginning before age 40, usually in their 20s, whereas late-onset drinkers exhibit the first alcohol-related problems later in life (Atkinson 2004). Both early- and late-onset problem drinkers use alcohol almost daily, outside of social settings, often alone at home or a bar. Both are more likely to use alcohol as a self-medicating measure in response to losses and stress than as a socializing agent. Most older patients in treatment are early-onset drinkers who have used alcohol to cope with personal, psychosocial, or medical problems and have continued their drinking patterns into later life. Psychiatric co-morbidity is common, especially major affective disorders and thought disorders (Devanand 2002).

About one-third of older adults who have a drinking problem are late-onset abusers,

and they are psychologically and physically healthier than early-onset drinkers. Late-onset drinkers are more likely to initiate or increase drinking in response to a significant loss (Satter et al. 2003). They are usually more willing to seek treatment than early-onset drinkers and often have insight into why they began drinking (Atkinson 2004). However, because late-onset drinkers have a shorter history of problem consumption and fewer health problems, health care professionals frequently miss the signs of at-risk or problem drinking.

Intermittent Problem Drinking

Intermittent problem drinking is characterized by a history of periods of heavy drinking (i.e., binge or weekend drinking) beginning between the ages of 20 and 30. Some individuals consume alcohol daily for weeks or years at a time and may have been abstinent for weeks or years at a time. The intermittent pattern may recur in response to losses, isolation, or health problems in later life. The drinking may also occur in conjunction with bipolar disorders, other psychiatric problems, or noncompliance with medication.

Older intermittent problem drinkers frequently have medical problems reflecting the severity and chronicity of their heavy drinking and the frequency and length of periods of abstinence. Some of these individuals may not present with serious medical conditions but report that the intensity of hangover symptoms has become more distressing.

The negative consequences of drinking binges may include strained or disrupted relationships with family members and friends, financial difficulties, and actions that cause legal problems. It is not unusual for family, friends, and colleagues to seek help for the abuser during the periods of heavy drinking, but once the episode has passed, they frequently will not continue to press for ongoing treatment to prevent relapses. After a period of time, they may believe that nothing can be done and tolerate the binge drinking. The abuser is especially difficult to get into treatment because the long history of drinking bouts has reinforced a strong denial system that a problem exists.

The prognosis depends on many factors: availability and accessibility of age-appropriate drug rehabilitation programs; the ability of abusers to have some understanding of their drinking patterns and the consequences; and the support of family and friends. People who have intermittent problem drinking fare better than those who have early-onset problem drinking, but their prospects of recovery and maintenance are not as good as those for late-onset problem drinkers.

Problem-Focused Drinking

The term *problem-focused drinking* characterizes individuals who have specific personal, health, psychosocial, or legal issues associated with alcohol consumption. Health problems such as hypertension and diabetes mellitus may become management challenges, because misuse and abuse of alcohol lead to hypertension, alter glucose metabolism, and modify the effects of prescription and OTC medications. If allowed to consume alcohol, individuals who have dementia become more impaired and their behaviors more difficult to manage. Loss of social inhibitions from heavy drinking may lead to inappropriate language and behavior, irritability, angry outbursts, being arrested for driving, or domestic violence.

Problem drinkers may consume large amounts of alcohol on an intermittent or regular basis such that they exhibit mild dependence or meet diagnostic criteria for alcohol abuse. Some abusers do not manifest sufficient symptoms to be diagnosed. The critical factor for a good prognosis is to target the issues specific to the focal problems quickly and appropriately.

Risk Factors
Gender

About 10 percent of men report a history of heavy drinking at some point in their lives, which places them at high risk for serious health problems in later life, including a five-fold risk of late-life psychiatric illness (e.g., dementia and depression), despite cessation of heavy drinking. A high percentage of veterans receiving long-term care have a history of substance abuse problems (Klein and Jess 2002). However, findings from the National Nursing Home Survey revealed that residents who had a history of alcohol disorders did not differ in overall functioning and health service use from residents who did not have alcohol abuse disorders (Brennan 2005).

Epidemiological and clinical research studies consistently report later onset of problem drinking among women (Satre et al. 2004). There are other differences between older male and female alcohol abusers. Women are more likely to be widowed or divorced, have had a problem-drinking spouse, or have experienced depression. Women also report more negative effects of alcohol, greater use of prescribed psychoactive medication, and more time spent drinking with a spouse or others.

Loss of Spouse

Alcohol abuse is more prevalent among older adults who have been separated or divorced and among men who have been widowed. Some researchers have hypothesized that a serious, destructive triad of disorders may be triggered among older men when their wives die: depression, alcohol problems, and suicide. The highest rate of completed suicide among all population groups is in older white men who become excessively depressed and drink heavily, often following the death of the spouse (Conwell et al. 2002; Sher 2006).

Other Losses

Advancing age is often associated with multiple losses, including the deaths of family members and friends. Retirement may bring economic insecurity, loss of meaningful social support systems, and loss of purpose defined by the workplace. Other losses include diminished mobility, impaired sensory capabilities, and declining health.

Medical Care Setting

Because prevalence rates for alcoholism are high in inpatient and outpatient settings, clinicians following patients for other conditions should screen them for possible substance abuse problems (Blow et al. 2007). The rates range from 2 to 15 percent among older persons residing in the community, in contrast to 18–44 percent among general medical and psychiatric inpatients (O'Connell et al. 2003).

Premorbid Alcohol Abuse

There is a robust association between having a substance use disorder early in life and a recurrence in later life (Stueve and O'Donnell 2005). Even recovering alcoholics who have sustained long periods of sobriety may relapse in later life after a major loss or from being bored and isolated (Satter et al. 2003; Moos et al. 2009).

Co-Morbid Psychiatric Disorders

Primary mood disorders, which occur in 12–30 percent of older persons who are alcoholic, may be precipitating or maintenance factors affecting late-onset drinking. Depression appears to be a risk factor for drinking, especially among women (Devanand 2002; Blow et al. 2007). Men and women who have problem drinking may not meet the clinical criteria for depression but often report feeling depressed before consuming the first drink on a drinking day. Late-onset alcohol abuse is probably related to significant losses in later life more than to psychiatric problems per se, with the exception of people, such as intermittent drinkers, who have been sober until alcohol or psychiatric problems occur again later in life.

Family History

Although genetic factors appear to be more important in early- than later-onset problem drinking, the results of several studies with older cohorts provide strong evidence that drinking behaviors have a genetic component throughout the lifespan (Schuckit 2000).

Misuse and Abuse of Medication

More than 25 percent of all prescribed medications in the United Stated are used by older adults, often for pain, insomnia, or anxiety (Culberson and Ziska 2008). Second to alcohol, the substances older adults most commonly abuse are nicotine and psychotropic medications. Both are prevalent among older adults who also abuse alcohol, and lifetime use of illicit drugs or nicotine contributes to poorer treatment outcome (Mason and Lehert 2009).

A substantial number of older adults are prescribed psychotropic drugs, especially benzodiazepines, sedatives, and hypnotics, despite the well-known adverse effects and without appropriate clinical management (Voyer et al. 2004; Cook et al. 2007). Patients may not understand the instructions and unintentionally misuse these medications (Simoni-Wistila and Yang 2006).

Abuse of narcotics is uncommon in the older population, and older narcotic abusers are usually people who abused opiates early in life (Han et al. 2009). Abuse of prescriptions for opioids is also rare. About 2 to 3 percent of noninstitutionalized older adults receive prescriptions for opioid analgesics, usually for severe pain, and the proportion that become dependent is negligible. Although little is known about the use of heroin, cocaine, and marijuana in the older population, the numbers presenting with symptoms of illicit drug abuse are predicted to increase as the baby boom generation ages (Crome et al. 2009; Johnson and Sung 2009).

Risks Associated with Medication Abuse/Misuse

Serious risks associated with the misuse and abuse of prescription and OTC medications can be prevented with appropriate interventions (www.samhsa.gov/OlderAdultsTAC). Adverse consequences include problems caused by age-related changes in metabolism, drug-drug interactions, drug-disease interactions, drug-nutrient interactions, and adverse drug side effects (Lindblad et al. 2006). Medication problems may be caused by many factors: abuse of recreational drugs, misuse and abuse of sleep and antianxiety medications, incorrect dosage, OTC overuse, harmful side effects, noncompliance with medication schedules, or changes in physical activity levels. Adverse results may include impairments in alertness, language, cognition, affect, mood, and functional effectiveness, as well as sensory and motor skills. Other negative sequelae may include delirium, insomnia, appetite changes, incontinence, agitation, anger, falls, intentional and unintentional injuries, and premature relocation to living situations requiring more supportive care.

Indicators of Drug Misuse

Circumstances considered diagnostic of medication misuse may include:

- Using drugs or alcohol when contraindicated
- Using drugs and ignoring dietary precautions
- Not adhering to prescribed medication schedules
- Taking medications that have not been prescribed
- Failing to follow instructions
- Using outdated drugs
- Continuing to take a drug when side effects are distressing and not reporting effects to the prescribing physician
- Not storing drugs properly
- Sharing or borrowing drugs
- Taking all medications prescribed for the day at one time for fear of forgetting to take all the medications as prescribed
- Supplementing prescribed drugs with OTC medications
- Engaging in contraindicated activities while taking the medications (e.g., driving, drinking, spending time in the sun)
- Not informing all physicians about other prescribed and OTC medications

Risk Factors for Drug Misuse

One of the most important factors is multiple physicians prescribing multiple prescriptions for older people in the community as well as long-term care facilities (Fick et al. 2004; PJ Barry et al. 2008). It is estimated that 50 to 75 percent of older patients may be vulnerable to dangerous drug-drug interactions (Tulner et al. 2008). Many older adults also do not tell their physician about OTC medications, alcohol use, and herbal supplements (Sleath et al. 2001).

Multiple drugs and complex medication regimens may create serious risks:

- Medication errors may increase when dosage schedules are more complicated.
- The risk of adverse drug reactions increases with each drug a person takes.
- The patient's caregiver may be confused about the dosing schedule or even be less capable than the patient.

Sensory impairment increases the risk of misuse of medications:

- A person with a hearing problem may not hear instructions for taking medications correctly.
- Poor vision and small print may make it difficult to read warning labels.
- Physical ailments and disabilities pose problems such as difficulty opening bottles.
- Some people may have problems swallowing tablets or capsules and may need a liquid or a skin patch.

Screening Tools for Misuse of Alcohol and Other Substances

Two of the most useful alcohol screening tools validated on older adults are the CAGE Questionnaire (Ewing 1984) and the Michigan Alcoholism Screening Test-Geriatric Version (MAST-G; Blow et al. 1992). Less than half of all older patients score positively on both instruments, suggesting that they are measuring different dimensions of unhealthy drinking behaviors (Moore et al. 2002). Before administering the CAGE, the MAST-G, or any other screening instrument, clinicians should clarify, without being condescending or disrespectful, whether patients are consuming alcohol.

The CAGE questionnaire, which may also be adapted for medication misuse, consists of four questions:

- Have you ever felt you should cut down on your drinking?
- Does criticism of your drinking annoy you?
- Have you ever felt guilty about drinking?
- Have you ever had an "eye opener" (a drink first thing in the morning) to steady your nerves or to get rid of a hangover?

Two or more "yes" answers suggest a serious alcohol problem. The CAGE is less effective for women problem drinkers than men. Many older persons who are not dependent on alcohol but who drink heavily enough to cause health problems are unlikely to be detected by the CAGE. Additional questions should be asked about the quantity and frequency of alcohol use, the type of alcoholic beverage consumed, and what the patient defines as a drink. Clinicians should also probe for symptoms of alcohol abuse and negative effects of drinking.

The MAST-G, developed specifically for older adults, has excellent psychometric properties (Allen and Wilson 2004). Another screening test, the Alcohol Use Disorders Identification Test (AUDIT; Babor et al. 2001) has not been assessed for its adequacy among older adults, although it has been validated cross-culturally and is recommended for identifying alcohol problems among older members of minority groups (Frank et al. 2008).

Validated substance abuse assessment tools can be helpful for clinicians because they provide a structured checklist to be reviewed during a patient's psychiatric interview. The TIP Consensus Panelists (Blow et al. 1992; www.ncbi.nlm.nih.gov/bookshelf/br.fcgi?book=hssamhsatip&part=A48302) recommend the use of two structured assessments with older adults: the Structured Clinical Interview for DSM-III-R (SCID, www.scid4.org; Spitzer et al. 1992) and the Diagnostic Interview Schedule (DIS) for DSM-IV (Robins et al. 1981; Robins and Cottler 2004). The SCID interview covers the full range of psychiatric disorders, and it takes a trained clinician about 30 minutes to administer the 35 SCID questions that probe for alcohol abuse or dependence. The DIS is a structured interview that does not require clinical judgment and therefore can be used by nonclinicians. It examines current and past symptoms and is available in a computerized version.

Treatment

The Treatment Improvement Protocol (TIP) Consensus Panel recommends that clinicians follow these general guidelines:

• Older adults who have substance abuse problems need to be motivated to collaborate in a treatment or rehabilitation plan by emphasizing that they can improve their health, avoid unnecessary disability and loss of independence, and prevent economic insecurity.

• Clinicians need to evaluate the extent to which the pattern of substance abuse may reflect medical problems, including delirium, seizures, suicidal ideation and behaviors, failure of outpatient/inpatient treatment, and psychosocial factors, including caregiver strain and depression, social isolation, and disconnectedness.

• A minimalist approach to treatment may be appropriate for older adults who admit to misusing alcohol and have insight into their problem. They may profit from brief interventions, including counseling, but if this strategy is not effective, more intensive interventions are indicated.

• Older abusers may have special personal and health issues that are often not addressed in formalized addiction treatment programs, and they are frequently uncomfortable in groups of predominantly younger patients. Often older people do not respond well to the confrontational and self-disclosing techniques of programs such as Alcoholics Anonymous. Engaging the older abuser as a partner in treatment and individualizing the care plan to address specific developmental and health needs are important strategies for a successful outcome.

• Motivating older adults to control their behaviors and limit the patterns of alcohol and substance abuse may be more effective than confrontation and insistence on immediate abstinence. Although abstinence may be the goal, short-term goals of reducing consumption slowly can be effective.

• With the older person's permission, it may be valuable to include family members in treatment. Adult children, who may be in denial or unsure of how to help, can be educated to be supportive during the treatment process and after. Older late-onset problem drinkers frequently feel guilty, requiring that family be carefully involved in nonthreatening ways.

· Addiction is similar to many chronic illnesses with ongoing cycles of improvements and setbacks. Different tactics and strategies are needed to intervene effectively over time.

· Home-based treatment programs are effective and can be combined with health and social service visits.

· All treatment strategies must be culturally appropriate. Beliefs, expectations, attributions, and practices among different racial and ethnic groups influence help-seeking behaviors, communication, acceptance of a diagnosis, treatment adherence, family involvement, and social support.

The TIP Protocol recommends an approach to facilitate brief interventions with the acronym FRAMES:

· *Feedback* regarding personal risks
· *Responsibility* for personal change
· *Advice* about ways to change
· *Menu* of change options to find an appropriate treatment strategy
· *Empathic* counseling
· *Self-efficacy* reinforcement of client during treatment and follow-up

The clinicians' roles are as partner, motivator, coach, and, if needed, a guide to more intensive treatment. Enjoining with patients in this process is critical to successful outcome.

Treatment of substance abuse among the older population has an excellent record of success. With the availability and accessibility of appropriate interventions, therapeutic optimism for a sustained recovery is warranted (Naegle 2008). The challenges for treating older abusers include dealing with their special needs and circumstances of later life and managing health conditions caused or exacerbated by their substance misuse/abuse.

Detoxification

Detoxification procedures can usually be done in outpatient or residential programs unless co-morbid medical conditions dictate inpatient care. Detoxification should follow the "low and slow" guidelines, with careful monitoring of vital signs, hydration, and treatment with vitamins for people who have longer-term alcoholism. Medications may be indicated for treating older patients during withdrawal: (1) short-acting benzodiazapines (e.g., oxazepam, lorazepam) for alcohol withdrawal; (2) clonidine and methadone for opiate withdrawal; and (3) phenobarbital for barbiturate withdrawal. These medications need to be decreased daily, and patients should be closely monitored.

Psychotherapy

Group therapy appears to be effective for older adults, especially those who have late-onset abuse and mild to moderate abuse behaviors (Simoni-Wastila and Yang 2006). The emphasis of a supportive group milieu is on self-acceptance and the support of others to reduce guilt, self-blame, and feelings of worthlessness. Different approaches, from psychodynamic to cognitive, may be used if individuals have some insight and are able to express themselves. It is essential that the group leader avoid using jargon and pressuring participants to reveal too much before they are ready. Groups provide an environment to educate patients about addiction and the consequences of addictive behaviors. They provide opportunities for older adults to examine and cope better with real life stresses of later life that affect substance misuse, including caregiving, loss of friends, role loss with retirement, and social isolation.

Individual therapies, short and long term, can be effective in conjunction with group therapy or educational programs, or they may be useful alone as an initial therapeutic intervention (Schonfeld and Dupree 1999). Individual psychotherapy can help explore life stresses or recent unresolved life crises and is an appropriate strategy to treat psychopathology associated with substance misuse (e.g., PTSD, depression). Privacy and confidentiality about substance abuse and other psychiatric problems are often very important to older adults.

Preventing a Relapse of Substance Abuse

Schonfeld and Dupree (1999) developed a brief group intervention that uses the principles of cognitive behavioral therapy to help older alcohol abusers analyze and self-manage substance abuse behaviors. This intervention is based on recommendations in the Treatment Improvement Protocols (TIP) Series 26 and 34 issued by the Substance Abuse and Mental Health Services Administration's Center for Substance Abuse (DHHS 1998, 1999b). The treatment approach consists of three stages over 16 sessions. Treatment begins with an analysis of the antecedents and consequences of using alcohol to create a "substance abuse behavior chain" for each individual. The next stage is to teach the older adult to recognize the components of the behavior chain in order to understand the high-risk circumstances leading to the use of drugs and/or alcohol. In the third stage, individuals are taught specific skills to deal with these high-risk situations to prevent relapse. For example, if high-risk situations include social pressures, loneliness, or anger/frustration, skills taught might include refusing a drink, rebuilding a social network, and assertiveness training.

Screening and Brief Intervention for Substance Misuse among Older Adults

The Brief Intervention and Treatment Project (BRITE) offers an effective approach to helping the older population with substance abuse problems (Schonfeld et al. 2010). The brief intervention consists of screening, followed by one to five sessions of motivational interviewing, advice, and education, and its effectiveness in reducing alcohol problems has been demonstrated in medical, aging services, and home settings (Blow and Barry 2000; Barry et al. 2007).

Medications

Medications have been an important component of substance abuse treatment, and most are well tolerated and effective with older adults. Methadone management has been practiced for years as an alternative to illicit drug use, and of the estimated 160,000 persons in the United States on methadone maintenance, 4–5 percent are age 55 or older (Firoz and Carlson 2004). Acomprosate, a glutaminergic drug that has been effective with younger patients, is under active investigation for efficacy in older patients (Zisserson and Oslin 2003; Boothby and Doering 2005). Naltrexone has also been shown to effectively reduce alcohol cravings (Streeton and Whelan 2001).

Persons who have dual diagnoses (i.e., a distinct diagnosed psychiatric condition in conjunction with the substance abuse) may need psychotropic medications. The clinician should prescribe appropriate medications (e.g., antidepressants, antipsychotic mood stabilizers), depending on the psychopathology, and should monitor patients carefully.

Family Involvement

Family members, who are critical support systems for the older abuser, should be involved in treatment strategies as appropriate and with the patient's permission (Dufour and Fuller 2003; DHHS 2004b). Family informants often provide critical information to assess the accuracy of patients' reports regarding their behavior, and family relationships may be causing the alcohol and substance abuse. Depending on the circumstances, family members may be educated to be allies to support the person in treatment, or they may be participants in family therapy with their relative. Family members may also be enablers, and clinical evaluation of their role is merited.

Case Management

Case management involves the organization of community, health, social, and mental health services on behalf of the patient (TIP 26, DHHS 1998). It is particularly valuable because older persons and their families may be frustrated trying to access the array of private and governmental agencies, services offered, and requirements to qualify for services. Case managers are experienced in facilitating and coordinating the appropriate mix of interventions, ranging from home-based care, supportive housing, and transportation, to legal assistance (Vanderplasschen et al. 2004).

Religiosity and Spirituality

Faith and religion may play a powerful role for many older people, and contacts with professionals in the religious community can be a valuable element of treatment success (Pardini et al. 2000). Religious and spiritual support may be effective not only for persons who have a history of religious attachment, beliefs, and practice, but may also provide comfort and hope for those with no prior religious affiliation.

Co-Occurring Substance Abuse and Mental Health Disorders

It is estimated that at least 10 million Americans have a dual diagnosis (i.e., a substance abuse disorder coupled with another mental health problem) and 2.8 million of these are age 65 or older (Kessler 2004; Buckley 2006). Older adults who have a dual diagnosis usually have low self-esteem; difficulties regulating thoughts, affect, and behaviors; and poor compliance with care plans (Natan et al. 2007).

The evaluation of co-morbid psychiatric symptoms and disorders is an important component of treatment. Depression, schizophrenia, and schizoaffective disorders should be considered as part of the differential diagnosis of older persons who have alcohol and drug abuse problems, and they should be treated expeditiously. The risk for suicide is high in these patients.

Psychotropic medications are usually needed for those who have dual diagnoses, and appropriate medications (e.g., antidepressants, antipsychotic mood stabilizers) should be prescribed, depending on the psychopathology, but the prescribing physician should monitor patients closely.

Principles of Managing Alcohol and Substance Abuse

1. Assessment of the presence and severity of possible alcohol and substance abuse should be part of the regular clinical examination of older patients.

2. Clinicians should tailor detoxification and treatments to the medical and sociocultural characteristics of individual patients, and patients must be closely monitored.

3. A wide range of treatment strategies, including psychotherapies, group therapies, family therapies, support groups, medications, and alternative strategies such as religion can be effective.

4. Medication management may include medications to reduce addictive craving as well as psychotropic drugs appropriate to the patient's psychiatric diagnoses.

5. Family members have roles as informants and allies in the treatment process, but they also should be evaluated to determine whether they are facilitating the substance abuse. Because patients' behaviors frequently alienate family members, education and re-establishing positive interactions become a critical component of therapy.

6. Case managers, other professionals in the aging network, and religious leaders may be valuable contributors to treatment and rehabilitation.

7. Therapeutic optimism is warranted if clinical resources are available and used appropriately.

14

Other Psychiatric Disorders and Behavioral Conditions

Relatively little research exists for several psychiatric and behavioral conditions in older adults: eating disorders, somatoform disorders, personality disorders, sleep disorders, and sexual disorders. This chapter reviews the clinical literature and emerging areas of knowledge likely to transform future practice patterns.

Eating Disorders

With the aging of the population, more middle-aged and older adults, primarily women, are being seen with eating disorders (Mangweth-Matzek et al. 2006; Lapid et al. 2010). These conditions are usually associated with adolescents and young adults, with a 10:1 female/male gender ratio (Pritts and Susman 2003). Older adults may seem to develop an eating disorder for the first time in later life, but most have been undiagnosed or misdiagnosed since adolescence and have grown older. This is not surprising, because an estimated 50 percent of young persons who have eating disorders are not diagnosed. A study of Canadian middle-aged and older women showed that high levels of stress, physical health problems, co-morbid mood and anxiety disorders, preoccupation with body image, and excessive dieting were associated with eating disorders, all known to be associated with eating disorders in younger people (Gadalla 2008).

A literature review of these disorders in older adults revealed that the average age was 69 years, with a range of 50 to 94 years, and 88 percent were women (Lapid et al. 2010). Co-existing psychiatric conditions, especially depression, occurred in 65 percent of cases. Treatment was successful in only 42 percent of cases, and the mortality rate was high (21 percent).

The following case illustrates some of the issues associated with later-life eating disorders.

RH, a 55-year-old university professor, had been obsessed with her weight since she was in her teens. A gifted child, she entered college at age 15, finished graduate school in three years, and became internationally recognized in economics. RH married and was devoted to her husband and three children. She maintained an active lifestyle, with a vigorous exercise regimen and a strict diet.

RH's husband joked about her strange eating habits, and her mother was upset that she prepared dinners for her family but only ate salads. When RH turned 54, her family noticed that her dieting had become extreme. They did not know she had become addicted to laxatives, which led to serious weight loss, and her 5 foot 2 inch frame gradually went from 118 to 80 pounds.

Only after RH was taken to the emergency room with chest pains was her eating disorder diagnosed. She did not have a heart attack, but the results of a careful history, an interview by a consulting psychiatrist, and a medical work-up revealed that RH had a long history of anorexia and had developed serious systemic complications.

RH rejected the diagnosis, refused to remain in the hospital for treatment, and would not discuss it with her husband or other family members. RH believed she was fine and insisted that 80 pounds was her ideal weight. If she were less than 80 when she weighed herself in the morning, she would eat, and if she were more than 80, she ate little or nothing. RH had another medical crisis several months later and was finally persuaded by her physician and family to enter a specialized inpatient program.

According to DSM-IV-TR, the hallmarks of eating disorders include refusal to maintain body weight at 85 percent of desirable body weight, fears of gaining weight or beliefs about being overweight in spite suboptimal weight, denial of the seriousness of the low-weight condition, and impaired self-image. The major eating disorders currently include anorexia nervosa, bulimia nervosa, and nonspecific eating disorder. There are two subtypes of anorexia: the restricted type, in which the patient has not engaged in binge eating and vomiting, and the binge-eating/purging type. Bulimia may also appear in two forms: the purging type, in which the individual induces vomiting and/or uses laxatives, diuretics, or enemas to compensate for binges, and the nonpurging type, which involves bingeing followed by fasting and/or continued exercise.

Epidemiology

Limited data exist about the prevalence and correlates of eating disorders, although it is estimated that more than 5 million people in the United States have an eating disorder (Becker et al. 1999). Lifetime prevalence estimates of anorexia nervosa, bulimia nervosa, and binge eating disorders from the 2001–2003 National Comorbidity Survey Replication are 0.9, 1.5, and 3.5 percent among women and 0.3, 0.5, and 2.0 percent among men (Hudson et al. 2007). The lifetime prevalence of these eating disorders in men and women in six European countries was 0.48 percent, 0.51 percent, and 1.72 percent, respectively (Preti et al. 2009). Eating disorders affect people of all socioeconomic classes and minority groups but appear to occur most often among Caucasians living in industrialized nations (Becker et al. 1999; Mehler and Andersen 2000). The prevalence in older persons is unknown. Most studies report average ages, and the few that report age ranges do not specify the proportion of older patients.

Etiology

Little is known about the etiologies of abnormal eating behaviors, but they are probably multifactorial (Jacobi et al. 2004; Dubnov and Berry 2006). Findings from twin studies for anorexia and bulimia are mixed, but there is some evidence for their cross-transmission in families, suggesting the possibility of a shared familial/genetic diathesis (Bulik et al. 1999; Strober et al. 2000). The social and cultural roles of food as well as influences on body image also likely are powerful influences on eating disorders in younger and older people (Peat et al. 2008). Younger individuals who participate in activities emphasizing the importance of being thin (e.g., modeling, certain sports) may be at risk for developing an eating disorder (Byrne and McLean 2001; Jacobi et al. 2004; Bonci et al. 2008).

Eating disorders should be considered serious illnesses with significant medical complications and a high mortality rate, usually due to heart attack or suicide (Keel et al. 2003; Hoek 2006; Crow et al. 2009). Malnutrition secondary to eating disturbances affects every organ system in the body, and although physical damage may be reversible, persistent malnutrition will have adverse effects in the body, especially the brain, and these may be permanent. People who have an eating disorder also have a higher prevalence of self-injurious behavior (Paul et al. 2002; D Stein et al. 2004). The crude mortality rate in anorexia nervosa for all causes of death in patients who have anorexia is 6 percent, and there is some evidence that the risk of death may be higher in older adults (Millar et al. 2005; Papadopoulos et al. 2009).

Diagnosis

Eating disorders do not have to be lifelong illnesses, but most individuals do not seek medical care, and those who do are often ambivalent about treatment and therefore difficult to treat (Steinhausen 2002; Geller et al. 2003). Although the DSM-IV-TR diagnostic criteria for anorexia and bulimia are different, both eating disorders are characterized by an impaired perception of body size and self-image. However, individuals who have significant symptoms but do not meet diagnostic criteria may need treatment as well.

The hallmark of anorexia is the refusal to

sustain a body weight at or above 85 percent of the standards defined by age-specific body mass index charts. Affected individuals are terrified of becoming overweight, and they restrict calories or exercise excessively to remain thin. Individuals who have bulimia have uncontrollable binge-eating episodes, which are typically followed by vomiting or the excessive use of laxatives, and persons diagnosed with the binge-eating/purging subtype of anorexia also manifest these behaviors. The weight range for patients who have bulimia ranges from underweight to overweight, in contrast to patients who have the binge-eating/purging type of anorexia, who are underweight.

A comprehensive interview, medical history, physical examination, nutritional assessment, and laboratory tests are essential for an accurate diagnosis (Lapid et al. 2010). The interview needs to include late life issues such as menopause, bereavement, major life stressors and losses, changes in eating and nutrition, financial security, marital conflict or divorce, and a history of sexual or physical abuse as possible contributors to abnormal eating habits.

There are no specific guidelines for geriatric practice, but the American Psychiatric Association has published general practice guidelines for eating disorders (APA 2002). The differential diagnosis needs to exclude medical conditions known to affect weight, such as Addison disease, cancer, chronic infections, diabetes, hyperthyroidism, immunodeficiency, and inflammatory bowel disease. Medically ill patients who have eating problems are usually concerned about their weight loss, in contrast to patients who have eating disorders, who have an altered perception of their body and want to be underweight despite being emaciated.

Psychiatric co-morbidities occur frequently. Major depressive disorder is the most common co-morbidity in people who have anorexia, with a lifetime risk of 80 percent (Devanand 2002). Anxiety disorders also occur frequently, and obsessive-compulsive disorder has a prevalence of 30 percent (Godart et al. 2003). The prevalence of substance abuse is estimated to range from 12–18 percent in people who have

anorexia and from 30–70 percent in people who have bulimia (Holderness et al. 2006). Personality disorders are also common, occurring in 21–97 percent of these patients (Sansone and Levitt 2006). Eating disorders and other eating disturbances are observed in older women and men who have chronic schizophrenia (Yum et al. 2009).

Management and Treatment

The American Psychiatric Association consensus guidelines for the management of patients who have eating disorders make only a brief reference to older patients (Yager et al. 2006). Regardless of age, patients need to be treated by a team of professionals, including a psychiatrist, an internist, a registered dietitian, a cognitive psychologist, and a family therapist (Robins and Chapman 2004; ADA 2006). The decision about outpatient versus inpatient treatment needs to be based on the severity of the weight loss and the patient's medical status. Careful monitoring of co-morbid psychiatric conditions is also necessary to help manage the patient's medical status. Nutritional interventions are essential during treatment, especially to avoid the risks of a heart attack in the "refeeding" stage as the patient's body shifts from metabolizing fat to carbohydrates. Cognitive psychotherapy teaches patients to restructure thoughts and behaviors around eating and self-care. Family therapy may enable spouses and other family members, who have often been detached or in denial about the seriousness of the disorders, to work through dependency issues and participate in the care plan.

The prognosis for successful treatment can be favorable for both anorexia and bulimia if patients are compliant, but improvement takes time. There is significant variability in patient outcome, with less than one-half recovering, about one-third showing improvement, and one-fifth remaining chronically ill (Steinhausen 2002). Unfortunately, empirical studies of treatment outcomes are limited (le Grange and Locke 2005).

A longstanding eating disorder often becomes an integral part of an individual's identity, and therapeutic interventions can be a destabilizing threat (Stein 2007). In contrast to people who have other psychiatric conditions and want relief from their symptoms, people who have eating disorders are often not motivated to give up their low weight and thinness. Not eating over many years has become a control mechanism, and therapy threatens to take away the only effective way the individual has managed the world around them for decades.

Unfortunately, most people of all ages do not seek treatment, and most health care professionals are not trained to recognize, diagnose, and treat them. With the urgent public health concerns about obesity and the simultaneous images of ultra-thin fashion models and media personalities, eating disturbances are set in a social context. Clinicians should be alert to patients who overuse dietary supplements and have repeated liposuction and cosmetic surgeries to maintain weight reduction and a youthful appearance.

Somatoform Disorders

Somatoform disorders are characterized by a syndrome of physical symptoms that in the aggregate suggest a medical disorder but cannot be explained by the existence of physical illness, substance abuse, or other psychiatric problems. However, the symptoms are so emotionally distressing that patients contact many medical providers in their search for relief (Leiknes et al. 2008). The overall prevalence is about 16 percent (De Waal et al. 2004).

DSM-IV-TR describes five somatoform disorders: (1) somatization disorder; (2) conversion disorder; (3) pain disorder; (4) hypochondriasis; and (5) body dysmorphic disorder. However, current diagnostic and treatment approaches are limited by the lack of research (Wigeratne et al. 2003; Janca 2005).

Somatization disorder is a chronic condition, has a prevalence of 1 to 5 percent, and is seen most commonly in older women (Yates 2010). Diagnosis requires that the person have an extensive history of numerous physical symptoms beginning at least by age 30, but with no objective medical disorders to account

for the symptoms. Patients must complain of symptoms in at least four categories: pain symptoms in at least four different locations, at least two gastrointestinal symptoms, at least one sexual symptom, and at least one neurologic symptom.

Undifferentiated somatoform disorder, a less severe form of somatization disorder, may occur more frequently than somatization disorder (Agronin 2004). The central feature is a complaint of one or more physical symptoms without objective findings that persist for six months. The presenting symptom(s) do not have to include the four categories identified for somatization disorder, but they must cause significant distress or functional impairment. The most common symptoms are chronic fatigue, loss of appetite, abdominal pain, and genitourinary symptoms.

Conversion disorders, which are more common in women, almost always develop during adolescence or early adulthood. They may occur at any age but are rare in older adults. Symptom onset is usually associated with a stressful life event, and the symptoms are the result of the patient's effort to resolve the distress. Symptoms usually mimic those associated with neurologic disorders, including impaired coordination, balance problems, weakness, limb paralysis, loss of sensation anywhere in the body, blindness, deafness, or swallowing problems.

Pain disorders are characterized by reports of pain in one or more parts of the body that are caused by psychological factors. They are relatively common in younger and middle-aged persons but are rare in older adults. Although psychogenic pain is common in many psychiatric disorders, acute or chronic pain is the principal complaint in pain disorders. Any part of the body may be affected, but the head, chest, abdomen, and back are the most common areas. Although underlying physical disorders may account for the location of the reported pain, the medical problem does not account for the severity and duration of reported pain or its disabling impact.

Hypochondriasis is characterized by a patient's preoccupation with fears or beliefs about having a serious disease. Although specific symptoms may vary over time, hypochondriacal concerns may persist for six months or more even when individuals have been assured that the medical examinations and tests are negative for pathology.

Several behavioral disturbances may occur as a result of the hypochondriasis: anxiety and agitation, sleep disturbances and fatigue, constant inspection of parts of the body, obsessive attention to and misinterpretation of bodily functions, ruminations about physical complaints, rigid exercise and diet patterns, avoidance of certain activities, and repeated medical consultations or requests for diagnostic tests. Patients frequently spend much of their daily life obsessing about their presumed illnesses.

Diagnosis

The differential diagnosis is usually difficult in older adults because of the mixture of symptoms (Wutzler 2007). Somatization disorder and undifferentiated somatoform disorder differ in the number, types, and severity of symptoms. Somatization disorder is characterized by complaints about multiple symptoms, whereas somatic pain disorder is focused on pain, usually in one location. Hypochondriasis is distinguished by a preoccupation with the underlying cause of the symptoms. In all these disorders, the individual's concerns are the presence of symptoms, not the occurrence of an underlying disease and its consequences.

Somatoform disorders must be distinguished from intentional attempts to appear physically ill that are observed in factitious disorders or malingering. In factitious disorders, which are extremely rare in older adults, the conscious motivation is to assume the sick role to obtain medical attention. In malingering, which is more common, external gain is experienced by rewards associated with remaining ill, such as financial gain or avoidance of responsibilities.

Medical disorders must be ruled out, and although extensive testing should be avoided, clinicians need to be aware that older patients presenting with a somatoform disorder may indeed have serious undiagnosed medical conditions. Depression in later life is often associated with somatic complaints, but it can be ruled out when other depressive symptoms are absent. People with a depressive disorder may become obsessed with beliefs about a serious illness, or the depression may be secondary to the hypochondiasis. Beliefs associated with hypochondriacal disorder are not as intense and should be distinguished from the somatic delusions that may occur in major depressive or schizophrenic disorders. Individuals who have been hypochondriacal for a long time may also have been misdiagnosed with a personality disorder as a result of expressed dissatisfaction and anger toward clinicians who would not take their problems seriously. The challenge lies in the fact that a disorder may exist, albeit not on the basis of the hypochondriacal symptoms.

Treatment

Treatment strategies for somatoform disorders are similar, and the goals are to improve the patient's quality of life and manage their use of medical services (Agronin 2004; Rabinowitz et al. 2006). These patients are a challenge, because medications and psychotherapies are generally not effective. The recommended approach is to maintain a supportive, directive relationship with patients, provide symptomatic relief, and protect them from unnecessary diagnostic or treatment procedures by working with their medical practitioners. Most randomized clinical trials have focused on somatization disorders where cognitive-behavioral therapy is the most effective treatment (Kroenke 2007).

After the diagnosis, patients should be monitored regularly with careful attention to their behavior. Appointments should be limited to 10 to 15 minutes, and patients should be informed about the time limit when treatment begins. It is important to end appointments on time, even when patients want to continue, and to limit the discussion of medical issues to the scheduled visit, discouraging telephone calls and e-mails. When patients identify prior medical encounters with other physicians, refocus them on their present concerns.

Although specific management strategies depend on an individual's particular problems, there are several general guidelines.

• Establish a trusting relationship and communicate support.
• Acknowledge the individual's distress.
• Explore the person's beliefs and fears about her or his health.
• Listen to the individual's specific complaints and present alternative explanations to her or his beliefs.
• Encourage individuals to develop new interests or activate previous ones to refocus attention away from their somatic concerns.

Cognitive behavioral approaches may successfully treat the patient's preoccupation with specific symptoms, body-checking behaviors, and misinterpretation of the seriousness of symptoms. Inspecting the body repeatedly may decrease anxiety for a short time, but the overall impact is to intensify the person's attention on the symptom and increase fears about what symptoms mean. After educating patients, instruct them to cease checking their body or seeking reassurance. Although this may increase anxiety for a short time, it may break the cycle. Finally, work out an agreement that individuals will not seek more medical care visits until some appropriate time in the future.

Patients who have somatoform disorders frequently refer themselves to many clinics and physicians in a pattern described as doctor-shopping, because they feel that their complaints are not being addressed. There is a danger, much like the "boy who cried wolf," that when a serious condition occurs, the voluminous patient chart will bias the clinician to ignore new symptoms and their underlying causes, possibly with fatal consequences. This is a serious dilemma.

Personality Disorders

Personality traits are patterns of perceiving, thinking, reacting, and relating that are relatively stable over time and in different situations. Individuals who have healthy personalities are able to cope with normative life stresses and form effective relationships with others within the cultural norms. Personality disorders occur when traits are so maladaptive that they interfere with affective stability and interpersonal functioning. The core hallmarks include maladaptive patterns of perceiving and responding to other people and stressful life circumstances as well as extreme emotional distress and / or social dysfunction.

Personality disorders are usually identified during adolescence or early adulthood. However, little is known about the course of illness of these disorders into later life or whether there are later-onset forms (Abrams and Bromberg 2006; Segal et al. 2006; Van Alphen et al. 2006; Zwieg et al. 2006). The prevalence of personality disorders ranges from 2.8 to 13 percent in older persons living in the community, from 5 to 33 percent in older outpatient populations, and from 7 to 62 percent in older inpatient populations (Van Alphen et al. 2006; Lenzenweger et al. 2007). A higher prevalence, approaching 60 percent, may be seen in long-term residential populations, reflecting an aggregation of vulnerable individuals who manifest symptoms of personality disorders as a result of poor adaptation to the stresses of long-term care environments.

Diagnosis

DSM-IV-TR recognizes ten personality disorders that are grouped into three hierarchical clusters referred to as A, B, and C as well as an eleventh condition referred to as a personality disorder not otherwise specified (i.e., does not fall under the three clusters). The cluster organization was intended to make personality disorders with similar symptoms easier to remember and does not reflect any theoretical framework or empirical evidence.

Cluster A: Cluster A, the odd / eccentric cluster, includes schizoid, paranoid, and schizotypal personality disorder (Parnas et al. 2005). Schizoid personalities are withdrawn, solitary, and emotionally distant from other people. Individuals who have paranoid personality disorder are untrusting and display inappropriate, angry outbursts because they believe other people are disloyal, patronizing, or dishonest. Schizotypal personalities have problems forming relationships and become extremely anxious and inappropriate in social situations. Individuals may be diagnosed with more than one cluster A disorder because of the overlapping symptom criteria.

Most empirical studies have focused on schizotypal personality disorder (Blashfield and Intoccia 2000), which has a symptomatic and genetic relationship to schizophrenia (Parnas et al. 2005). Schizotypy is not a distinct personality diagnosis in ICD-10, but it is recognized as a syndrome and listed after schizophrenia (Parnas et al. 2005). Paranoid personality disorder appears to be a component of the range of schizophrenic disorders. Schizoid personality disorder is seldom seen in clinical settings and does not have any apparent genetic association with schizophrenia.

According to DSM-IV-TR, cluster A disorders have an age of onset in adolescence or young adulthood, develop gradually, and are stable, although they may manifest with brief psychotic episodes. A small proportion of patients with schizotypal personality disorder will progress to develop schizophrenia or another psychotic disorder (Roach 2004). However, there are few empirical studies of the course of personality disorders (Parnas et al. 2005; Segal et al. 2006) The prevalence of the cluster A disorders in patient populations varies widely across clinical studies, a function of the nature of the populations studied and use of different methodologies (Abrams and Bromberg 2006).

Cluster B: Cluster B, the dramatic/erratic cluster, includes antisocial, borderline, histrionic, and narcissistic personality disorders (Maj et al. 2005; Segal et al. 2006). Borderline personalities are volatile and impulsive and do not form stable relationships; antisocial personalities show no regard for the needs and rights of other individuals and display a pattern of disruptive, delinquent, and criminal behavior; histrionic personalities are intensely emotional and display attention-seeking

behavior; and narcissistic personalities are characterized by grandiose, self-centered thinking and behaviors (Cloninger 2005; Ronninghamstam 2005; Stone 2005).

The prevalence of antisocial personality disorder varies from 30 to 80 percent in convicted felons, depending on the setting (Cloninger 2005). The lifetime prevalence, derived from epidemiological studies of the general population, is 3.3 percent in men and 0.9 percent in women, and prevalence decreases with increasing age. DSM-IV-TR emphasizes behavioral criteria to make the diagnosis and a history of recurrent disruptive behaviors beginning about age 15. The number and severity of antisocial behaviors in childhood predicts adult antisocial behaviors. By middle age, a significant proportion of those with antisocial behavior disorder either burn out (i.e., show a decrease in the number and severity of antisocial behaviors), are incarcerated or die, or develop a productive lifestyle and cease their criminal activity.

The literature on borderline personality disorder is more extensive than any of the other personality disorders (Stone 2005; Segal et al. 2006). The disorder has a prevalence of 2.5 percent in the general population. The phenomenology of borderline personality disorders varies across cultures and includes a heterogeneous constellation of nonspecific symptoms associated with a pattern of instability in self-identity, impaired interpersonal relationships, and significant impulsivity beginning at a young age. As a result, borderline personality disorder has the highest rate of co-morbidity with Axis I disorders and the other Axis II disorders in DSM-IV-TR. The heterogeneity of this disorder has been a serious barrier to studies of its course.

Histrionic personality disorders are characterized by a pervasive pattern of exaggerated emotionality and attention seeking (Stone 2005; Segal et al. 2006). The prevalence rates vary significantly, from 3–12 percent in the general population to 10–15 percent in clinical populations. Histrionic personality disorder frequently co-occurs with borderline personality disorder, and the rate of co-morbidity with

Axis I disorders and other Axis II disorders is also high.

Narcissistic personality disorder refers to a pattern of pathological grandiosity, self-aggrandizing reactions to criticism, difficulties with regulation of affect, and feelings of shame and low self-esteem (Ronningstam 2005; Segal et al. 2006). The severity of symptoms and the effects on functioning vary considerably, and the clinical presentation may vary across cultures. The prevalence in the general population is less than 1 percent and ranges from 1 to 20 percent in clinical populations. These disorders are usually diagnosed from adolescence to young adulthood, and although many individuals shed their symptoms as they grow older, narcissistic personality disorder may be exacerbated in middle age.

Cluster C: Cluster C, the anxious/inhibited cluster, includes avoidant, dependent, and obsessive-compulsive personality disorders (Costa et al. 2005; Tyrer 2005; Segal et al. 2006). Individuals manifest some form of anxiety that causes emotional distress and interferes with interpersonal encounters, including those with clinicians. Avoidant personalities are characterized by inhibition and inadequacy; dependent disorders are characterized by clinginess and submissiveness; and obsessive-compulsive personality disorders are characterized by rigidity and perfectionism.

The cluster C disorders are the least clearly defined of the three clusters, and symptoms overlap with depressive and anxiety Axis I disorders. There is consensus that symptoms of timidity, anxiousness, fearfulness, lack of confidence, and the persistent apprehension about the future coupled with help-seeking behavior are distinguishable from depression and anxiety disorders (Tyrer 2005). Most research has focused on avoidant personality disorder, and the few available epidemiological studies suggest that the prevalence of avoidant personality disorder is about 5 percent, and of dependent personality disorder, about 2.5 percent. Less is known about the prevalence of obsessive-compulsive personality disorders because of definitional and diagnostic problems (Costa

et al. 2005). There is some evidence that cluster C disorders become more prominent with advancing age, but this finding remains to be replicated (Segal et al. 2006).

DSM-IV-TR Diagnosis: The categorical organization of personality disorders in DSM-IV-TR is useful for clinical assessment and treatment. Each of the 10 personality disorders is defined by a range of seven to nine symptoms, and the diagnosis is made if an individual meets a cut-off score for the number of symptoms present to meet criteria for one or more personality disorders.

Despite the pragmatic usefulness of this categorical diagnostic framework, personality disorders may not be distinct diagnostic entities. The significant overlap of symptomatology and co-morbidity suggest that the classification system is not efficient or reliable, and existing assessment instruments are poorly conceptualized and operationalized. Furthermore, although personality disorders are considered lifelong patterns of traits, their stability may not be as enduring as conceptualized.

Personality disorders are assumed to be chronic conditions, and individuals who have these disorders may manifest maladaptive patterns of behavior and coping for the rest of their lives, although this is not always the case. Axis I psychiatric disorders may also develop with symptoms similar to those of a personality disorder, but these symptoms usually have a defined onset and improve with appropriate treatment. A change in personality from a previously adaptive level in older adults may indicate the onset of a dementia or other psychiatric disorders and medical conditions, particularly if there is no evidence of a major trauma precipitating the change.

Treatment

Treating individuals who have a personality disorder(s) is a long, difficult process, and treatment interventions are not well developed at this time. Personality traits take many years to develop, and as a result interventions to change them are difficult. At this time there are no medications for these disorders unless they co-exist with Axis I disorders (Maj et al. 2005).

Cluster A: There is little research about stability or treatment effects with cluster A disorders, because few individuals who have these disorders are seen in treatment settings (Parnas et al. 2005; Segal et al. 2006). It is widely believed that these individuals do not seek mental health treatment, but it is difficult to support or refute this conclusion. There are no evidence-based studies of treatment with psychotherapy. Treatment with appropriate psychotropic medication of patients who have cluster A disorders and co-occurring depression or bipolar disorder may lead to symptomatic relief (Maj et al. 2005). Symptomatic improvement may also be observed in younger persons who have schizotypal personality disorder, suggesting that type A disorders overlap with schizophrenic spectrum disorders. However, data on older patients have yet to be reported.

In the clinical setting, these patients are usually emotionally distant, interact in odd ways, manifest bizarre ideas about their illness, and are difficult to engage in treatment. Efforts of a clinician to inquire about personal issues are construed as intrusive and distance patients even more. The appropriate clinical management strategies are to respect the need for interpersonal distance by assuming a respectful, reserved professional manner and to communicate medical information clearly. When patients who have paranoid and schizotypal personality disorders exhibit distrust or strange ideas, it is essential not to directly challenge these ideas or become too involved in discussions about personal or psychosocial issues.

Cluster B: A larger literature exists for cluster B disorders (Agronin 2004). There are a wide range of effective treatments for antisocial behavioral personality disorders (Cloninger 2005; Stone 2005). Small treatment effects have been shown for structured behavioral interventions, moderate treatment effects with psychotherapy among more verbal individuals, and moderate effects with medications targeting specific symptoms (e.g., lithium for aggres-

siveness). Treatment approaches to borderline personality disorder are moderately successful. Dialectical behavioral therapy and psychodynamic therapies are equally effective in reducing suicidal behaviors within the first year of treatment, and SSRIs are effectual in the treatment of depression, anger, and impulsiveness.

There are no controlled studies of psychodynamic, cognitive-behavioral, or supportive interventions for the treatment of histrionic personality disorders (Stone 2005; Segal et al. 2006). The clinical approach should be characterized by a firm but fair interactive style, including limit-setting for acting out behaviors, emphasis on the importance of keeping appointments, and direct discussions about the meaning of emotional displays.

Cognitive-behavioral therapy, group and family therapy, and therapeutic milieu interventions have been effective with narcissistic personality disorder (Ronninghamstam 2005; Segal et al. 2006). The clinician faces challenging transference and countertransference issues because patients treat clinicians as an extension of themselves. The different countertransference concerns that emerge can help clinicians understand patients' thinking processes and develop treatment strategies. Short-term interventions should focus on setting goals and treating specific areas of functioning (e.g., alternatives to grandiose beliefs). Cognitive interventions, such as schema-focused therapy, identify narcissistic behaviors or schemas for treatment and focus on the individual's close relationships, vulnerable moods (e.g., emotional deprivation), and subjective experiences (e.g., feelings of superiority and need for approval). The clinician's goal is to help the patient identify and tolerate strong feelings and prevent him or her from shifting between different schemas.

Cluster C: There are no evidence-based therapeutic interventions for older adults (Segal et al. 2006). Pharmacologic treatment of co-existing anxiety disorders in cluster C has been reported to be successful in some patients, and cognitive-behavioral approaches have limited effectiveness. However, there are no clearly definitive approaches to manage this cluster of disorders (Costa et al. 2005; Tyrer 2005).

. . . .

Personality disorders remain an important but poorly understood group of conditions. The overlap of symptoms among the eleven disorders as well as the Axis I disorders can easily create a confusing clinical picture. Furthermore, the stability of a specific condition may be questionable. The virtual absence of data about the etiology, diagnosis, and treatment of personality disorders in the geriatric population represents an important research opportunity.

Sleep Disorders

Changes in sleep patterns occur naturally in later life, especially after age 75 (Ancoli-Israel 2009). Significant disturbances of sleep may be caused by pathologic anatomic conditions, psychosocial stressors, physical health problems, psychiatric disorders, medication side effects, bereavement, and circadian changes.

Alterations of sleep with advancing age include changes in sleep stages, time in bed, total sleep period, sleep efficiency, and other changes (Ancoli-Israel and Cooke 2005; Ancoli-Israel and Ayalon 2009). The amount of time spent in rapid eye movement sleep (REM), associated with dreaming and diminished muscle tone, is maintained until very late life, at which time there may be some decline. Marked changes occur in non-REM sleep. The duration of time spent in light sleep (i.e., stages 1 and 2) and the number of shifts into stage 1 sleep increase. Decrements occur in deep sleep stages (i.e., stages 3 and 4) with advancing age, and in those 90 years or older, they may disappear. Some studies have shown that older women have normal or increased stage 3 sleep in contrast to older men who have normal or reduced stage 3 sleep.

Older people spend more time in bed to get the equivalent amount of sleep obtained when they were younger, although some may show small decreases in total sleep time as well as increased nocturnal awakenings and daytime napping. There is considerable variability in sleep latency (i.e., time period from going to bed to onset of sleep), and this is attributed to factors such as physical discomfort, the need to urinate, pain, restless leg syndrome, dyspnea, a snoring partner, lack of exercise, and daytime naps.

Insomnia and Sleep Disorders

Symptoms of insomnia include difficulty falling asleep or staying asleep and early morning awakening, and they result in daytime tiredness, irritability, and impaired concentration (Buysse et al. 2005). Almost every medical disorder and many drugs can cause insomnia, which may be transient, short-term, or chronic. Transient insomnia, which usually lasts a few days, is often the result of an acute stress, changes in temporal rhythms, or environmental changes. Short-term insomnia, which usually lasts one to three weeks, can result from a significant ongoing stressful situation or the initiation/discontinuation of a medication. Adjustment sleep disorder is a sleep disturbance associated with acute stressful circumstances, conflicts, or environmental and life changes. Chronic insomnia, which lasts more than three weeks, is the result of chronic stress medical disorders, drugs, poor sleep behaviors, or primary sleep disorders. Chronic insomnia is associated with psychiatric disorders, most frequently depression, in 30 to 50 percent of people who have insomnia.

The schedules within hospitals and long-term care settings can make healthy sleep difficult. Nursing homes residents are usually required to retire based on organizational routines rather than individual preference. Hospitalized patients are often monitored throughout the night, and some patients find it difficult to resume sleep without hypnotic medication. Other factors affecting sleep include high levels of ambient noise, lack of privacy, uncomfortable beds, uncomfortable room temperatures, boredom and inactivity, lack of daytime exposure to light, excessive daytime napping, and bladder retention.

The prevalence of sleep disturbances and insomnia is high in the older populations (Ancoli-Israel 2009; Ancoli-Israel and Ayalon 2009; Pandi-Perumal et al. 2010). Older women are more likely to experience sleep disruptions than older men, and more than 50 percent of people 65 years or older living at home, and two-thirds of older people in long-term care facilities are estimated to have some form of sleep disturbance. At least 5 million older adults have severe disorders of sleep, and most of them do not receive treatment. Two primary sleep disorders that increase with advancing age, sleep apnea and periodic limb movements, not only impair quality of life but also are associated with increased mortality.

Sleep apnea, the momentary lack of breathing during sleep, occurs in three forms: obstructive sleep apnea, caused by occlusion of the upper airway; central sleep apnea, caused by a neurodegenerative disorder; or mixed obstructive/central sleep apnea (Ancoli-Israel 2007; Norman and Loredo 2008). Symptoms include waking up gasping, confusion and wandering in the night, and restless motor thrashing during sleep. The prevalence in healthy community-residing older adults is about 30 percent in men and 20 percent in women, in hospital patients 33 percent, and in nursing home residents who have dementia 42 percent. Sleep apneas may cause daytime drowsiness, systemic hypertension, cardiac arrhythmias, enlargement of the right ventricle (i.e., cor pulmonale, and sudden death).

Periodic limb movements in sleep or nocturnal myoclonus, is characterized by recurring leg jerks that only occur during sleep and awaken the individual, although most people are not aware of waking up (Cooke and Ancoli-Israel 2006). The incidence increases with age and occurs in up to 45 percent of older adults in the community. Sleep complaints are a function of the frequency and intensity of leg movements that usually manifest as unilateral or bilateral flexion of the big toe, rapid flexion of the ankle, partial flexion of the knee and hip, as well as some movement of the upper extremities. Movements last several seconds and usually occur throughout the night.

Two other parasomnias occur more frequently in older persons than younger persons, although their occurrence does not increase with advancing age: restless legs syndrome and REM sleep behavior disorder (Allen et al. 2003; Wolkove et al. 2007). Restless legs syndrome refers to a condition where individuals experience uncomfortable sensations described as an overwhelming need to move the legs (Clardy and Conner 2004). It usually occurs before bedtime or while the patient is lying in bed. Although the condition may abate with rubbing and moving the legs, symptoms reappear when the legs are motionless again. REM sleep behavior disorder, which is more common in older men than women, is a condition where patients experience vivid dreams and violent body movements during sleep that may cause injury (Schneck and Mahowald 2002).

Circadian rhythm sleep disorders, characterized by alterations in sleep and wake cycles, occur more frequently in older persons than younger persons (Ancoli-Israel and Ayalon 2009). The increased incidence suggests age-related loss of circadian control of sleeping. Older people also take longer to recover from circadian rhythm sleep disorders, which include jet-lag, delayed sleep phase syndrome (i.e., falling asleep and waking later than desired), advanced sleep phase syndrome (i.e., falling asleep and waking earlier than desired), non–24-hour syndrome (i.e., sleep-wake cycles that are shorter or longer than 24-hour cycles), and irregular sleep-wake patterns (i.e., erratic patterns of falling asleep and waking).

Sleep changes occur with Alzheimer disease and related dementias (Bliwise 2004; Comella 2008). Parkinson disease impairs the individual's ability to fall asleep and stay asleep, and levodopa may affect REM and deep sleep as well as cause nightmares. Alzheimer disease affects many brain areas that control sleep. Patients experience lower sleep efficiency and more awakenings, and they spend more sleep time in stage 1 sleep and less time in stage 3 and stage 4 NREM sleep than older persons who do not have dementia. Sleep problems become more evident and the percentage of REM sleep decreases as the dementia progresses.

Diagnosis and Treatment

A detailed clinical history, physical examination, medication review, psychiatric interview, and psychosocial interview are essential components of the differential diagnostic evaluation (Mai and Buysse 2009; Pandi-Perumal et al. 2010). The clinical history should include a thorough assessment of sleep behaviors, and it is desirable to interview the patient's spouse or partner, when available. The detailed sleep history should include the number of hours asleep, temporal pattern of going to bed and getting up, sleep latency, number of times awake during the night, comparability of sleep patterns during weekdays and weekends, napping patterns, daytime somnolence, use of bed for other activities, snoring or breathing problems, and kicking patterns as well as use of hypnotic medications, alcohol, and nicotine. Having patients keep a sleep diary for several weeks before the medical visit not only gives the clinician a valuable perspective about the individual's sleep patterns but also educates the patient about their sleep behaviors and patterns.

Consultation with an ear, nose, and throat specialist should be considered for individuals who snore or have other nasogastric problems. When insomnia cannot be explained or a patient is not responsive to treatment, or when sleep apnea, periodic limb movements in sleep, and other sleep disorders are suspected, individuals should be referred to a sleep center for a polysomnogram This procedure records night-time brain waves, eye movements, chin muscle tension, leg movements, heart rate, and blood oxygen saturation levels. A second option is to monitor the individual with a portable recorder to sleep with at night.

If sleep disturbances are secondary to a medical condition, the intervention strategy is to first treat the medical problem. However, if evaluations do not identify a significant cause of the sleep disturbance, the recommended approach is to educate the patient about sleep changes and sleep hygiene and engage them in a program of improved sleep behaviors, including:

- Going to bed and getting up at the same time
- Relaxing before bedtime
- Using the bed for only sleep and sex
- Maintaining a quiet, dark bedroom and a comfortable temperature
- Avoiding daytime naps, although a single nap may be restorative
- Exercising daily but not before bedtime
- Being in bright light daily, preferably outdoors
- Avoiding large meals before bedtime
- Eating snacks that promote sleep
- Avoiding alcohol, caffeine, and nicotine before bedtime
- Avoiding arguments before bedtime

Clinicians should prescribe sedative-hypnotic medications cautiously for older adults (Pandi-Parumal et al. 2010). Even the few medications recommended for older adults provide only brief relief of symptoms and should be used only for brief periods of time. Long-term use leads to tachyphylaxis (i.e., diminished drug response), resulting in persistent or increased sleep disturbances. Barbiturates, chlordiazepoxide, and meprobamate should not be prescribed, because they have serious side effects, significant interactions with other medications, high potential for abuse and dependence, dangerousness if the patient overdoses, and severe withdrawal reactions. Chloral hydrate is also not recommended because of its side effects, and antihistamines should not be used because they have strong drug-drug reactions and quickly lose effectiveness.

Certain benzodiazipines (e.g., temazepam, estazolam), may be the medications of choice for very short periods of time, except with patients who have sleep apnea, severe depression, and untreated alcohol or drug abuse, and the lowest effective dose should be used. Routine use should be limited to 2 to 4 weeks, and in circumstances in which longer-term use is indicated, the medication should not be taken more than 2 or 4 times/week. Benzodiazepines vary in half-life: short-acting (e.g., triazolam) and intermediate-acting (e.g., temazepam, estazolam) are less likely to cause daytime sedation than long-acting ones. Short-acting benzodiazepines have a decreased risk of drug-drug interaction but are more likely to result in rebound insomnia when discontinued. Undesirable side effects of triazolam include confusion and retrograde amnesia. Long-acting benzodiazepines (e.g., flurazepam, diazepam, chlordiazepoxide, quazepam) should not be used, because their effects will persist into the daytime hours and may alter cognitive functioning. In addition to adverse side effects, the long-acting benzodiazepines are associated with a high risk of falls and hip fractures.

Before treatment, the clinician should carefully evaluate individuals who have been using a sedative-hypnotic for long periods of time, because adverse sleep disturbances caused by the medication may be impossible to differentiate from the symptoms of insomnia. Patients should be monitored carefully for adverse effects as they are weaned off the medication, and they should be informed that withdrawal may cause sleep to worsen before it improves. Individuals who decline to withdraw from the sedative-hypnotic medication should be counseled about the negative consequences of continuing use, and they need to be supported in considering the initiation of short-term psychotherapy to help them withdraw.

Sexual Function and Dysfunction

There is a small and growing literature about the nature and frequency of sexual activity in the older population. A large-scale study of sexuality and health in older adults showed that many are sexually active, but the proportion declines with age, especially among women because of the lack of an available partner (Lindau et al. 2007). Sexuality and intimacy are important physical and emotional experiences for many older adults when they have an available partner and are in good health. Lack of sexual activity is not the consequence of aging (Laumann et al. 2008; DeLamater and Karraker 2009). This is true for all older people, regardless of their sexual orientation.

A sexual history and assessment of current sexual functioning and activities is an important component of a clinical evaluation, and clinicians should interview patients in a direct and respectful professional manner. The sexual history should address the individual's interest in sex, self-esteem, beliefs about attractiveness to others, past and present relationships, frequency of sexual thoughts and fantasies, frequency of masturbation, dyspareunia, erectile dysfunction, and ability to achieve an orgasm. The interview also gives clinicians the opportunity to discuss safe sex practices and sexually transmitted diseases. Sexual functioning should be evaluated within the context of sexual orientation and practices, physical and psychiatric disorders, use of medication, social networks, environmental circumstances, partner concerns, and frequency of sexual activity and satisfaction. All forms of sexual activity should be discussed, including intercourse, oral and anal sex, use of sex accessories, masturbation, touching and fondling, kissing, and holding.

Some older persons may be reluctant or refuse to discuss sexual issues because of embarrassment, anxiety, or fear of being rejected. Older adults may also be misinformed about healthy sexual behaviors or have false beliefs about sexual functioning and practices in later life. Still others may have chosen not to exercise their sexuality. Clinicians need to be nonjudgmental about sexuality and use verbal and nonverbal expressions of acceptance and reassurance to help older persons express their sexual needs or sexual problems. Clinicians should avoid expressing opinions about what are acceptable sexual behaviors.

Residents in long-term care facilities have sexual needs and problems as well. Those residents who are not cognitively impaired, are living apart from a spouse or partner, or are single and have formed an intimate relationship should have privacy and opportunities for a sexual relationship in the facility. The guiding ethical principles should be that no harm be done to either party and that the intimacy should enhance well-being. If residents have the capacity to understand, consent to and form a relationship, and express enjoyment with each other without coercion, they should be allowed to have sexual relationships. This may challenge the staff to carefully reconsider institutional policies, balancing the ethical rights of residents to independence and quality of life with protection from harm and abuse. Facilitating discussions with the administrative and nursing staff members as well as relatives most closely related to the resident may be helpful but also has the potential to create conflict.

About 25 percent of nursing home residents manifest several types of inappropriate sexual behavior: sexual talk that affects others; individual sexual acts (e.g., undressing, exposure of genitals, masturbation); touching staff; touching other residents (e.g., fondling, intercourse); and repeated requests for unnecessary genital care. Residents who have dementia or other psychiatric problems often display sexually assertive behaviors, but these behaviors can usually be resolved with comprehensive assessment and management strategies (chapter 9).

Testosterone levels diminish with age in men because the production and metabolic clearance of testosterone decreases, and this in turn causes decreased libido, muscle strength, energy, and well-being (Harman et al. 2001). Although lower testosterone influences the frequency of nocturnal erections, it does not affect erections stimulated by erotic stimuli. Older men show few signs or symptoms of testosterone deficiency in contrast to those seen in women at menopause.

Erectile dysfunction, an inability to develop and maintain an erection for adequate sexual intercourse in 50 percent or more attempts, may occur at any age for many different reasons, but persistent erectile dysfunction increases with age (Kupelian et al. 2006). The prevalence is greater than 50 percent among men 40 to 70 years of age and even higher in older men, especially those who have medical disorders. One or more of the following factors may cause erectile dysfunction: vascular, neurologic, and endocrine disorders; structural abnormalities of the penis; negative drug side effects; and psychiatric disorders.

Vascular disorders and diabetes are the most common cause of erectile dysfunction among older men, followed by medications, which cause about 25 percent of cases (Fazio and Brock 2004; Thompson et al. 2005; Wyllie 2005). The most common medications include certain antihypertensives, antipsychotics, antidepressants, lithium, hypnotics, estrogen, progesterone, and alcohol (Lowy 2006). Many drugs may also decrease libido, inhibit ejaculation, or delay/inhibit an orgasm (e.g., SSRIs), all reasons for men's failure to adhere to treatment. Discussion about side effects with the prescribing clinician often leads to adjunctive care using other medications or varying the timing of the SSRI. Unfortunately, many men are too embarrassed and will simply stop taking the medication. Clinicians need to ask specifically about changes in libido and sexual performance and reassure patients that these are common side effects that are usually manageable.

A number of neurological conditions and disorders may also contribute to erectile dysfunction, such as multiple sclerosis and strokes as well as peripheral and autonomic neuropathies (Lue 2000). The most common endocrine disorder affecting sexual functioning in older men is a syndrome called Androgen Deficiency in the Aging Male (ADAM), but other endocrine conditions, such as hypo- or hyperthyroidism or Cushing disease, may also have an effect. Although psychiatric disorders by themselves account for only 10 percent of cases of erectile dysfunction, psychological and medical factors are frequently contributing factors. Anxiety about a medical disorder frequently causes erectile dysfunction. Depression can cause erectile dysfunction, and, in turn, erectile dysfunction can worsen depression.

Clinicians need to explain that erectile dysfunction is common and that effective treatments are available. In private, patients should be asked if they would like to discuss the matter with or without their sexual partner present. It is valuable to have the partner's perspective and to understand how partners deal with the resumption of sexual function. Because many men would not otherwise seek medical attention, physicians and other clinicians can use this opportunity to also focus on the management of related disorders such as diabetes, hypertension, cardiovascular disease, high cholesterol, smoking, and alcohol abuse. Urologic consultation should also be considered.

The treatments for erectile dysfunction include several approaches, and the choice should be based on the individual's goals and preferences (Morales 2003). Sildenafil (Viagra), which was approved by the FDA in 1998, is effective in older men (Wagner et al. 2001; Marshall 2006). Two other medications have since been approved: vardenafil hydrochloride (Levitra) and tadalafil (Cialis) (Eardley and Cartledge 2002; Morley 2004). Vardenafil hydrochloride is effective in a smaller dose and works faster than sildenafil. Tadalafil stays active in the body for 24–36 hours, much longer than the other two drugs, which last 4–5 hours. These medications help cause an erection, but the individual must be sexually aroused and stimulated.

Rubber constriction rings may help men who are able to attain but not maintain an erection, because the ring decreases venous blood outflow at the base of the penis (Holmes 2000). Vacuum tumescent devices, which consist of a plastic cylinder placed over the penis and a pump, create a vacuum to draw blood into the penis, and after the erection occurs, a constriction ring is applied and the vacuum device is removed. Penile prostheses or implants may help when other treatment approaches are not successful. When psychological distress is prominent, ongoing support and encouragement may be helpful, and when affective disorders are causative and treated, sexual functioning will usually be restored (American Association of Clinical Endocrinologists 2003; Lowy 2006).

Little is known about sexual functioning in older women, but decreased libido and arousal, inhibited orgasm, and dyspareunia are the most common disorders (Hayes and Dennerstein 2005). It is likely that a combination of biological, emotional, social, and environmental factors mediate an older woman's sexual interest and/or responses (Dennerstein et al.

2001). Libido is dependent on testosterone in both women and men, and, in older women, changing levels of ovarian hormones and adrenal androgens in the years before menopause also contribute to reduced libido. Alcohol and certain medications, such as anticonvulsants, anticancer drugs, and SSRIs may affect libido. Incontinence also may decrease libido and inhibit arousal and the ability to achieve orgasm.

Sexual arousal disorder may occur during or after menopause as the result of decreasing estrogen levels that cause changes in vaginal lubrication and elasticity (Avis et al. 2009). Women who have frequent sexual intercourse sustain vaginal lubrication and tissue elasticity even without estrogen replacement therapy more than women who are not as sexually active. Women undergoing chemotherapy or pelvic surgery and using certain medications (e.g., anticholinergic or tricyclic antidepressants) that influence vaginal dryness may develop a sexual arousal disorder (Raina et al. 2008). The effects of vascular diseases on sexual functioning are not well understood, and although sildenafil may improve blood flow in the vagina, it does not necessarily improve sexual satisfaction (Alatas et al. 2004). Menopausal and post-menopausal women with vaginal dryness may benefit from oral or transdermal estrogen, water-soluble lubricants, or an intravaginal estrogen ring (Genazzani et al. 2007). Finally, erotic books and movies as well as vibrators and other sex objects may enhance arousal and sexual fulfillment.

Pain associated with intercourse or attempted intercourse occurs in about one-third of women age 65 or older who are active sexually (Hayes and Dennerstein 2005). Dyspareunia may be caused by many factors, including irritation and dryness of the vagina and external genitalia, vulvovaginitis, urethritis, anorectal disease, a retroverted or prolapsed uterus, lesions and scarring, as well as arthritis. Diagnosis depends on a thorough physical and pelvic examination, medical and sexual history, and an understanding of when dyspareunia occurs during sexual encounters.

Treatment is a function of the underlying cause. Because dyspareunia is frequently the result of atrophic vaginitis, the clinician should consider recommending a trial of topical estrogen or an estrogen ring if local lubrication does not suffice. Discussions about sexual practices and the effects of medical disorders on sexual functioning as well as education about modified sexual techniques may be helpful. Urologic consultation may be appropriate as part of the evaluation and management of this problem.

15

Family Caregiving

The family provides a complex multidimensional system that may support or disrupt healthy interactions between and among the generations. Family ties usually continue throughout a lifetime, and with increasing life expectancy, people are living longer and living longer together. Longevity has created new opportunities for family members to interact with each other and also has made family caregiving a normative experience in most societies.

Although family members usually accept responsibility for the care of older relatives, this may vary as a function of cultural influences and available resources. The demands of caregiving have been increasing as more people are living longer, technological advances allow families to provide complex care at home, the rates of dementias and unrecognized behavioral health problems increase in the older population, the burden of chronic illnesses grows in our communities, and health policy changes shift greater burden onto families. Changes in health care, such as shorter inpatient hospital stays and increased involvement of managed health care, have created fiscal advantages to governments and insurance companies but have increased financial and emotional pressures on family caregivers.

The increasing demand for home-based care caused by these trends has created an urgent public health and policy agenda for the twenty-first century (Tally and Crews 2007; CDC 2008). Spouses and adult children are the backbone of our country's systems of health care, and the more than 44 million adult caregivers provide $375 billion worth of unpaid services annually, twice the amount ($158 billion) spent on nursing home and home care service combined (Arno 2006; AARP 2007).

A growing body of literature has emerged recognizing the prevalence and impact of family caregiving by children under age 18 (Siskowski 2006; Becker 2007). Although it is considered appropriate for adults to assume unpaid family caring roles, children are not expected to assume substantial ongoing caregiving responsibilities. However, research in the United Kingdom and several other countries indicates several findings: children and adolescents provide considerable unpaid family caregiving; those who have extensive involvement experience adverse effects in their development, educational attainment, and emotional health; and national policies, programs, and services can be implemented to effectively support youth caregivers (Becker 2007).

In the United States, research on child caregivers is almost nonexistent. The only national survey indicated that 1.3–1.4 million children ages 8–18 have substantial caregiving responsibilities and may be at risk for emotional, social, and educational problems (NAC/UHF 2005). This is probably an underestimate. A 2004 U.S. survey of adult caregivers estimated that there were 22.9 million caregiving households in which 37 percent (8.5 million) also had children under age 18 years living at home (NAC/AARP 2004). The report did not provide data about the children and excluded families in which the primary caregiver was a youth.

Adult family caregivers are at high risk for depression, diminished immune competence, physical health problems, work/family disruptions, a deteriorating quality of life, and death (Schulz and Martire 2004; Feinberg et al. 2006). Families provide more than 80 percent of the needs of impaired relatives, and they need supports and services to maintain their health and caregiving responsibilities. Caregiver and family assessment and intervention are not only appropriate but also clinically indicated, for, as the saying goes, "When the caregiver goes, so goes the patient!"

This chapter reviews the challenges family caregivers face, the importance of clinician-family partnerships, the strengths and vulnerabilities of family caregivers and the family system, and the efficacy of caregiver interventions. Understanding the roles and impact of family caregiving is made more complicated by many changes in the nature of the family itself. Divorce rates are high, remarriage is common, and blended families with children from prior marriages and new marriage(s) have become more common in contrast to the nuclear family of previous generations.

Families as Informants

One of the most important resources for clinicians is a valid, reliable source of information about the older patient's history, current circumstances, medication use, and changes in health and behavior. Family members are arguably the best source when they have been involved in the patient's care and are relatively well informed about their relative's medical conditions, emotional, cognitive, functional, and social status.

Clinicians should cover several areas during informant interviews: the structure and dynamics of the family, the historical and present relationship of each informant with the patient, and their attitudes, beliefs, and emotional maturity. Family members are active interpreters during interviews, and they may distort the nature of the information they provide. Given the complexity of caregiver-care-recipient and family system relationships, the more the clinician understands about these interactions, the higher the likelihood of developing an effective care plan (Lingler et al. 2008).

Depressed family caregivers often overstate the patient's functional losses, and cultural values may influence whether family members deny or diminish the nature and severity of impairments in an older parent. Spouses may complain about the dependency of their part-

ner but deny specific incapacities because they are fearful of receiving a diagnosis that may be perceived as leading to the institutionalization. Adult children may become angry with an impaired parent and/or the caregiving parent because either or both have become a burden. Relatives who have a legal or financial agenda are not likely to be unbiased reporters. Thus, although informed family members are usually excellent sources of information, they are rarely unbiased, and the clinician must appreciate the magnitude of partiality and prejudice when interpreting the information obtained.

Clinicians face serious ethical barriers when the patient does not want family members interviewed or involved. This may occur when there are longstanding conflicts and estrangements within the family or the patient's psychiatric status interferes with insight and the importance of others helping them. This can be especially challenging when older parents/relatives and the involved family members are geographically distant and the clinician does not know the family members who are making contact, such as during a medical emergency.

Health Insurance Portability and Accountability Act (HIPAA) regulations protect a patient's privacy with regards to individually identifiable health information, and clinicians cannot provide health information without the express permission of the patient. However, there are circumstances in which family members perceive a risk of violence by the identified patient or caregiver and want to communicate with a clinician despite the patient's objections. Clinicians have a responsibility to listen to family members and evaluate the information without revealing medical data that would violate the patient's privacy.

Assessment of the Family

The clinician's role is to create a working partnership with families and guide them through the process of recognizing and dealing with the many challenges of caregiving. Clinicians need to assess what is going on in the family system and understand each member of the family. Beliefs that family members hold about illness, treatment, physicians, mental health, life, and death can interfere with their motivations and desire to cooperate with health care professionals. The elements to be assessed include:

- The degree of organization/disorganization of the family
- Family members' knowledge and sophistication about medical and psychological issues
- The disruption in the family caused by the patient's needs
- The degree of cooperation or conflict in the family
- The presence of medical problems in any family member
- The status of the marriage and the dynamics of the couple
- Racial and cultural beliefs and practices
- Recent crises
- The nature and severity of the patient's condition and how family members perceive her or him
- Reserve capacity and burden on very old caregivers
- Needs of children with caregiving responsibilities

Degree of Organization or Disorganization in the Family

Families have different ways of working together that affect caregiving styles and efficacy. Families characterized by effective collaborative and partnership inter-relationships may be more effective because they share the burden of caregiving responsibilities over time. Some families are tightly enmeshed, and although they work closely together, the family system may become overwhelmed by the ongoing stress of caring and be unable to function. Chaotic and poorly organized families are usually minimally effective if at all, unless there is a single family member who takes on the caregiving responsibilities.

Medical and Psychological Sophistication of Family Members

Educational attainment does not always correlate with the medical and psychological

sophistication of family members to deal with an older relative's health care. The strain of caregiving often interferes with understanding the nature and severity of a particular problem and making decisions even when family members are professionally accomplished. It is important to identify the educational level of different family members, and when there is significant disparity, to determine how this may affect the ways family members are involved in the patient's care.

Several other factors influence the ability of family members to deal with medical, psychological, and legal issues. These include personal biases, cultural beliefs and practices, religious or spiritual beliefs, and ethical/moral orientations. Health care discussions will be even more difficult when these factors are a source of family disagreement and conflict.

Older persons and family caregivers who are prejudiced against seeing physicians or using medications are difficult to engage in health care discussions. Likewise, persons who refuse to see mental health professionals, deny the necessity to be hospitalized for clinical care, or fail to consider the necessity of alternative housing or a nursing home require ongoing emotional support coupled with factual information about the clinical care plan.

Family Disruption Caused by the Patient's Needs

Caregiving disrupts the normal routines and rhythms of family life, and when several caregivers are involved, many families are affected. Furthermore, when caregiving continues over many years, the demands inevitably disrupt the dynamics of even the healthiest families whose members are coping with many instrumental, social, and emotional demands that change over time.

Clinicians need to help the family decide about the distribution of caregiving responsibilities assumed by family members such as:

- Providing direct assistance with personal care
- Supervising daily medical care and medication use

• Making appointments and transporting the patient
• Supervising diet, exercise, and other lifestyle needs
• Finding/interacting with home and community services
• Communicating with other family members

To minimize disruption, it may be necessary to help family caregivers redistribute caregiving responsibilities or hire home aides as circumstances change.

Understanding the Pattern of Conflict

Conflict is not unusual in any family, especially given the strains of caregiving. Even when families are successful in resolving disputes, seemingly insignificant personal beliefs and memories can fire disagreements among family caregivers: "Mom always liked you more; you stole my boyfriends; you went to college, while I had to stay home and work." Clinicians need to focus everyone on the needs of the patient and redirect caregivers from emotional antecedents that compromise problem solving. Clinicians should be aware of personal rescue fantasies to save the family and maintain the clinical focus on the best interests of the identified patient.

Resolution of conflicts may require family meetings to assess the basis for discord and determine how issues can be resolved in ways that maximize the well-being of the older patient without disrupting the entire family. Clinicians should not fall into the trap of siding with one person or faction within the family, but if family conferences are not effective and referrals are not possible, the focus should be on the best interests of the patient. When the patient has a legally empowered surrogate, that person's decisions must prevail.

Psychiatric or Physical Illness in Other Family Members

The presence of a mental or physical health condition in primary caregivers may compromise their ability to be effective, and the demands of caregiving may exacerbate a previous condition. Caregivers' health status needs to be evaluated and considered in care planning, especially when older caregivers deny their difficulties and insist on maintaining primary responsibilities.

When other family members are compromised by serious chronic illnesses and other disabling conditions, the drain on financial, physical, and emotional resources needs to be carefully evaluated. Clinicians have a valuable role to play in assessing the realistic needs of the patient and the resources as well as in dealing with the frustration, anger, and guilt of caregivers who need to revise their caregiving investments.

Status of the Marriage and Marital Dynamics

Marital functioning can be one of the earliest casualties of caregiving burden, even when the marriage has been a longstanding and fulfilling one. Caregiving dynamics are especially complicated by a late-life marriage. If the patient's children are resentful of a stepmother or stepfather or are concerned about the eventual disposition of the estate, they may play a disruptive role. These issues are becoming more frequent as the older population ages and the desire for companionship among widowed and single older persons leads to marriage or stable, intimate relationships outside of marriage. Unique problems arise among same-sex relationships and partnerships because unsupportive relatives may challenge the legal status of the partner.

Racial, Ethnic, and Cultural Beliefs and Practices

Race, ethnicity, and culture affect the knowledge family caregivers have about a particular disease or condition, coping styles, and willingness to seek help as well as the ability to access information and services. In the case of families that have emigrated from other countries (and cultures), distance from the dominant culture or acculturation to the new culture affects motivations and approaches to caregiving. When multiple generations differ in their cultural integration, intra-familial discord may occur. Clinicians, who often have an orientation to work more closely with younger or more culturally assimilated family members, need to be attentive to their professional role as family counselors in order not to further alienate generations and impair caregiving effectiveness. The goals are to be culturally competent, to maintain a focus on patients' needs, to be responsive to caregiver needs, and to support involvement of other family and social supports as well as to educate and refer families to culturally responsive community agencies.

Recent Traumatic Events in the Family

Family trauma changes the way family members allocate financial, emotional, and time resources and also changes the delicate equilibrium of family commitments. It may also compromise the primary caregiver's ability to provide for the patient's needs. Clinicians need to maintain professional contact for emotional support and help the primary caregiver and others to meet the patient's needs until the crisis is past and the family has reconstituted itself, at least to the extent possible. Recovery from severely disruptive circumstances (e.g., the off-time death of children) may take a long time. The clinician's responsibility is to refer the families to community and social resources to assist with basic necessities of life, make referrals when relocation occurs, and provide referrals to bereavement support services.

Family Members' Perceptions of the Patient

The patient's personality, family responsibilities, and accomplishments before the illness affect the way family members view the patient as well as the quality of care provided. The older person who was financially or personally successful may be seen as revered and beloved or may be resented for ignoring family members in pursuit of personal success. Thus, family members may vary in their motivation to provide care.

Clinicians who understand the perceptions of family members, including those who are not participating in caregiving, may help family members balance the needs of the patient with those of everyone else, facilitate discus-sions about the need for changes in roles and responsibilities as the illness progresses, and help individuals come to terms with negative affect and thoughts about the situation.

Age of Caregiver and Care Recipient

When caregivers or care recipients are in their 80s or older, clinicians may face special challenges helping them make decisions and implement care plans in ways that do not overwhelm them. Caregivers of advanced age may have health problems, and even if in good health, often have a decreased physical and emotional reserve that may make caregiving activities more taxing. Many aspects of daily life seem relatively easy to accomplish, but in the world of older caregivers, normal chores become overpowering and increase the level of caregiver stress to the extent that they cannot make decisions easily or provide the necessary care.

Older caregivers may be stressed by the technical aspects of caring. Medication management with multiple drugs of different dosages administered at different times throughout the day can be stressful, especially when both parties are taking medications. Making or changing appointments with physicians can be nerve-racking with the telephonic menu systems that make it virtually impossible to access a human being. When there are multiple physicians, keeping a calendar of doctor visits as well as other clinical appointments and therapeutic services can tax the most organized individual.

Stress models of caregiving refer to the phenomenon of caregiver captivity, because the needs of the care recipient during the rituals of daily life dominate the caregiver's schedule. Older spousal caregivers are especially vulnerable to fatigue, poor nutrition, disrupted sleep, and not having time for their own health and personal needs, all of which increase the risk of emotional and physical problems.

Clinicians can be helpful in many ways: being available, making time to listen and talk, giving praise for what the person is doing, assisting in the contact of referrals, talking with adult children and other informal caregivers, and helping the caregiver to take care of him- or herself. Clinicians also need to appreciate the essential supportive roles they play when older caregivers are making critical health care decisions about themselves or the care recipient as well as when arranging transitions to and from hospitals, rehabilitation, home care, and other care settings.

Needs of Youth Caregivers

Children under age 18 may be hidden caregivers, and some may assume a caregiving load similar to adults. It is important to identify and assess the nature and intensity of their effort, clarify whether they had a choice about being a caregiver, evaluate how they feel about what they are doing, and determine what resources are needed to help them at home or school. As the level of responsibilities increase, there is greater risk for physical injuries, depression and anxiety, fatigue, impaired school performance, and reduced time to enjoy being a child. If the demands are not overwhelming, children may also derive great satisfaction and develop a sense of pride and enhanced self-esteem from their involvement.

Phases of Family Caregiving

An assessment of family members and their interactions with the patient provides information about the adequacy of the patient's support system and a framework to help family members cope with successive changes (Cohen and Eisdorfer 1995), including the ability:

- To recognize and prioritize problems
- To overcome denial
- To manage emotion
- To build collaborative relationships with family and professionals
- To balance needs and resources
- To move on after the patient has died

Ability to Recognize and Prioritize Problems

Caregivers may be so overwhelmed by caregiving that defining and prioritizing problems is impaired. Many other factors also affect the ability to recognize problems: the caregiver's past relationship with the patient; the caregiver's worldview and attributions; the caregiver's knowledge about the patient's condition(s); the caregiver's fear of aging, illness, and death; and the way the family system operates (i.e., the beliefs and rules families use to deal with problems).

Ability to Overcome Denial

Denial of the nature and expected course of the patient's illness can serious impair effective caregiving. Denial is a natural response to upsetting, painful situations, and, in the short term, can be adaptive, giving individuals time to cope with unpleasant or difficult situations. If denial persists, however, it prevents caregivers from recognizing and dealing appropriately with a relative's care needs and may even harm the patient's health. Caregivers who experience serious, persistent denial are a challenge for clinicians who help them work through the denial, confront their deeper feelings, and begin to deal realistically with a painful situation.

Ability to Manage Emotions

Effective caregiving is emotional business under the best of circumstances. It is often characterized as a roller coaster, ranging from feelings of satisfaction and pride to anger, resentment, and frustration. Caregivers, especially those with a prior history of depression, may find themselves overwhelmed, and when negative emotions persist, they may be at high risk for clinical depression. Depression not only compromises the caregiver's ability to function but also usually has a direct impact on the care recipient. Clinicians should evaluate the caregiver's emotional functioning and intervene as necessary.

Some persons who view themselves as the patient's best caregiver assume total responsibility for the care recipient and may become defensive and resist alternative suggestions for the patient's care. These caregivers have made the care recipient their raison d'être and perceive any other individual's help as an intrusion and an insult to their integrity.

Ability to Build Collaborative Relationships

Successful caregiving involves maximizing the resources available to meet the patient's needs and support family caregivers. Collaborative partnerships with other family members, professionals, and religious and cultural groups as well as with community support groups are necessary to reduce caregiver isolation and the burden of care. Failure to build bridges across these networks increases the strain of caregiving and consequently the risks of negative health and psychosocial effects.

Ability to Balance Needs and Resources

Many challenges occur throughout the course of the caregiving, and all require a flexible, adaptive response to balance resources to respond effectively to changing circumstances. The central issue for the clinician is to evaluate the decision-making effectiveness of caregivers in the family and extended support system, even when family preferences and solutions are not congruent with the clinician's advice and recommendations.

Maintaining control in the face of numerous and changing challenges involves the effective use of a range of coping strategies and support from professional and community sources. Loss of control will inevitability compromise the most vulnerable member of the family—the care recipient.

Moving On and Letting Go

Neither institutional placement nor death provides a clear end of the caregiver's relationship with the patient. Caregivers may need assistance to review what they have done and recognize that they have done the best they can. Helping caregivers deal with their worries and consolidate the past will facilitate a journey into a healthy and productive future.

The availability of women to care for aging parents, which has been the traditional norm, is changing. With cultural shifts in the marketplace and their ascendancy in the workplace hierarchy, women have less time for roles as traditional homemakers, caregivers, and other family responsibilities, which may or may not

be shared with a spouse. With more women working, fewer married women, and fewer children per family, the available family support system for the baby boom generation and future generations will likely diminish. Unfortunately, clear solutions have yet to be developed to deal with the increasing challenges of family caregiving and the economic costs for society.

The Clinical Challenges of Caregiving

Health care professionals face complex clinical and ethical challenges in balancing the needs of patients and family caregivers. Because family members who are primary care providers are at heightened risk for physical and mental illnesses, clinicians have a crucial role in enhancing the family's continuing ability to provide care. Caregiving tests the resilience of even the most resourceful family members, who often become captives of their caregiving roles and responsibilities.

Depressive symptoms and disorders are the most common mental health consequence among family caregivers (Schulz and Martire 2004). Clinical depression interferes with personal, family, and social functioning, and if undetected and untreated, leads to personal suffering, decreased effectiveness, family disruption, abuse, neglect, death wishes, and occasionally to violence reaching extremes such as suicide, homicide, and homicide-suicide.

Caring for a family member who has Alzheimer disease or a related dementia has greater negative consequences than caring for a relative who has another chronic debilitating condition (Ory et al. 1999). Although the time for both caring for someone who has dementia and caring for someone who does not averages about five years, dementia caregivers are usually spouses, whereas other caregivers are usually adult children. Dementia caregivers spend significantly more hours per week in care activities, and a higher proportion provide 40 or more care hours a week. The negative impact in terms of work disruptions, mental and physical health problems, family conflict, and other problems is significantly greater for dementia caregivers. Twice as many dementia caregivers took early retirement, quit work or cut back hours, lost job benefits, and gave up promotions.

The risk factors that mediate caregiver depression include the following variables:

- Gender
- Relationship to the patient
- Racial group/ethnicity
- Cultural adaptation
- Patient's behavioral and emotional changes and ADL impairment
- Level of religiosity/spirituality
- Caregiver's coping style
- Family/psychosocial support
- Use of community services
- Caregiver's psychiatric history
- Alcohol misuse/abuse

The best predictor is gender. Currently, studies show that women are more likely to be adversely affected, but kinship has an interactive effect: wives are the most likely to have a diagnosable depression, followed by husbands, daughters and daughter-in-laws, and sons: 60 percent of wives, 40 percent of husbands, 33 percent of daughters and daughter-in-laws, 25 percent of sons, and 15 percent of other relative caregivers (Cohen et al. 1990). The lower prevalence of male depression may reflect their task-oriented caregiving style (Bookwala and Schulz 2000; Narumoto et al. 2008). Men are more likely to delegate responsibility, while women are more likely to use a nurturing role, with the likelihood that the patient's inevitable decline will have a greater emotional impact on them.

Racial, ethnic, and cultural factors also play an important mediating role, and the Alzheimer's Association has a Diversity Toolkit to help clinicians and other professionals work with diverse population (www.alz.org/professionals_and_researchers_11194.asp). The availability of an extended social family system among African Americans serves to diminish depression among daughters, whereas strong expectations of family involvement such as exist among Cuban Americans enhances the risk for depres-

sion in wives and daughters (Pinquart and Sorenson 2005). African American caregiving daughters reported less depression than Cuban American and Caucasian daughters, with Cuban American wives and daughters having the highest prevalence of depression (Eisdorfer et al. 2003; Mitrani et al. 2006).

The patient's emotional and psychological state and declining physical/emotional functioning can have a significant detrimental impact on caregivers' mental health (Covinsky et al. 2003; Nelson et al. 2008). In contrast, spirituality and religiosity have a positive impact on caregiver's well-being (Yeung and Chan 2007). Among African Americans, strong religious beliefs and affiliations are thought to be the most potent contribution to the low prevalence of depression in this population (Roff et al. 2004).

The level of instrumental and psychosocial support within the family, the existence of a strong marital relationship, the network of friends and intimates, as well as family support groups and community agencies, provide lifelines to caregivers who, even in the best of circumstances, are strained by the burdens of caregiving (Toseland et al. 2002; Chrisakis 2004; Mittelman et al. 2007). Among African Americans, fictive kin, persons who have no genetic relationship to the family but have strong emotional and social ties, are powerful forces to mitigate the risk for perceived isolation depression and other negative consequences. These lifelines maximize feelings of being connected to others and having access to supportive help, whereas a history of psychiatric problems, including alcohol misuse/abuse, in caregivers enhanced the risk of depression.

Although caring for relatives takes its toll, there are unique circumstances, pressures, and stresses associated with dementia caregiving (Ory et al. 1999; Yee and Schulz 2000). These include, but not limited to, watching the patient's progressive loss of self, living with the uncertainties of the rate of deterioration, managing behavioral problems, the constant vigilance to ensure safety, and the patient's changing dependency. Dealing with behavioral and psychological symptoms in the patient has a great impact on the caregiver's mental health. It is likely that other factors will affect family members in the future, with the introduction of new cognitive-acting drugs, earlier detection, genetic screening, and extended care as patients live longer.

Undetected and untreated depression in caregiving men, who feel helpless and hopeless, can be lethal, resulting in homicide-suicide or homicide/mercy killing (chapter 18). Most older homicide-suicides involve couples who have been married a long time, and men are almost always the perpetrator. At least half of the perpetrators have depression that has not been detected. A subset of older men retain strong beliefs about their roles and responsibilities, often are unwilling to seek or accept help, and are particularly prone to violence. Men do not have or use social networks the way older women do, and they become withdrawn and disconnected from others, despite the potential availability of family and friends. Depressive beliefs that there is nothing more they can do to make their spouse better, can lead to homicidal or homicidal-suicidal plans and actions.

Family Interventions
Forging a Working Partnership with Family Caregivers

Working with family members requires a commitment to accept and partner with family members in care planning. It is essential that clinicians recognize family caregivers for the social capital they bring to the working relationship and provide the information they need to improve their knowledge and skills during the many transitions in the caregiving journey. The United Hospital Fund of New York developed a unique resource website to integrate family members into health practice settings: www.nextstepincare.org. The website provides 16 family caregiver guides in English and Spanish to help with situations such as hospital admission and discharge, visits to the emergency room, medication management, and planning for post-hospital care. It also provides guidelines for health care professionals to communicate effectively with family members and evaluate their needs.

Types of Family Caregiver Interventions

Many different family caregiver interventions have been used with varying degrees of success (Schulz et al. 2002, 2005; Sorensen et al. 2002; Gitlin et al. 2003; Martire et al. 2004; Gallagher-Thompson and Coon 2007; Lopez et al. 2007; CA Thompson et al. 2007). No one approach has been shown to be consistently effective in reducing distress or enhancing emotional well-being in family members caring for individuals who have different chronic illnesses, although most studies have focused on dementia caregivers. There is an emerging literature examining differences in coping, resources, and outcomes in caregivers who have different ethnic and cultural backgrounds and different sexual orientations (Dilworth-Anderson and Gibson 2002; Coon 2003, 2007; Pinquart and Sorensen 2005; Yao and Gallagher-Thompson 2006; Borrayo et al. 2007).

The various categories of caregiving interventions include:

- Education and training
- Psychoeducational/skill-building programs
- Clinical therapeutic strategies for patients and/or caregivers
- Service system interventions
- Technology-based interventions
- Combinations of the above

Education and training approaches include information and referral, empathic listening and advice, community workshops and forums, lectures followed by discussions, and support groups. Psychoeducational interventions teach caregivers how to identify and prioritize problems as well as to adopt specific solution-focused strategies and skills. Skill-building approaches can target patients (e.g., social and cognitive skills training) and caregivers (e.g., stress management, behavioral management, and environmental management). Clinical interventions include individual counseling, psychotherapy, family counseling, family therapy, and dementia effectiveness therapies as well as service interventions (i.e., case coordination and management). Technology-based interventions include computer-enhanced telephones, videos, and robotic devices to enhance communication and interaction among everyone involved in caregiving.

Effectiveness of Interventions

Although all these approaches may be helpful, most research has focused on interventions based on psychological theories and stress models (Schultz and Martire 2004; Gallagher-Thompson and Coon 2007). A review of caregiver interventions from 1980 through 2006 indicates that three types of interventions are considered evidence-based: (1) psychoeducational/skill-building programs (Pinquart and Sorenson 2005); (2) psychotherapy/counseling (Gallagher-Thompson and Coon 2007; Lopez et al. 2007; Selwood et al. 2007; CA Thompson et al. 2007), and (3) multicomponent strategies (Eisdorfer et al. 2003; Gitlin et al. 2003; Mittleman et al. 2004, 2007). However, there is significant variation in the nature of the intervention and outcome measures used within each of these categories (Gatz 2007).

Psychoeducational and skill-building approaches are the most effective in reducing depressive symptoms, anxiety, and anger as well as improving adaptive coping skills, self-esteem, and effectiveness. Five intervention subtypes met evidence-based treatment criteria: (1) depression management, (2) behavior management, (3) anger management, (4) management programs targeting problem behaviors in the care recipient, and (5) multiple-component interventions. The largest average effect sizes were seen in studies using psychotherapeutic techniques, and the most effective therapy for reducing depression was cognitive-behavioral therapy (Gallagher-Thompson and Coon 2007).

Given the complex, ongoing challenges of caregiving, it is not surprising that programs using multiple approaches are currently the most effective caregiver interventions (Sorensen et al. 2002; Schulz et al. 2005; Gallagher-Thompson and Coon 2007). However, it is important to emphasize that no single "one size fits all" intervention or combination of interventions helps everyone. The selection of intervention(s) depends on many variables: the setting, caregiver characteristics and needs, presence of psychiatric and other medical condition(s) in caregiver, presenting problem(s) of care recipient or family member(s), caregiver's coping styles, and the severity of dementia or other health conditions in care recipients.

Diversity Considerations in Family Interventions

The results of two large multisite studies, Resources for Enhancing Alzheimer's Caregivers Health (REACH I and II), demonstrated the efficacy of interventions with a diverse group of caregivers (Steffen et al. 2008). REACH recruited sizeable numbers of black/African American and Hispanic/Latino caregivers in addition to Caucasian/Anglo caregivers (Schulz et al. 2003; Wisniewski et al. 2003). In the first REACH study, the minority focus at the Palo Alto, California, site was Mexican Americans, and the minority focus at the Miami, Florida, site was Cuban Americans. Both the psychoeducational intervention used in California and regular telephone support in Florida were effective in reducing depression and enhancing adaptive coping in Hispanic/Latino and Caucasian caregivers (Eisdorfer et al. 2003). The minority focus at the Birmingham, Alabama, and Philadelphia, Pennsylvania, sites were African Americans. The psychoeducational intervention used in Alabama (Burgio et al. 2001, 2003) and the occupational therapy home safety intervention in Pennsylvania were also effective with both minority and Caucasian/Anglo caregivers (Gitlin et al. 2003).

In the second REACH study, a single multicomponent intervention created from the most successful interventions used in the first study was tested in all sites. The intervention included teaching skills for stress management and problem behavior management, modifying negative thoughts about caregiving, and increasing daily pleasant activities. The racially and ethnically diverse caregivers in the treatment condition showed considerable improvement in quality of life compared to a control group. This was the case for Hispanic/Latino and Nonhispanic Caucasians regardless of kinship. In African American caregivers, spouses improved more than adult children and other relatives.

Interventions for Dementia Caregivers

Patient-oriented regimes (e.g., exercise, daily routine, music and dance activities, environmental modifications, and, when necessary, medication management) enhance patient well-being and reduce psychological and behavioral problems when implemented consistently over time. Recent studies using cognitive rehabilitation techniques with people who have dementia show some promise of improving some areas of cognitive and behavioral functioning, with the consequent effect of reducing caregiver burden (Spector et al. 2003; Loewenstein et al. 2004; Knapp et al. 2006; Logsdon et al. 2007; Logsdon 2008; Londos et al. 2008).

Since the 1990s, the Seattle Protocols (Teri et al. 2005a, 2005b, 2005c, 2008; Logsdon et al. 2006, 2007) have been developed as a systematic approach to train family caregivers in the community to improve the quality of life of their relatives who have dementia. This approach has been successfully applied to the treatment of depression, agitation, physical inactivity, and sleep disturbances (McCurry et al. 2004, 2005, 2006).

Interventions for Children and Adolescents

There is no intervention research focused on children under age 18, many of whom have a level of caregiving responsibilities similar to adults. The only youth caregiver intervention in the United States is a school-based program in several middle schools in Palm Beach County, Florida (Siskowski 2004, 2006).

Evidence-Based Caregiver Interventions Resource Center

The Rosalynn Carter Institute for Caregiving has developed an extensive program of online caregiver supports for professionals and caregivers, including evidence-based interventions (www.rosalynncarter.org/evidence_based_resources/). This resource center lists a brief description of each study and its outcome variables. The outcomes range from reduced anxiety, stress, and depression to reduced patient agitation and improved quality of life for caregivers. This is a valuable resource for keeping track of new interventions for family members.

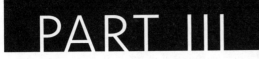

PART III

SPECIAL CLINICAL ISSUES

16

Assessing the Capacity of Older Persons

Clinical opinions about the capacity of older adults to function and legal determinations of competence disrupt the lives of patients and their families. Although true for people of all ages, especially those who have mental health problems, older adults are particularly likely to be evaluated for capacity (Lai and Karlawish 2007; Moye and Marson 2009). The concepts of capacity and competency embody complex value systems about liberty, personal choice, autonomy, and aging as well as clinical, ethical, and legal concerns (Moye and Marson 2009; Walaszek 2009). The process of determining whether a person will lose personal freedom because of criminal actions occurs within a legal framework, reflecting a specific society's laws and political culture. The legal decision to evaluate the competency of an older person often transcends the individual's wishes and control, even though the person has not committed any civil violations or criminal acts.

Competence is a legal construct, and the law acknowledges that many different competencies exist. The standards for competency to write a will are different from those for managing finances, living independently, making medical decisions, or standing trial. Moreover, many studies suggest that specific skills can be measured for different competencies. Appelbaum and Grisso (1998) identified four basic legal categories for the determination of competence, and each addresses different skills: (1) the ability to maintain and communicate stable choices; (2) the ability to comprehend information presented; (3) the ability to appreciate the consequences of a decision for the individual; and (4) the ability to manipulate information rationally.

When it is suggested that an individual has lost certain abilities and is so deficient in specific aspects of decision-making, independent functioning, and emotional control, a competency hearing is a legal mechanism intended to protect the individual and/or others. This is accomplished by imposing the responsibilities and authority of government to protect the safety of individuals and the greater society. Because legal definitions and standards of competence vary across governmental jurisdictions, it is important to know the relevant state statutes and federal regulations. Competency standards also vary according to the circumstances. The requirements to be competent to sign or change a will (i.e., testamentary capacity) are different from those to consent to medical procedures, manage financial affairs, consent to participation in research studies, or to stand trial.

Clinicians evaluate medical conditions and mental status to assess an individual's capacities—abilities and skills (ABA/APA 2008a). The evaluation typically involves a clinical interview of mental status and a capacity assessment test. It may also involve interviews with family members and other appropriate informants, neuropsychological testing, and sometimes a home visit. Results of the clinical evaluation of an individual's capacities are presented to a court. The court, in turn, considers the rights of the person while recognizing that certain impairments may render the individual unable to make reasoned decisions or function adequately according to criteria set by law. A decision about competence and a judgment to deprive or restrict freedom is not clinical; it is based on the law and judicial determination. The protection of personal freedom is counterbalanced by the need to protect the impaired individual and society from the faulty exercise of that freedom.

Individuals who have mental impairment, particularly older adults who are frail and dependent, are vulnerable to having their rights challenged. This is often exacerbated when there are moral and financial incentives influencing others who may wish to deprive an older individual of their ability to exercise independent judgments. This is also the case when an older person's decisions run contrary to the beliefs of others about what is in that individual's best interests. Such circumstances may include a decision to avoid surgery, invest in risky financial transactions, be a victim of economic scams, or marry a much younger person without a pre-nuptial agreement.

The specific capacity of older citizens who have dementia to vote in elections has become a major policy issue (Karlawish 2008). Some general guidelines have been established to allow healthcare professionals, family members, and long-term care staff to decide which individuals should be excluded or assisted in casting a ballot (Karlawish et al. 2004; Kohn 2007). A 2002 federal court decision specified the first clear criteria that are simple to administer and reliable—the DOE voting capacity standard (www.med.uscourts.gov/opinions/singal/2001/gzs_08092001_1-00cv206_doe_v_rowe.pdf). Individuals who have very mild to mild cognitive impairment were found to be capable of voting, whereas the capacity of those with moderate impairment was highly variable. Individuals who have severe impairment were determined not to have the capacity to vote (Appelbaum et al. 2005).

Significant ethical and legal issues remain to be analyzed, including the autonomy of persons who have dementia, integrity of the election process, and prevention of fraud (Wislowski and Cuellar 2006). Furthermore, methods to evaluate the capacity to vote, clarification of acceptable types of assistance, and development of policies for voting in long-term care facilities are important issues for modern society.

There are several excellent books and references in this area, including the classic edition *Evaluating Competencies,* by Grisso (2003), which reviews conceptual models, the state of the art of forensic mental health evaluations for legal competency, specific areas of legal

competency, and available forensic assessment instruments. The American Bar Association and the American Psychological Association have published three reports for the assessment of diminished capacity in older adults for psychologists, lawyers, and judges (ABA/APA 2008a, 2008b, 2008c). The Mental Capacity Act 2005 in the United Kingdom specifies a legal framework for evaluating capacity within the Code of Practice 2005 (Church and Watts 2007; Singhal et al. 2008).

Assumptions about Age and Competence

Legal standards exist for the special treatment and protection of children and adolescents under age 18 because it is assumed that they are vulnerable and require special attention. However, there is no scientific or legal basis to treat older adults any differently from younger adults. This may seem clinically irrelevant, but it is not. Ageism is a destructive influence that undermines the rights of older persons striving to maintain responsible roles in society. Widespread beliefs that advancing age inevitably leads to a general decline in the abilities to function independently are fueled by assumptions that older adults will inevitably become intellectually compromised and cognitively incompetent. Ageism also negatively affects the expectations of older persons themselves to participate actively in productive roles, and some may not even trust their judgment, relying on others and, on occasion, being unduly influenced or victimized.

A fundamental and flawed assumption in the evaluation of capacity is the unfounded belief that at some point all older persons will lose basic skills necessary for the exercise of acceptable judgment. Because some older persons are indeed likely to lose some capacities, the clinical examiner has to approach each evaluation as a neutral party (i.e., has no interest in the outcome) and with an open mind. The role of the examiner is to fairly assess an individual's capacities with regard to the circumstances and the requirements of the law. This chapter reviews the capacity to consent to medical care, capacity to consent to participation in research, testamentary capacity, substituted judgment associated with the need for guardianship or conservatorship, and competency to stand trial.

Measurement Issues

Several factors must be included in the evaluation of capacity, and if they are ignored, may lead to erroneous conclusions about individual's ability to function effectively. These variables include:

- The person's physical and mental state
- Medication effects
- The individual's attitude
- The setting of the examination
- The attitude and approach of the examiner

Older adults should be examined when they are functioning at their best. Sensory changes, if uncorrected, may significantly alter the outcome of an evaluation. Visual impairment can significantly degrade performance on many neuropsychological tests, leading to inaccurate test results. Hearing loss is common, particularly among men and women who experienced combat or who worked in noisy work settings, yet many older people choose not to wear hearing aids, forget to change batteries, or are too vain to admit that hearing loss is a problem. Not hearing a question carries a high probability that a person will not answer it correctly. Furthermore, hearing-impaired individuals, especially if they are socially isolated, are also at increased risk for exhibiting increased suspiciousness and will often give "I don't know" answers to extricate themselves from the "interrogation."

Physical illnesses and medications play a decided role in the assessment. Infections, heart disease, metabolic conditions, endocrine disorders, and other problems can impair cognitive status and performance, but the impairment is often reversible with proper treatment. Many medical conditions can cause discomfort or pain, such as arthritis, emphysema, impaired bladder control, as well as back, neck, and joint problems. An older person sitting

through a long examination in an uncomfortable room may become irritable, angry, hostile, and answer abruptly or incompletely, all of which could be misinterpreted by the examiner.

Medications can interfere with communication during the interview and compromise test performance. Psychotropic medications in particular can cause sedation, anxiety, or drug-related cognitive impairment. Older people also frequently self-medicate with alcohol, pain medications, or over-the-counter medications, any of which can have a pattern of side effects deleterious to the assessment process and outcome.

The attitude of the older person toward the examiner may influence response patterns, particularly if they are stressed or suspicious about the intent of the examination (e.g., "My children want to put me away"). Rather than risk being wrong, the older individual is likely to say nothing or shrug their shoulders. This pattern of errors of omission, particularly among older men, is often a sign of feeling stressed by the examination or just wanting the examination to be finished. Older people who have clinical depression or anxiety may be apathetic in responding and inhibiting responses to questions. They may also say, "I don't care," as a way to terminate the interaction as quickly as possible, without appreciating the consequences.

The physical setting in which the examination takes place has a potent affect on response patterns. Such basic issues as the lack of privacy, the presence of distracting interruptions, the impact of background noise on hearing, and the lack of adequate lighting can all serve to diminish the measured, as opposed to actual, capacity of the individual. When older adults are evaluated at home, family members or other caregivers should not be present in order to give the person freedom from interruptions by others.

Examiners need to work toward establishing a collaborative relationship with the patient. This process begins with the first meeting, in which the examiner explains the purpose of the interview and requests that the patient sign a consent form, so that, to the degree possible, the patient fully appreciates the importance of putting forth their best efforts during the evaluation.

The attitudes and biases of the examiner are likely to create a psychological environment that facilitates or impedes good interactions. An examiner who is rushed, gruff, not interested in the individual's responses, or unduly influenced by the family's presentation of circumstances may be more likely to lose objectivity. In medical settings, pressures from a surgeon or other physician for the patient to agree to be treated, despite protests from the patient, may precipitate an evaluation for capacity. In these situations the examiner must guard against pressure from colleagues or those above them in the medical hierarchy. The examiner's role is to assess capacity, not to prove competence or incompetence.

Capacity to Consent to Treatment

The criterion for capacity to consent to treatment is informed consent, and there are significant ethical, clinical, and legal issues, especially for individuals who have mental illness (Rao and Blake 2002; Roberts et al. 2002; Jeste et al. 2003b; Buchanan 2004; Appelbaum 2007). The three components to informed consent include information, decisional capacity, and voluntarism (Roberts 2003; Sugarman and Paasche-Orlow 2006). The patient/subject has the right to be given an explanation of the procedures involved, the rationale for the procedures, the risks and benefits and the likelihood of adverse reactions, alternatives to the proposed interventions/procedures, and choices available in the future. It needs to be established that the individual has the capacity to make decisions (i.e., is cognitively intact and can communicate, understand, and appreciate the procedures) and is aware of the consequences of accepting or deferring treatment on her or his health and well-being. A voluntary decision refers to the act of making an authentic choice without coercion due to illness-related, psychological, cultural, and contextual factors.

Patients may elect to refuse treatment, in which case the examiner has the responsibility to assess the rationality of this decision in the context of the patient's mood and judgment, medical status, and her or his explanation for refusal. Refusing medication or surgery to postpone death is not per se an indication of impaired decision-making capacity. A patient may choose palliative care in hospice rather than the prospect of extended terminal care. When clinical depression or severe cognitive impairment exists, the clinician may need to approach the patient's guardian or court-appointed guardian as a surrogate decision maker.

Although clinicians assess the medical decision-making capacity of patients during every encounter, there are at least four situations in which a careful assessment of capacity is merited (Tunzi 2001): (1) when the patient has a rapid change in mental status; (2) when the patient refuses to give consent and is unwilling or unable to give a rational explanation for her or his decision; (3) when the patient consents to a risky procedure in haste and does not seem to understand the risks and consequences; and (4) when the patient has a documented health condition that may impair decision-making. However, several issues need to be considered during the assessment process. Abrupt changes in mental status may be temporary and resolve with treatment. Patients may have reasons for refusing a treatment that may be uncovered after a probing discussion. Patients may also give a quick consent because they are content to follow what the physician has recommended. Finally, even patients who have psychiatric and neurologic conditions may have the capacity to make certain decisions about their care.

The evaluation should be carried out using a semistructured interview, a competency assessment measure, and appropriate ancillary tests to determine the patient's decision-making abilities and functional effectiveness and the potential for improvement (Appelbaum and Grisso 1998). The checklist below describes domains to be considered in determining an individual's capacity to participate in treatment:

- Patient is awake and alert
- Patient is able to communicate
- Patient relates to the interviewer appropriately and is able to have a conversation and focus on issues
- There is no evidence of delirium, psychosis, or depression that impairs judgment
- Patient understands the nature of her or his disorder/condition
- Patient understands what may happen without treatment
- Patient understands the treatment proposed as well as alternative treatments available
- Patient understands how the information presented applies to her or his situation
- Patient can incorporate the medical information and discuss the implications with regard to her or his values with regard to medical procedures and outcomes
- Patient can communicate choices clearly
- Patient appreciates her or his right to refuse treatment
- Patient makes a decision
- Patient's decision is not affected by mental state
- Patient's decision and reasons for the decision are stable over time

Assessment tests are useful adjuncts to a clinical interview (Dunn et al. 2006). The Aid to Capacity Evaluation (Etchells et al. 1999) and the MacArthur Competence Assessment Tool for Treatment (MacCAT-T; Grisso et al. 1997; Appelbaum and Grisso 1998) both use standardized questions and scoring systems to derive a more objective assessment of capacity than an interview. However, the abilities assessed are the same as those assessed in a clinical interview, and the scores need to be interpreted. The Aid to Capacity Evaluation is a brief clinical test that can be administered and scored in five to 10 minutes. The MacArthur Competence Assessment Tool for Treatment is a comprehensive measure designed for patients who have psychiatric or neurologic conditions in which capacity determination may be challenging. It examines four domains of capacity: (1) understanding of the disorder and treatment, including attendant risks and benefits; (2) appreciation of the disorder and appropriate treatment; (3) reasoning about decision-making, including comparison of alternatives; and (4) the ability to express a choice.

Capacity to Consent to Research

Institutional review board procedures for subject participation of all ages in clinical research have been closely scrutinized in recent years to examine the adequacy of informed consent processes (Yank and Rennie 2002). Empirical studies of advance directives for patients who have mental illness, involuntary hospitalization of persons who have mental illness, and the disease-related vulnerabilities of patients being treated for alcohol abuse, schizophrenia, or dementia have demonstrated the need to improve ethical safeguards (Carpenter et al. 2000; Dunn and Jeste 2001; Flory and Emanuel 2004; Dunn et al. 2006; Stocking et al. 2006).

When individuals who have Alzheimer disease or a related dementia are recruited for clinical drug trials, the patients' ability to give voluntary and informed consent must be established (Quereshi and Johri 2008; Vorm and Rikkert 2008; Mayo and Wallhagen 2009). When patients have moderate to advanced dementia, family members are often used as surrogate decision makers. However, family members do not have complete authority for decisions. They may make decisions consistent with a patient's interests, but neither family or court-appointed guardians can give permission for treatments that will not benefit the patient or those that the courts consider extraordinary (e.g., electroconvulsive therapy and sometimes psychotropic medication).

Geriatric professionals have usually sanctioned the practice of asking family members to give consent for research. The Ethics Committee of the American Geriatrics Society issued a statement that took the position that researchers should be able to access family members or appropriate surrogates who have intimate knowledge of the patient's wishes or value system (Sachs 2007). Appelbaum (2002) argued that this is acceptable practice when research projects are similar to current clinical care and when the risk is minimal. However, a great deal of research goes beyond standard care in many ways (e.g., choice of treatment, use of a placebo, examinations designed only for research purposes) (Mayo and Wallhagen 2009). Some states have limited the rights of surrogates to enroll incompetent persons in any study in which the person is unlikely to benefit personally (Appelbaum 2002).

Evaluating capacity will become even more important with increasing numbers of patients being detected and diagnosed earlier and the increasing number of intervention trials—drug, behavioral, and psychosocial. A number of scales are available, but the relationship between a performance score or profile of scores and consent-giving capacity has not been elucidated. The Mini-Mental State Examination is of limited value in establishing capacity in cognitively impaired patients (Kim and Caine 2002), and many investigators use independent expert panels to help screen research subjects. Clinician evaluations of capacities are fairly reliable, and the use of a structured interview to examine capacities increases the reliability of expert judgments (Kim et al. 2001). The MacArthur Competence Assessment Tool for Treatment appears useful for older patients who are not cognitively impaired but may have psychiatric symptoms (Appelbaum 2007).

Family members may be consulted to identify whether the treatment choices appear to be consistent with the patient's values and beliefs. Consultations are useful when there is evidence of impairment. After evaluating the patient, the clinician should document in the medical record that the patient's capacity was evaluated, tests used, and the basis of the determination.

Testamentary Capacity

Testamentary capacity refers to the ability of an individual to sign a legal instrument, such as a will or trust, disposing of personal assets and possessions after death (Gutheil 2007; Shul-

man et al. 2009). There are four widely used requirements, but they may vary in different state statutes. These tests operationally define the concept that the testator be "of sound mind" when the will is signed. The testator must be able to comprehend: (1) know that she or he is making a will; (2) know the nature and extent of the resources or the extent of the resources or "bounty" involved; (3) know the natural objects of her or his bounty; and (4) understand the consequences of the will as a legal document.

The first and last stipulations address the legal qualities of the instrument. Does the individual know that she or he (and her or his lawyer) are drafting and signing a legal instrument (i.e., the will) and how this disposes of the estate? The second prong requires that the person have a reasonable idea of the extent of her or his wealth, and the third requires that the person know her or his heirs. Although people with mental illness such as paranoia may not have the capacity to make a binding will, these criteria do not rely on diagnostic labels. Individuals diagnosed early in a dementing illness may be fully able to make a will.

Wills are usually challenged in the following circumstances:

- Significant money is involved
- An earlier will(s) is changed with different beneficiaries
- The amendments are perceived as detrimental to members of the family who expected to become beneficiaries
- An older person remarries or has a new partner to whom at least some members of the family object, particularly if this individual becomes a major beneficiary
- The older person shows, or family members perceive, evidence of mental problems or behavioral changes before signing the will, a change in patterns of spending money, or altered relationships with other family members
- The older person is believed to become unusually dependent on someone who is felt to be exerting undue influence, an issue discussed in chapter 17

- The testator refuses medical intervention or life-prolonging procedures, initiating questions of impaired judgment
- An unhappy beneficiary has a lawyer in the family

The existence of dementia or mental illness per se is not sufficient to assume lack of capacity or incompetence. In general, courts lean toward preserving the wishes of the testator, and the burden of proof lies with the party(ies) challenging the will. A diagnosis of dementia also does not necessarily mean that a person lacks testamentary capacity. It is inappropriate to assume that a patient who lacks capacity in one domain also lacks capacity in all areas. Many people with dementia are capable of knowing how much money they have and what they want to do with it as well as making other decisions about medical, legal, and personal issues (Shulman et al. 2007).

Conservatorship and Guardianship

Every state and territory has laws governing the assignment of a guardian or conservator for adults when they are considered to be unable to care for themselves and their assets. Guardianship refers to guardianship of a person, and the court appoints an agency or individual to be a substitute decision maker for all day-to-day activities (ABA/APA 2008c). Some states have two forms of guardianship: a guardianship of person for medical decision-making and a guardianship of property, essentially equivalent to a conservatorship. Conservatorship usually refers to guardianship of the estate only, and the court appoints a substitute decision maker for finances (Wilber et al. 2001).

Every aspect of a person's life can be evaluated to make a determination regarding the need for a guardianship, and if the older person is found to be legally incompetent, he or she will lose total control of personal choices about a residence, marriage, health care, voting, use of leisure time, driving, and decisions regarding assets. Guardianship and conservatorships can be valuable mechanisms to care for an impaired

individual, but they have also been criticized as compassionate ageism at best and as a legal mechanism for robbing older persons at worst. These mechanisms of substituted judgment are based on the principle of *parens patriae,* the protection of an individual by the state to help those unable to manage their affairs.

Legal decisions about the need for these mechanisms usually involve older persons who have severe psychiatric and neurological illnesses, alcohol or drug abuse problems, or persons who have grown old with developmental disabilities. Family members usually petition the court for guardianship when they are concerned about impaired relatives, but courts may also appoint a person who has a reputable guardianship practice. With the increasing number of older persons without close relatives available or willing to serve as guardians or conservators, many states have established guardianship commissions or expanded the responsibilities of state programs for adult protective services.

Guardianship is an important mechanism to protect the rights of older persons who have decisional impairments (Morgan 2007). However, it must be undertaken carefully, with protection of the individual's rights through due process, a clear standard to determine incapacity, and the availability of trained guardians. The courts also need to have the time and resources to monitor guardians. There have been many national studies and reports to develop recommendations for guardianship reform in order to develop the best systems to care for impaired individuals and still protect their rights for self-determination (Teaster et al. 2005, 2007). The website of the American Bar Association Commission on Law and Aging provides the most up-to-date information about guardianship jurisdiction, laws, and practice (http://new.abanet.org/aging/Pages/default.aspx).

Assessing Older Persons for Guardianship

Many states have replaced the concept of generalized legal incompetency, which implies a general loss of ability, with the concept of specific incompetency. This allows the legal option of limited guardianships for behavioral and functional limitations, medical care decisions, or living arrangements. The evaluation of capacities should not focus on advancing age and frailty, but rather on the number and severity of specific functional impairments under consideration.

Recommended guidelines for guardianship assessment include:

• Clarification of the reason for referral, including specific problems in question and appropriateness of guardianship vs. other alternatives
• Ability to understand consequences in order to make an informed consent
• Clinical interviews with the individual patient, family members, and professionals involved, including clarification of the patient's values, needs, and preferences as well as a psychiatric examination, if needed
• Cognitive evaluation
• Direct assessment of ADLs and IADLs
• Synthesis and communication of findings
• Evaluation follow-ups to determine the impact of the interventions, especially when limited third-party guardianships exist (e.g., medical decision-making, living arrangements)

An individual's functional effectiveness is the central issue in the legal determination of competence and the need for substituted judgment. However, state statutes vary in criteria for determining competency to make decisions about finances (managing assets and writing a will), health care (consenting to treatment and managing health care), independent living, transportation (continuing to drive) as well as other transactions, such as the ability to vote or marry. For example, California law requires judges to consider:

• Alertness and attention, including orientation to time and place
• Ability to process information, including the ability to remember and recognize others
• Integrity of thought processes, including the interference of presenting delusions and hallucinations
• Ability to control mood

Alternatives to Guardianship

Guardianship is based on an adversarial legal process laced with economic and emotional costs, and the process in the United States accentuates differences between the parties rather than a constructive dialogue to resolve differences. In reality, guardianship often involves conflicts among the parties petitioning for guardianship and the older person alleged to need a guardian. Longstanding sibling and other family rivalries may play out in guardianship proceedings, and after the guardian is appointed, family conflict may escalate, leading to even greater and more divisive economic and emotional turmoil.

Most petitions for guardianships are granted, and usually after brief hearings (Burress et al. 2000). As a consequence, advocates for the aged have been trying to implement alternatives that will provide greater involvement and protection of the older person, including appointment of special judges (Hurme and Wood 2002). There are at least two alternatives to guardianship. The first is mediation to help parties address problems and disagreements that precipitate guardianship petitions and discuss alternative solutions (Larsen and Thorpe 2006). The second is advance planning, using tools such as advance directive and durable power of attorney so that individuals decide who will make certain decisions for them well in advance of any challenges to their competence (Emanuel et al. 2000). Both of these alternative mechanisms are less restrictive of individual rights than guardianship (Butterwick et al. 2001; Whitton 2007–2008).

Mediation

Mediation is a discussion among parties conducted by a certified mediator that may occur before a guardianship is filed, while it is pending, or after a guardian has been appointed. The mediator does not make decisions but is trained to guide a process to facilitate understanding by clarifying issues, cultivating options for conflict resolution, and building consensus for a mutually acceptable solution.

There are many advantages to mediation. It is less formal and intimidating, provides the opportunity to move away from the legal issues to examine underlying dynamics driving the conflict, is confidential (unless abuse of an older person is uncovered), provides a forum to examine options, provides opportunities to agree on mutually acceptable solutions, minimizes polarization, and allows the older person to be an active participant in the process.

Mediation needs to be used judiciously. It does not deal with the legal issue of competency, which is the court's domain. Furthermore, mediation is not the preferred option in all guardianship cases, and not all cases need mediation. Cases most suitable for mediation are those involving domestic violence or substance abuse and when one or more parties are hostile, coercion of a vulnerable person is suspected, or the court needs an emergency decision.

Advance Planning/Advance Directives

Adults of all ages need to prepare for the possibility that another person may have to take over decision-making for them in the event of incapacitation. Without legal documents in place specifying wishes and decisions, guardianship is likely to be imposed if capacities are questioned. Advanced planning mechanisms include health care decision-making alternatives and property/financial management alternatives.

Advance directives for health care decision-making are legal documents that provide a way for persons to determine health care decisions in the event that she or he becomes incapacitated or unable to give informed consent. They include living wills and a durable power of attorney, but state statutes vary in technical requirements for these instruments. A living will is a written document by a competent individual specifying her or his wish about whether life-sustaining treatment will be withheld or withdrawn if the person is terminally ill. Some states also permit the inclusion of a persistent vegetative state in a living will. A durable power of attorney for health care, also referred to as a health care proxy health care agent, is a legal instrument whereby an individual appoints someone, not necessarily an attorney, to make health care decisions if and when the person is incapacitated. These advance directives are useful even if an individual has a guardian, because many states limit a guardian's ability to make certain medical decisions, including the decision to refuse life-prolonging treatment.

The Patient Self-Determination Act (PSDA), which was passed by Congress in 1990, was the first Federal legislation to address medical decision-making. The PSDA requires that all entities that receive Medicare and Medicaid funds—including hospitals, nursing homes, HMOs, home health care agencies, and hospices—inform all patients in writing, at the time of admission, of several rights: (1) to accept or refuse medical treatment, including surgery, even if refusal would result in death; and (2) to make or not make an advance directive for health care.

Health care providers must document whether a patient has an advance directive, but they cannot make admission contingent on executing one.

There are several alternative strategies to guardianship or conservatorship to deal with the diminished capacity to handle financial affairs, such as bill payor services, durable powers of attorney, trusts, and joint property arrangements. Powers of attorney do not remove any of the principal's power, and a competent principal can always revoke the power of attorney. The principal, who must be competent at the time, appoints a fiduciary agent and specifies exactly what that person can do. Jane Pollack presented the following story of her Aunt Molly Orshansky, in her February 2003 testimony before the U.S. Senate Special Committee on Aging (Pollack 2003; http://aging.senate.gov/hearing_detail .cfm?id=271872&).

Mollie Orshansky's saga is clear and convincing evidence that the rights of even the most accomplished and prepared persons can be abused. She was distinguished in economics and statistics and was best known for envisioning and creating the federal poverty line formula in 1963, which set national standards and empowered millions to obtain benefits for themselves and families. Over a 46-year career in public service Ms. Orshansky was sought out by congressional members and other politically influential figures for her advice, appeared regularly as a commentator on national media, and was the recipient of many prestigious awards.

Ms. Orshansky took steps to plan for her future if she ever became incapacitated. She named her niece as agent when she executed a health care proxy and established a trust in 1981 with all her assets and made her sister co-trustee. She also purchased a home in New York City to be close to her sister and other family members and would move when she felt it was time. However, even these well-crafted plans were to fail.

In 2000, the family noticed that Aunt Mollie was having some problems. She was not as well groomed, her apartment was no longer as clean, she lost mail, and she was not paying her bills. However, Aunt Molly refused to have anyone live with her or visit part-time, and she insisted it was not time to move to the new place she had bought.

The building manager contacted adult protective services because of his concerns about her appearance and confusion. The caseworker informed the family that she was bringing in home care services, but the caseworker did not inform the family when this did not work out. One day the caseworker took Aunt Mollie to the hospital in an ambulance against her will. The hospital began guardianship proceedings, even though both the hospital and caseworker were aware that she had several attentive family members.

When the family was finally notified, Ms. Pollack flew into Washington to present the health care proxy, and the rest of the family prepared her apartment in New York and arranged for full-time home care. When Ms. Pollack visited her aunt, she found her restrained in a geri-chair, heavily medicated, and disoriented. She was informed that her aunt had to be medicated and in four-point restraints because she was agitated and had

tried to elope from the premises. She was also told that the hospital was waiting for a nursing home opening for placement. Ms. Pollack's requests for her aunt's release were denied because of the guardianship hearings, which would not occur for seven weeks. Even after numerous meetings with the hospital administrator, Ms. Pollack, who had the legal authority to direct her aunt's care, was denied that right.

Over the next several weeks, Ms. Orshansky's mental and physical functioning deteriorated. She fell twice, developed a bedsore, had several urinary tract infections, was chronically malnourished and dehydrated, became incontinent, and was not able to stand or walk. In spite of the repeated refusal of the hospital to release her aunt, Ms. Pollack wheeled her out of the hospital at 6:00 pm on the night before Martin Luther King Day, and called the hospital after 10:00 to let them know where she was. The hospital was not even aware that she was gone.

Ms. Pollack retained attorneys in Washington, D.C., and New York, and her attorneys informed the D.C. court that they would begin guardianship hearings in New York to ensure Ms. Orshansky's well-being. However, the court-appointed D.C. attorney requested an emergency hearing and persuaded the judge to change his role from temporary guardian to Ms. Orshansky's attorney because there was a large account in a brokerage firm. The judge voided Ms. Pollack's health care proxy, froze Ms. Orshansky's accounts, and ordered the attorney to contact New York City police to have Ms. Orshansky returned to Washington, D.C. Ms. Pollack and the family were successful in getting the New York court to issue an order to prohibit Aunt Mollie's removal from their jurisdiction.

Ms. Pollack testified at a hearing in D.C., but she lost her counter-bid for guardianship. The temporary guardian, a stranger, was appointed as her permanent guardian and given control of her trust. Aunt Mollie's guardian, not her court-appointed attorney, represented her, and her attorney never spoke with Ms. Orshansky before the hearing, never advised her of the results, and never told her she could appeal.

The guardian diverted money from Ms. Or-shansky's trust and called the family repeatedly to harass them. Because of the dedicated involvement and ability of the family, the case was appealed. The Washington Appeals Court vacated the decisions of the lower court because of abuse of discretion.

Health Care Decision-Making for Unbefriended Elderly People

A 2002–2003 study by the American Bar Association Commission on Law and Aging (Karp and Wood 2003) described the following three criteria to define the unbefriended older patient:

1. The patient lacks decisional capacity to give informed consent for a specific treatment.
2. The patient does not have advance directives specifying wishes for the treatment at hand and does not have the capacity to do so.
3. The patient does not have a legally recognized surrogate decision maker and does not have family who can participate in the decision-making process.

Although these criteria may also apply to developmentally challenged and mentally retarded younger persons, this discussion focuses on older persons.

There are no data regarding the exact number of unbefriended older persons, given differing definitions and ascertainment difficulties, but it is estimated that 3–4 percent of nursing home residents, about 60,000 persons, are is this category (Karp and Wood 2003). Other scholars have used a broader definition of the unbefriended to include long-term care residents who may or may not have decisional capacity, but who have no responsible party named in the medical record, whose listed relative cannot be contacted or will not be involved in the resident's care, or who have not had a visitor in the past two years (Mathes et al. 2004; Meisel and Jennings 2005). As many as 30 percent of residents are isolated and unbefriended using these parameters.

Types of Health Care Decision

Older unbefriended patients have usually been isolated much of their lives and have fallen through the cracks of the social and health care systems. Most encounters occur in hospitals and nursing homes where these persons have major medical crises requiring immediate and difficult decisions. However, health care decisions include three other areas: emergency care, routine medical care, and end-of-life care.

Health care providers are able to treat unbefriended persons in emergencies and routine care. The consent for emergency treatment is implied under common law (i.e., the law assumes that a reasonable person would want medical care in an emergency). However, the definition of an emergency varies across states and is defined by state statutes in some instances. Consent for routine care is usually not required. Routine care refers to low-risk procedures and treatments that are widely accepted standards of care. For example, consent would be assumed, unless the patient objects, for noninvasive procedures such as taking a pulse, blood pressure monitoring, using a stethoscope, taking a temperature with a thermometer, or blood draws. Signature consent is required for HIV testing and other tests and procedures.

Major medical and dental care as well as end-of-life care are more problematic. Major medical care refers to any treatment that is associated with significant risk, pain, and/or invasive interventions. Examples include surgery, dialysis, chemotherapy, radiation treatments, and the administration of powerful drugs, such as psychotropics. End-of-life care decisions include many issues, including, but not limited to, resuscitation, use of a ventilator or feeding tube, artificial nutrition and hydration, use of antibiotics, and hospitalization for aggressive treatments.

Who Makes the Decisions and How

Making decisions for unbefriended patients is complicated because, by definition, they do not have a surrogate to make decisions for them. In some instances, it is possible to locate family and friends with significant effort, but frequently there is little time or the search is not successful. The crucial question then becomes, who should make the decisions? An American Bar Association report (Karp and Wood 2003) described the array of decision makers to include:

- Physicians, treating and consulting
- Judges
- Social workers
- Clergy, broadly defined
- Operators or employees of a long-term care facility
- Adult protective service (APS) professionals
- Ethics committees or ethics consultation teams in hospitals and long-term care facilities
- Regional ethics committees
- Guardians, public and private

Legislative Mechanisms

Karp and Wood (2003) identified four existing governmental mechanisms for surrogate decision-making on behalf of unbefriended persons:

1. At least ten states have statutes designating one or more decision makers (i.e., statutory consent of last resort). Most statutes specify the primary treating physician or the attending physician, in consultation with an ethics committee or independent consulting physician.

2. At least three states have laws empowering external professional committees to make health care decisions.

3. Many states as well as local jurisdictions have created public guardianship programs, but staffing and funding are often inadequate to meet the need. There are several models for public guardianships: an independent state agency, a state agency providing social services, contracts to private sector programs, and a state agency not providing social services (e.g., attorney general) (Schmidt et al. 1982; Teaster et al. 2007).

4. At least seven states have statutes enacting a judicial process to authorize treatment decisions. Health care providers, adult protective services professionals, or other interested parties may file a petition with the court to be granted decision-making authority or petition the court to make a treatment decision.

Institutional Mechanisms

Health care professionals and health care systems in states without specific laws face difficult choices in the process of surrogate decision-making in the absence of advance directives. Karp and Wood (2003) described three general strategies used by institutions when state law did not identify alternatives other than a guardianship:

1. Ethics committees in hospitals and long-term care facilities frequently review past cases, formulate policies, and act as advocates for patients, clinical consultants, or surrogate health care decision makers. The Joint Commission on Accreditation for Health Care Organizations has required approved member organizations to have a means to deal with ethical issues since 1992.

2. An informal surrogate system, developed at the Hebrew Rehabilitation Center in Boston, operates under the auspices of the in-house ethics committee. The Center cultivates an environment of close resident/staff/family relationships, such that when a social worker identifies a resident without a family member or proxy, the chair of the ethics committee appoints a committee member to be the informal surrogate for decisions in the nursing home.

3. In states where statutes for health care decision-making are lacking and the guardianship system is overtaxed, health care institutions and physicians may implement their own best practices, referred to as "flying below the radar screen." This reference does not imply that the practices are illegal, but rather that the practices may not be clearly specified by that state's laws. Examples include hospital administrative consent by the administrator or medical director, nursing home administrative consent for acute care, and physicians as "ad hoc guardians" (i.e., who do what is best ethically and medically at the moment of a critical medical decision).

Competence to Stand Trial

The concept of competence to stand trial recognizes that there are mental health conditions that may interfere with the right of a defendant to a fair trial. State statutes vary in the specificity of factors to be considered for competency evaluations and judicial decisions. For example, according to the rules of the State of Florida (Rule 3.210), "A person accused of an offense or a violation of probation or community control who is mentally incompetent to proceed at any material stage of a criminal proceeding shall not be proceeded against while incompetent." Florida law requires that the defendant meet the following six criteria:

1. Appreciate the allegations and charges
2. Appreciate the range and nature of possible penalties that may be imposed (e.g., length of prison sentence, definition of probation)
3. Understand the adversarial nature of the legal process (e.g., describe the role of the judge as well as the prosecuting and defense attorneys)
4. Cooperate with counsel and disclose information pertinent to the case
5. Behave appropriately in the courtroom
6. Testify in a relevant manner, based on cognitive and emotional functioning

Some states have a requirement that the defendant's impairments must be attributed to a mental condition or defect. However, the presence of mental illness per se is not sufficient for a court to find someone incompetent to stand trial.

If experts evaluating the defendant determine that a person is incompetent to proceed, the experts are required to report any treatment recommendations for the defendant to become competent. The experts are to report on several issues:

- The mental illness causing the incompetence
- Appropriate treatments
- The availability of acceptable treatment
- The likelihood of the defendant's becoming competent after the recommended treatment,

an assessment of the probable duration of treatment, and the probability that the defendant will become competent to proceed in the near future

Restoration to competence from successful mental health care involves the defendant's understanding of charges, the possible consequences of the charges, and ability to work with counsel. Restoration to competence does not deal with the defendant's guilt/innocence or sanity/insanity at the time of the offence.

TY, a 64-year-old divorced male with a seventh-grade education, shot his 64-year-old terminally ill ex-wife outside her oncologist's office. TY remained with her body, admitted his guilt to the detective who arrested him, and was charged with first-degree murder. Pursuant to a court order, two mental health professionals evaluated the defendant to address the issue of insanity at the time of the alleged offense. Subsequently, because of TY's outbursts and unusual behavior in the courtroom, the judge issued an order to evaluate his competency to proceed.

The two examiners interviewed the defendant, reviewed a videotape of the initial interrogation after the alleged offense, interviewed the defendant's relatives and a close friend, reviewed law enforcement investigative reports and statements of witnesses, and also reviewed medical examiner reports. Both examiners were of the opinion that the defendant was incompetent to stand trial as a result of mental illness (i.e., Major Depressive Disorder with Psychosis). TY was deemed to be potentially dangerous to himself and others, and he met criteria to be placed in a forensic hospital for treatment.

At the time of the competency examination, the defendant did not possess a rational or factual appreciation of the legal proceedings against him, and he did not have the ability to consult with his attorneys. TY understood that he was charged with shooting his ex-wife. However, he did not understand the seriousness of the charges, and he believed the justice system was over-reacting. His ex-wife had been terminally ill and in great pain, and he believed that she wanted to die, which in his mind, justified

killing her. After his confession to the police, TY assumed that he would be allowed to return home.

TY was paranoid about his counsel and believed that they were in collusion with the judge and not working on his behalf. He was abusive to his attorneys for not filing the appropriate papers to get him released from jail, and he believed that their incompetence was the reason he remained in jail. TY did not believe that he was being treated fairly by the legal system, and at the same time believed that he would be found not guilty. His ability to work with his attorneys and testify in a relevant manner were significantly compromised by his agitation and paranoia, his rambling speech and disjointed thought process, and his beliefs that he was not being treated fairly. During a bail bond court hearing, TY yelled at his attorney and attempted to approach the bench inappropriately. This lack of impulse control would likely occur again if he appeared in court.

TY would answer questions with fragmented speech and frequently wandered to different topics. He described visitations from God, Jesus, the Virgin Mary, the devil, and his ex-wife, where he saw them, heard their voices, and spoke with them. TY believed that he had a particularly close relationship with the Virgin Mary and that she gave him specific medical advice.

At the state forensic hospital TY was again diagnosed with psychotic disorder, not otherwise specified, and probable major depressive disorder, and he was given antipsychotic and antidepressant medications. After a week, TY refused to take these or any other medications.

The state psychologist reported that he had little insight, was paranoid and delusional, emotionally labile, and was coping poorly with the stress of incarceration.

After finally being successfully treated in the forensic hospital, TY was returned to the local jail. The court appointed two mental health professionals to evaluate TY, and the court found him competent to proceed. At that time, the state and TY's defense attorneys reached a plea bargain. TY pled guilty to second-degree manslaughter and was sentenced to 18 months in prison (with credit for jail time) and 5 years' probation.

Autonomy, Risk for Harm, and Capacity

Western cultures have always favored legal and ethical preferences for personal autonomy in the face of beneficent interventions by others (Beauchamp and Childress 2008). Adults, old and young, are presumed to be capable of making decisions, even if another person has different beliefs. Any action to limit a person's autonomy requires convincing evidence that an individual is so impaired in specific areas that serious and irreparable harm will result. Because harm is a difficult concept to define and varies among persons, tasks, and circumstances, an individual's capacities need to be evaluated for specific tasks, requiring specific decisions, with specific risks and benefits, and using a semistructured clinical interview, a competency assessment tool, and sometimes neuropsychological testing.

17

Elder Abuse

Elder mistreatment is now well recognized as a serious global public health challenge (Bonnie and Wallace 2002; WHO 2002; Lachs and Pillmer 2004). Elder abuse professionals recognize seven categories of elder mistreatment, and older persons may be subjected to more than one type simultaneously or over time (www.preventelderabuse.org):

1. Physical abuse, the intentional infliction of physical pain or injury
2. Sexual abuse, nonconsensual sexual contact
3. Psychological abuse, the intentional infliction of emotional distress
4. Financial exploitation, inappropriate and nonconsensual use of assets for another's benefit
5. Neglect, refusal or failure of caregivers to provide necessary care
6. Self-neglect, behaviors that threaten an older person's health, safety, and well-being
7. Miscellaneous forms of abuse, violation of personal rights (e.g., respect for dignity and autonomy, medical abuse, and abandonment)

Most victims of elder mistreatment are frail and chronically ill and depend on others to meet their basic needs (Lachs and Pillmer 2004; Joshi and Flaherty 2005). They are frequently socially isolated and therefore are not seen by others who might become suspicious of possible abuse or neglect. Family members, friends, acquaintances, strangers, and professionals may perpetrate hurtful actions in domestic and long-term care settings (Choi and Mayer 2000; Payne and Fletcher 2005).

Mistreatment occurs across all racial, cultural, socioeconomic, and religious groups. Some studies show that older women are more frequently abused than men, possibly because they are more likely to report mistreatment or because women usually sustain more serious injuries. If mistreatment, including neglect, is not detected and appropriate interventions are not implemented, these older persons are at a heightened risk for mortality (Lachs et al. 1998, 2000).

Surprisingly little is known about the characteristics, causes, and consequences of elder mistreatment or the most effective techniques for intervention and prevention. The first case report in the medical literature was an article in the *British Medical Journal* about "granny battering" (Burston 1975), and by the close of the 1970s, case-control studies verified that abuse was also a significant problem in the United States. However, precise epidemiological studies of the prevalence and clinical patterns have been hampered by many factors, including limited interest in this phenomenon, lack of standardized definitions of elder abuse types, and the different definitions used by state agencies charged with responding to elder abuse.

It is estimated that 1.5–2.5 million older persons in the United States experience mistreatment in any one year, and the prevalence has been reported to range from 3 to 11 percent, with 4 to 6 percent being the most common estimate (Bonnie and Wallace 2002; Cooper et al. 2008). Pillemer and Finkelhor (1988) were among the first to systematically operationalize three types of elder mistreatment—physical abuse, psychological abuse, and neglect—and to survey a stratified probability sample of older persons in Boston, where the prevalence was 3.2 percent. There have been studies in many other countries, including but not limited to Australia (Boldy et al. 2002); Israel (Lowenstein et al. 2009); the Netherlands (Comijs et al. 1998); Norway, Finland,

Sweden, and Denmark (Saveman et al. 1993; Erlingsson et al. 2005); Canada (Podnieks et al. 1990); and the United Kingdom (McAlpine 2008), where the prevalence of elder abuse ranged from 2 to 10 percent. Elder mistreatment is recognized as a significant social issue in many other countries where prevalence data are not available, including China (Yan et al. 2002) and other countries in Europe and Asia (Cooper et al. 2008).

The first national estimate of elder mistreatment in the United States, the National Elder Abuse Incidence Study, reported the following findings for 1996 (Tatara et al. 1998):

• 449,924 persons age 60 or older experienced abuse or neglect in domestic settings, and another 101,087 experienced self-neglect, for a total of 551,011 persons.
• Only 21 percent of the total cases were reported and substantiated.
• Older women were abused more often than older men.
• The oldest-old were at the highest risk.
• The perpetrator was a family member in 90 percent of cases, and two-thirds were adult children or spouses.
• Older persons who neglected themselves were cognitively impaired, depressed, or frail.

The National Elder Abuse Incidence Study validated the widespread belief that reported cases were the tip of the iceberg. However, the ratio of 1:4 reported versus unreported cases may be an underestimate, because many mistreated older persons are socially isolated (Wolf 1997). There are no national data about the incidence or prevalence of abuse and neglect in institutional settings, although it has been recognized in governmental hearings and ombudsperson reports.

Research on elder mistreatment is limited, in part perhaps, because it has not been recognized as an important social problem. In 2002, the National Academy of Sciences released a report reviewing the available information on elder abuse and developed recommendations for a national research agenda. In a legislative attempt to implement the recommendations

of the report, the 2003 Elder Justice Act (EJA) was introduced in Congress to improve knowledge about the prevalence, detection, intervention, and prevention of elder mistreatment as well as coordinate elder justice programs in the federal government. Although the EJA did not pass that year, it was reintroduced several times and finally passed as part of the Obama administration's 2010 Health Care Reform Bill (www.whitehouse.gov/health-care-meeting/).

States have laws for reporting, investigating and prosecuting abuse, and they implement these laws through a number of state and local social service, law enforcement, and legal government agencies and offices. Resources may be accessed on the websites of the National Association of State Courts (www.ncsconline .org/wc/courtopics/ResourceGuide.asp?topic =EldAbu) and the National Center for Elder Abuse (www.ncea.aoa.gov/NCEAroot/Main_ Site/Find_Help/State_Resources.aspx).

Adult Protective Service (APS) agencies exist in every state to investigate and intervene when abuse is suspected and reported (Dyer et al. 2005; Teaster et al. 2006). The funding to support investigative activities and prevention mainly comes from Federal Social Service Block Grants, Older Americans Act funding, and state legislative appropriations. Medicaid is used for investigating abuse in long-term care settings in some cases. The system for reporting and investigating abuse in nursing homes and assisted living facilities is different from that used in the community. Cooperation between the Long-term Care Ombudsman for nursing homes (www.ltcombudsman.org) and APS for home and community (www .apsnetwork.org) is necessary, because vulnerable older people frequently move between independent living, health care, and long-term care settings.

The Institute of Medicine released several reports with recommendations for the prevention of elder abuse in institutional care settings (IOM 1996, 2001b). The Joint Commission on Accreditation of Healthcare Organizations first identified the importance of recognizing and intervening when abuse was suspected in emergency and outpatient care settings in 1996 and published updated recommendations in 2005 (http://endabuse.org/section/programs/health_care/_jcaho). The American Medical Association (1992) also published diagnostic and treatment guidelines for various health care settings, reviewed strategies for managing and preventing mistreatment, and discussed clinico-legal issues.

Requirements for Reporting Elder Mistreatment

Almost every state has legislation requiring physicians and other medical professionals to report all cases of suspected elder abuse to a state agency. However, paradoxically, many physicians do not. Results of a 2004 APS survey revealed that physicians were the source of only 1.3 percent of cases reported (Teaster et al. 2006). There appear to be many reasons for this failure to report. Many physicians seem to be unaware of state laws or are not well informed regarding their obligation to protect vulnerable older adults (Rodriguez et al. 2006; Gupta 2007). Some physicians believe that only authenticated cases must to be reported or are misinformed about the necessity of obtaining a patient's permission to report mistreatment. Other explanations include concerns about lawsuits by angry patients and families, desire to avoid court appearances, not wanting to interfere with a patient's private life, or being cynical that state interventions will lead to a good outcome.

Physicians need to know the elder abuse laws in their respective states. All fifty states and the District of Columbia have adult protection statutes that establish a system for reporting and investigating abuse as well as, in some cases, providing social and community services (National Center for Elder Abuse, www.ncea.aoa.gov/Main_Site/Find_Help/State_Resources.aspx). Reports of suspected mistreatment must be made by specific categories of persons, except in six states—Colorado, New Jersey, New York, North Dakota, South Dakota, and Wisconsin. These states authorize reporting but do not require it. In general, elder mistreatment is reported to the state APS agency, although in some states reporters may be required to transmit their suspicions to a law enforcement agency or another organization in lieu of or in addition to APS agencies.

According to a statutory analysis conducted by the American Bar Association Commission on Legal Problems of the Elderly (http://new.abanet.org/aging/Pages/elderabuse.aspx), in eight of the mandatory reporting states (Delaware, Indiana, Kentucky, New Mexico, North Carolina, Rhode Island, Texas, and Wyoming) any person who suspects mistreatment is required to report it. In the other jurisdictions, the reporting obligation is directed to specific professional groups. Nine states use a hybrid approach, requiring any person and members of specific professions to report. The occupations commonly mandated to report include physicians, nurses, social workers, psychologists, and law enforcement officers.

Risk Factors

Research on risk factors has been based on a number of theories about the causes of elder mistreatment, none of which has substantial empirical support (Pillemer and Wolf 1986; Schiamberg and Gans 2000; Gordon et al. 2001; Fulmer et al. 2005). The transgenerational family violence theory assumes that violence is a learned behavior, and individuals who have been victims or have observed serious abuse are likely to be abusive. Several hypotheses propose that the stress of caregiving and caregiver psychopathology lead to an increased probability of harmful behaviors. Circumstances in which a care recipient is physically dependent on a caregiver, or a caregiver is financially dependent on a care recipient, have also been implicated. The latter may occur when relatives keep patients at home in order to maintain control of the patient's financial assets and money is not spent for outside help, thus victimizing the care recipient.

The Institute of Medicine's 2003 report described a framework to elucidate the multiple biopsychosocial, cultural, and environmental factors leading to elder mistreatment (Bonnie and Wallace 2002). The general model is based on the assumption that many interactive and multiplicative factors within the following macro- and micro-domains mediate the increasing risk and occurrence of mistreatment:

- Characteristics of potential victims
- Characteristics of responsible actors or perpetrator(s)
- Power dynamics between potential victims and actor(s)
- Contextual factors (e.g., living arrangements)
- Relationship factors (e.g., kinship, formal caregiver)
- Sociodemographic factors
- Cultural factors

Perpetrators' characteristics are more significant predictors of abuse than the characteristics of victims, but factors associated with the vulnerability of victims increase the risk of mistreatment (Bonnie and Wallace 2002). The most significant perpetrator characteristics include the presence of psychiatric problems; dependence on older person for money, housing, or other resources; and a history of aggressive or antisocial behavior. A national study of severe violence involving family members caring for a relative with dementia at home showed that 17 percent of households experienced severe violence (e.g., kicking, hitting, stabbing) and patients were violent toward caregivers in half of those cases (Paveza et al. 1992). The presence of depression in the caregiver, coupled with circumstances where the patient lived with family but without a spouse, increased the risk ninefold.

Many victim characteristics are associated with abuse: chronic illness, functional impairments and disabilities, cognitive impairment, psychotic symptoms, and social isolation. Medical problems and functional impairments affect the ability of older persons to defend themselves and seek help from others. Older persons who are living with relatives but are socially isolated are more likely to be abused because the isolation decreases the probability that the abuse will be detected.

Older women are more likely to be victims than older men for all forms of mistreatment except abandonment and financial exploitation (Prichard 2000; Roberto and Teaster 2005). The National Elder Abuse Incidence Study revealed that older women were victims in 76 percent of psychological abuse cases, 71 percent of physical abuse cases, 63 percent of financial exploitation cases, and 60 percent of cases of neglect (Tatara 1998).

Detection of Abuse

Recognition and clinical intervention are essential because of heightened mortality in mistreated older persons (Lachs and Pillemer 2004). Signs of abuse may be subtle, and frequently there is a cluster of indicators. However, caution is necessary because signs, which may appear to indicate abuse, do not always mean that the patient is being mistreated. Bruises and other signs of trauma may be the result of other causes of injury, often forgotten by the patient. Likewise, allegations of theft or other types of financial exploitation may be the unsubstantiated beliefs of paranoid and/ or cognitively impaired individuals. A comprehensive evaluation is necessary to determine whether physical injuries are the result of assaults or natural injuries (e.g., falls), whether weight loss is the result of medical conditions or neglect, or whether overuse/underuse of medications reflects a patient's dementia, a caregiver's inability to manage medications, or malice.

Because empirically validated scales to detect elder mistreatment are lacking (Fulmer et al. 2004; Nelson et al. 2004), the clinical examination needs to be conducted with care and sensitivity. Many factors contribute to the complexity of accurate detection: the lack of geriatric forensic expertise among many clinicians, ageism, the reluctance of victims to report abuse, and the difficulties in distinguishing mistreatment from other circumstances.

The possibility of elder abuse should be a routine consideration in geriatric clinical practice (Shugarman et al. 2003). SAMHSA maintains an online course for screening and assessing elder abuse (http://pathwayscourses .samhsa.gov/elab/elab_4_pg7.htm). Every clinician and health care setting should have a protocol to detect and assess mistreatment. Evaluation should include a thorough history from the older patient, the alleged perpetrator(s), and other family members and/ or close friends as well as a thorough physical examination. Understanding the complex factors underlying abuse may also require consultation with other health professionals and, whenever possible, the involvement of an interdisciplinary geriatric team.

The interview and physical examination of the older patient should always be done privately. Older adults may have strong feelings of shame, fear, and misplaced loyalty that make them reluctant to report that family members are mistreating them. They may also fear rejection, escalating abuse, or threats of being relocated if government agencies become involved. Furthermore, older persons feel safe and secure living at home or in familiar surroundings, and anxiety about the unknown (e.g., fear of being taken to a hospital or nursing home) may offset their longing to escape from hurtful circumstances.

Clinicians should routinely ask questions about elder abuse and neglect, even when the older patient is cognitively impaired, because some patients may still have the capacity to report being hurt or threatened (Vandeweerd et al. 2006). However, patients who have dementia or paranoid ideation may falsely accuse caregivers of physical or sexual assaults as well as threats to hurt or kill them. It is important to conduct a mental status examination and, if needed, to refer the patient for further evaluation.

When the older patient has severe dementia, it is often critical to find a knowledgeable informant other than the suspected perpetrator. However, this can be a challenging task for several reasons. Other informants may not be available, or, when serious conflicts are present in the family, relatives may falsely accuse the caregiver or other family members of abuse. It requires sensitivity to interview several persons and also maximize the privacy and confidentiality of interviewees.

AK, age 80, began to neglect her home and herself about six months after her husband's death. Despite the efforts of her two daughters, AK insisted that she needed no help and would live in her home until she died. The youngest daughter, CK, age 48, lived thirty minutes away, and JC, age 54, lived several hundred miles away. They had been attentive to AK over the years, but CK saw more of her mother because of the geographic proximity.

Both daughters noticed that their mother's memory problems were becoming progressively more prominent. AK also lost about 30 pounds over a two-month period and complained about being tired, not sleeping well, and having difficulty breathing. She spoke frequently about hearing voices from behind the back door and believed that poisonous gases were being pumped into her home.

Despite CK's attempts to talk her mother into seeing a physician, AK refused, and the discussions usually escalated into angry confrontations. AK repeatedly accused CK of wanting to take her money and property and then kill her by chopping her into pieces with a chain saw. JC did not believe what her sister was telling her about their mother's beliefs, and when JC visited, AK did not exhibit any unusual behavior.

One afternoon AK tripped going down the back porch steps and broke her right hip. However, additional tests showed that AK also had lung cancer. After recovering from hip surgery, AK began radiation therapy. CK asked her mother to move into her home for the duration of the treatments, and she re-arranged her work schedule to care for her.

CK and her mother continued to argue about many issues, and the combination of AK's memory impairment and CK's caregiver stress made the arguments worse. AK denied she had cancer and insisted that she could live alone in her home. Although AK complained about pain, she refused to take her pain medications when

CK reminded her, or when she forgot to take them, she accused CK of hiding the pills. AK complained daily to her other daughter that she was not being treated well and asserted that CK had threatened to kill her.

One morning, when CK accompanied her mother to a special health care team meeting at the cancer center, a team member informed her that they believed she was psychologically abusing her mother by threatening to kill her. CK was told that as required by state law, they had reported this to APS, and they were taking her mother into protective custody. CK could not know where her mother would reside and could not have contact with her.

CK was stunned by the alleged abuse and tried reaching her sister, who did not return her phone calls for a week. When CJ finally did call, she told CK that their mother said that CK was mistreating her, and she wanted nothing to do with her. CK contacted an elder law attorney who verified that physicians must report suspected abuse and that CK would likely be investigated by APS. She also advised her to contact the patient's advocate program at the cancer center.

CK was never contacted by the state, but she and her lawyer did meet with the cancer center's advocacy program representative and the chair of the cancer center's ethics committee. CK was upset that her mother's doctors and other team members did not understand that her mother had severe memory problems and a history of paranoia. She had never threatened or abused her mother.

After an internal review, the ethics committee concluded that AK's clinical team had not met an acceptable standard of care. Their errors not only affected her treatment as a cancer patient, because AK was determined not to be competent to consent to her cancer treatment, but also contributed to an inappropriate accusation of elder abuse. AK had not been given a mental status screening examination nor had she been referred for a psychiatric consultation, standard institutional protocol to assess elder abuse. The intake form CK had completed, noted that AK had a history of progressive cognitive problems and paranoid thinking but had refused to see

a doctor for a diagnosis. Documentation from staff at the cancer residential center documented that AK was often confused and paranoid.

Because AK was being treated at the cancer center after the committee's review, she was referred for psychiatric and neurological consultations. She was diagnosed with moderately severe Alzheimer disease, and additional psychological testing indicated that she did not have the capacity to understand and consent to her treatments. Her consent forms had been signed by the social worker, without a witness, and there was no evidence that anyone had tested her comprehension of the procedures to diagnose and treat her cancer.

The ethics committee recommended that the chief of geriatric oncology meet with AK and her two daughters to discuss guardianship. A court date was set, but AK deteriorated rapidly, became bedridden, and was transferred to hospice care. CK and JC repaired their relationship with ongoing psychotherapy, and they were able to care for their mother until she died.

Signs of Abuse, Neglect, or Mistreatment

When clinicians suspect abuse, the patient should have a thorough examination and the findings should be documented, including statements made by the patient (U of Maine Center on Aging 2007). Although financial exploitation may not be readily detectable, the patient's appearance, clothing, and interactions as well as canceling appointments or not paying bills may provide clues (Tueth 2000).

Elder mistreatment is classified as nonwillful when caregivers are unable or untrained to care for the care recipient appropriately. Family members, especially spouses, may be steadfast about keeping a loved one at home at all costs even when the patient's needs exceed what the family can do. Intentional abuse and neglect most often occur in domestic settings, and it is usually ongoing, not an isolated act by an overwhelmed caregiver.

Physical Abuse

Physical abuse may include acts of violence such as hitting, beating, stabbing, shoving, shaking, slapping, kicking, pinching, and burning. It may also refer to the inappropriate use of drugs and physical restraints, incorrect positioning, force-feeding, and physical punishment. Clues suggesting physical abuse may include:

• An older person's report of being hurt or injured
• Broken bones, bruises, burns, welts, lacerations, black eyes
• Physical signs of being restrained or punished
• Repeated unexplained injuries or accidents
• Sprains, dislocations, and internal injuries/bleeding
• Untreated injuries in various stages of healing
• Broken eyeglasses, walkers, canes, and other assistive devices
• Laboratory results verifying overdose or underuse of prescribed medications or over-the-counter medications
• Abrupt changes in the older person's behavior
• Indifference about injuries and an unwillingness to seek help
• Changes in affect, body language, and behaviors when older patients are questioned
• Caregivers refusing to let other people see the older adult
• Caregivers trying to prevent the patient from being examined alone

Sexual Abuse

Sexual abuse refers to any sexual act that is not consensual as well as sexual acts with persons incapable of giving consent. It may include any form of undesired touching as well as acts such as rape, sodomy, coerced nudity, or taking sexually explicit photographs. Signs of sexual abuse include but are not limited to:

• Bruising around the mouth, breasts, genital area, or anus
• Unexplained venereal diseases or genital infections
• Unexplained vaginal or anal bleeding
• Torn, stained, or bloody underwear
• An older person's report of being touched inappropriately or sexually assaulted

Emotional or Psychological Abuse

Psychological abuse includes a number of threatening behaviors, ranging from verbal assaults, insults, threats, intimidation, humiliation, and harassment to inappropriate behaviors that infantilize the person or isolate them from other persons and activities. Signs of psychological/emotional abuse in older persons include:

• Unusual fearfulness and agitation
• Uncharacteristic withdrawal from activities and other persons
• Evasive and unwillingness to communicate
• Report of being verbally or emotionally mistreated

Financial Exploitation

The improper exploitation of an older person's assets may include cashing checks without authorization; forging a signature; stealing money, property, or possessions; forcing or misleading an older person into signing any document; and the improper use of a conservatorship, guardianship, or power of attorney. Financial exploitation also includes a number of economic scams associated with services and products.

Signs of financial or material exploitation include:

• Sudden changes in financial management practices
• Addition of other names to bank or other financial accounts
• Unauthorized withdrawals from accounts
• Sudden unexplained changes in a will or other financial documents
• Unexplained disappearance of money or valuables
• Inadequate health or personal care despite the availability of adequate financial resources
• Discovery of a signature being forged for financial dealings or for the titles of possessions
• Emergence of previously uninvolved relatives claiming they have rights to be involved in an older person's affairs

- Unexplained, sudden transfer of assets to a family member or someone outside the family
- Situations in which unnecessary services are being provided and paid for
- An older person's report of being financially exploited

Neglect

Neglect is usually characterized by the refusal or failure to provide an older person with basic necessities as food, water, clothing, shelter, personal care, and medical care as well as to provide comfort and personal safety. Signs of neglect include:

- Dehydration and malnutrition
- Poor personal hygiene
- Untreated bed sores
- Untreated health problems
- Unsanitary or unsafe living conditions
- Older person's report of being mistreated

Self-Neglect

Self-neglect, which accounts for 66 percent of investigated mistreatment cases, is characterized by behaviors and actions where older persons place their health or safety at risk. They may also neglect themselves because of dementia, depression, and other health problems, including alcohol and drug abuse. Self-neglect does not include circumstances in which a competent older person makes a deliberate, voluntary decision to endanger his or her health or safety (e.g., a person is terminally ill and refuses food).

The signs and symptoms of self-neglect include:

- Dehydration and/or malnutrition
- Untreated or inappropriately treated medical conditions
- Poor personal hygiene
- Unsafe living conditions such as hazardous electrical wiring; absence of indoor plumbing; lack of heat, air conditioning, or running water
- Unsanitary home environment such as animal/insect infestation, dirty or nonfunctioning toilet, presence of urine and fecal matter

- Inadequate clothing
- Lack of the necessary personal items such as eyeglasses, hearing aids, dentures

An extreme form of self-neglect is the Diogenes syndrome, which usually affects seemingly well-adjusted and once-accomplished older people who deteriorate into conditions of profound personal neglect, domestic squalor, clutter, and social isolation (Reyes-Ortiz 2001). The syndrome is named after Diogenes of Sinope, the ancient Greek philosopher who shunned material things and lived in a barrel. Affected persons are usually from a high socioeconomic bracket, and although most live alone, the syndrome may also characterize spouses and siblings (Esposito et al. 2003).

It has an incidence of 0.5 per 1000 population, and approximately half of affected persons have significant psychopathology and serious medical conditions (Galvez-Andres et al. 2007; Snowden et al. 2007). Psychotic disorders and/or severe cognitive impairment are the typical causes of acute self-neglect in older persons who have been socially engaged in the past. However, extreme self-neglect behaviors may also occur in persons who are not psychotic or demented.

The Diogenes syndrome has been associated with "collectionism" or "syllogomania," the pathological collection of seemingly useless items. Attempts have been made to create diagnostic categories based on the presence and degree of intentionality in self-neglecting and hoarding behaviors (Gibbons et al. 2006). The forensic evaluation of these individuals can be difficult because of the squalor and disrepair in which they live as well as because of injuries and body decomposition (Byard and Tsokos 2007).

Violation of Human Rights

An older person's personal rights are desecrated when caregivers or professional providers ignore a competent person's rights to make decisions. This mistreatment, which may be reported by the older person or observed in family interactions, may take the form of:

- Denying the older person a home
- Forced nursing home placement
- Denying the older person's right to privacy
- Denying the person's right to make decisions about health care
- Denying the person's right to make personal decisions (e.g., marriage, divorce, living companion, voting)

Elder Abuse Interview Protocol

Interviews with patients should include several components:

- Sociodemographic data about the victim and family caregivers
- Family composition, including fictive kin, where applicable
- General inquiries about the patient's overall physical and emotional well-being
- Mini-Mental State Examination
- Specific questions directed to the patient about different forms of mistreatment

The AMA Diagnostic and Treatment Guidelines (1992) recommend that the following questions be asked:

- Has anyone at home (or long-term care facility) ever hurt you?
- Has anyone ever touched you without your consent?
- Has anyone ever made you do things you didn't want to do?
- Has anyone taken anything that was yours without asking?
- Has anyone ever scolded or threatened you?
- Have you ever signed documents that you didn't understand?
- Are you afraid of anyone at home (nursing home) (other family)?
- Are you alone a lot?
- Has anyone ever failed to help you take care of yourself when you needed help?

Every question that is answered positively should be followed by additional queries to clarify how and when the possible mistreat-

ment occurs, who perpetrates the actions, and how the patient copes with it. Clinicians need to evaluate the seriousness of the danger and engage the older patient in discussions about what can be done to protect them and prevent maltreatment from occurring.

Clinicians do not have the responsibility to prove that an older person was abused, but rather to document that there is "reasonable cause" that mistreatment occurred. When clinicians suspect abuse but do not have firm documentation, concerns can be reported to the state agency with a statement that the patient has health or personal problems and needs assistance.

Undue Influence

The legal definitions of undue influence lack clear operational definitions (Scalise 2008–2009). Undue influence refers to manipulation of a relationship between a perpetrator and a victim to serve the interests of the perpetrator. An assessment must examine the characteristics and motivations of the perpetrator and characteristics of the older person, including cognitive functioning, emotional status, physical health, dependency, and psychosocial and environmental circumstances (Blum 2003, 2005).

Undue influence is more than simply trying to persuade someone to take certain actions. It reflects a degree of fraudulent manipulations that are coercive in the decisions and actions of a victim (Shulman et al. 2007). Blum (www .bennettblummd.com) proposed a framework to evaluate victimization and financial exploitation, in which four psychosocial conditions must exist:

1. The victim is older and frail, has physical and/or mental illnesses, and is physically and/or emotionally dependent on the perpetrator.
2. The perpetrator acts to keep the victim isolated from important social contacts and information.
3. The perpetrator manipulates and pressures the victim.

4. The perpetrator gains control of the victim's money and property.

State statutes vary in the definition of undue influence, but the common criteria usually demand clear and convincing evidence that the victim is personally and emotionally vulnerable, that the perpetrator has the disposition to exert influence, that the perpetrator has opportunities to exert influence, and that the perpetrator benefited financially.

The perpetrator often manages household finances, meals, transportation, and overall care or support for the person over a period of time. In the course of these activities, the perpetrator creates and/or takes advantage of the victim's dependency with behaviors and actions that encourage and enhance dependency. This psychological bondage, coupled with control of the victim's access to other people and the outside world, creates an environment that for all practical purposes maintains the victim as a captive who is afraid to lose the perceived life-sustaining care of the perpetrator.

Older people are rarely kidnapped and restrained, although this sometimes occurs. The most common situation involves someone who takes advantage of a person already isolated and needy because of health, frailty, family estrangement, geographic distance from family, or a combination of these circumstances. Perpetrators restrict or cut off contact with family, friends, or professionals by controlling the flow of information to the victim. This may include discarding mail, limiting telephone access, restricting visits into or out of the home, and not leaving the victim alone when others are around.

The perpetrator may lie to the victim about the greedy or evil motivations of others who are not acting in the victim's best interests. The perpetrator creates a fantasy world for the victim, manipulating her/him to believe that the perpetrator is the only one who can or is willing to take care of him or her. Sometimes the perpetrator assembles associates to persuade the victim. It is not unusual for the victim to become fearful and anxious about the situation as well as the possibility that the perpetrator-

protector will desert her or him. The older person may accept this version of the perpetrator's world and lie to keep family members and friends as well as Adult Protective Service professionals away. In some circumstances, the victim may feel a genuine sense of attachment to a perpetrator who cares for all her or his needs.

Assessment of Patient Safety and Care Planning

After the clinician has reported the suspected abuse to APS or the appropriate state agency, the timing of an assessment depends on whether the patient is in immediate danger.

Immediate Safety

If persons are in imminent danger, they may need to be hospitalized, relocated to a shelter, or assisted with a court protective order. If there is no immediate danger, options to protect them need to be considered (e.g., involvement of other family members, home health care). Many older persons are ashamed and embarrassed about being mistreated by family, and they may resist taking the actions necessary to protect themselves, fearful of further mistreatment. It is important to educate, counsel, and support them about the risks and consequences of any decisions to enhance their safety and well-being.

Health and Need for Treatment

It is essential that the clinician determine whether mistreatment could have caused or exacerbated a patient's medical problems and whether the patient's functional impairments interfere with her or his ability to self-protect. In addition to the specific signs and symptoms listed above for the different forms of elder abuse, the following factors should raise the index of suspicion: (1) the explanation of an injury or condition is vague or peculiar, inappropriate for the nature and severity of the injury, or inconsistent between patient and caregiver; (2) patient and/or caregiver deny injury despite clear wounds; (3) there have been previous reports of a similar or related injury; and (4) there is no good reason for a delay in seeking treatment.

Accessibility of Resources

Clinicians may need to access other persons and resources to assess the older patient who is resistant to participation in the assessment. A trusted relative, clergy, or friend may be an effective ally to engage the patient in an honest discussion of the situation. Other valuable resources include APS programs and agencies as well as elder law attorneys and legal advocacy groups.

Cognitive Functioning

Having an accurate assessment of the patient's mental status is fundamental to assessing and intervening when elder abuse is suspected. The Mini-Mental State Examination as well as other cognitive screening tests should be used to screen for cognitive impairment (chapter 3). Cognitive impairment may be reversible or partially reversible. Patients may have delirium if there is an acute fluctuating change in mental status with an altered level of consciousness and if the patient has difficulty focusing and is unaware of the environment.

Patients who have dementia may still be able to participate in a discussion about their situation unless the dementia is severe. Family members who are not suspected perpetrators, clergy, APS departments, elder law attorneys, and professionals in the aging network may provide helpful resources.

Psychological Functioning

It is not unusual for older patients to deny mistreatment. Older people who are being financially exploited frequently do not understand that they are being victimized, or they may have deep feelings of loyalty to certain individuals or causes, such as religious organizations, and believe no one else needs to know their business. The clinician needs to carefully probe for the reasons behind a patient's reticence.

Denial is a complex thought process to overcome because it has unconscious components. It is a defense mechanism that shields a person from feeling distress, and abuse can certainly be categorized as stressful, painful, and hurtful. The process of denial distorts unwanted, unpleasant, or painful facts and feelings by revising them to partial truths or untruths or eliminating them altogether. Thus, mistreated older adults may minimize or rationalize family conflict or violence.

Elder abuse creates a chronic threatening environment that impairs the patient's motivation and ability to pay attention as a protective mechanism to avoid facing reality. Individuals show depressive affect, impaired attention span, anxiety, and insensitivity to changes in their body, including injuries. It is a clinical challenge to help patients shift their attentional set to perceive the dangerousness of the environment and circumstances. The clinician needs to recognize the potential signs of harmful denial in order to orchestrate an effective interview. Impaired attention, altered consciousness, impaired information processing and thinking, blocked emotions, physical distress beyond any physical injuries, and behavioral changes may all be indicators of denial (GR Horowitz 1988).

The inability to remember details or sequences of mistreatment is common and may be confused with a conscious reluctance to disclose. Many abused adults are not able to think or communicate clearly and may frequently lose their train of thought or become inflexible about other options available to them. It is as if they cannot make associations between obvious contingencies (e.g., my son's girlfriend wants money and hurts me to get it from me).

Although some abused older persons will appear emotionally flat during an interview, others will manifest depression and anxiety or express shame, guilt, humiliation, and/or anger without admitting mistreatment. These psychological reactions make it difficult to establish and maintain their trust to obtain necessary information to evaluate or treat them, particularly if victims believe that you are allied with those who are abusing them.

Some abused patients manifest psychotic features, lack of insight, inappropriate thoughts, and disconnectedness from reality. Mistreated patients frequently distort memories of abusive encounters, create fictitious stories, and minimize or exaggerate the reality of their situation. Using fantasy is a way of not facing the danger inherent in their situation.

Abused older adults may display a wide variety of somatic symptoms that are the result of emotional reactions to the stress of being mistreated. These may affect every part of the body, including, but not limited to the head (e.g., dizziness and lightheadedness, shooting pains in the face or head, headaches); hearing (e.g., ringing in the ears, deafness, noises in the head); sight (e.g., eye tics, blurred vision, eye sensitivity); touch (e.g., tingling, numbness, pain); mouth and stomach (e.g., bloating, swallowing problems, nausea, abdominal distress); arms and legs (e.g., tingling, rashes, muscle twitches); and chest (pains, heaviness, discomfort, tachycardia).

Suspected Perpetrator(s)

The clinician needs to assess many characteristics of the suspected perpetrator, including relationship to the patient, health status and history, psychiatric health and history, and cognitive and emotional status. The person's attitude as well as observed behavior and interactions with the patient and other family members, ability to cope with the stress of caregiving, economic stability, beliefs and perceptions about the patient, and possible motivations for abuse should also be assessed.

Social and Financial Resources

It is important to identify whether the patient has family and/or friends who are prepared to help if needed. Likewise, if the patient has adequate financial resources for their living situation and care, are they being used appropriately?

Summary and Care Planning

Many questions need to be asked, including the nature and frequency of abuse, the consequences, duration of the problem, and triggers for abuse, as well as what the patient does when abuse occurs, what the perpetrator does when abuse occurs, what can be done to prevent the abuse, and whether the patient and abuser want help to change the pattern.

Intervention and Case Management

The intervention and management of older patients who have been determined to be mistreated include immediate care, long-term assessment and care, education, and prevention. The central principles for intervening are to follow the state reporting requirements and to choose alternatives that impose the least restrictions on the older person's independence and decision-making. When available, a multidisciplinary team should be involved in the investigation of reported mistreatment (Dyer et al. 2007).

After the immediate needs of the patient have been met, and if the patient is willing to accept voluntary services, it is important to educate her or him about many different issues relevant to self-protection and getting appropriate help; to develop an ongoing safety plan; to provide appropriate services that will diminish the ongoing risks of abuse (e.g., mental health treatment for substance-abusing caregivers, home- and community-based care for stressed caregivers); and to refer the patient and/or family members for supportive services such as counseling and legal assistance.

If the patient lacks the capacity to consent to assistance, the clinician needs to discuss the following possible needs with APS or the appropriate state agency: assistance with financial management, guardianship or conservatorship, or special court actions (e.g., protection orders).

Educating older adults who refuse help about their safety options is essential, because the abuse will continue and likely escalate. It is important to leave written information with the names, addresses, and phone numbers of agencies in the area that can provide help. Give the patient a contact name for each agency, and ask the patient if she or he would consider making a phone call at the time of a home visit. If possible, help the older person think through and develop a safety plan to leave the home. Work with other professionals or team members to create a follow-up plan.

The long-term assessment and care of mistreated older adults depends on the patient's needs. The use of a multidisciplinary team is especially helpful during home visits to evaluate the older person's functional effectiveness, the living environment, the condition of the caregiver or caregivers, and other friends and neighbors who serve as part of the patient's psychosocial support system. The team also provides a range of expertise to develop and implement an ongoing care plan for the patient.

Mistreatment in Long-Term Care Settings

Any number of persons may mistreat residents in nursing homes, assisted living residences, and other senior living facilities, including staff, other residents, visitors, or trespassers. Although the types of abuse and neglect that occur in long-term care settings can be the same as those in home settings, the failure to carry out an appropriate care plan is a major concern. Examples include unnecessary or inappropriate use of physical and chemical restraints for staff convenience or as a substitute for behavioral, psychological, or environmental treatments, poor quality care or ongoing neglect for physical and emotional disorders, neglect of nutritional care or skin care, and neglect of adequate pain control. Medical directors, private practitioners, nurses, and other professionals have a responsibility to develop and maintain a documented care plan, which will be scrutinized along with other clinical records to determine whether actions/inactions resulted in substandard care, abuse, or neglect.

Long-term care residents are particularly vulnerable to abuse and neglect for several reasons. The presence of multiple physical, cognitive, and functional impairments make residents dependent on others, and many do not have family members or friends who monitor care closely. Many staff members lack training in behavioral management, time management, and stress management, increasing the vulnerability of residents. Structural and organizational problems, such as staff shortages, high staff turnover, inadequate supervision, and inadequate resources increase the overall environmental risk for mistreatment.

Resident-to-Resident Aggression and Violence

Available data suggest that resident-to-resident violence is a serious emergent problem, and the number of incidents may be increasing (IOM 2001b; Glock 2005). An analysis of 1997–2002 data from the National Ombudsman Reporting System (NORS) showed that reported rates of abuse, gross neglect, and exploitation across states ranged from 0.4 to 158.0 per 1,000 nursing home beds. Physical abuse and resident-to-resident abuse were the highest reported types of abuse (Jogerst et al. 2005).

The first statewide study of nursing home resident-to-resident violence was done in 2000 in Massachusetts using data from the Minimum Data Set (MDS). Approximately one in four incidents resulted in serious injuries such as bruises, fractures, or hematomas, but there were no deaths (Shinoda-Tagawa et al. 2004). This study and a few others suggest that resident characteristics associated with physically aggressive and violent behavior include male gender, dementia, active paranoia and psychotic symptoms, and pain. Facilities with a higher proportion of residents who have dementia have more episodes of resident violence. Residents who are injured by another resident's aggressive behavior are more likely to be cognitively impaired and have physical infirmities that increase their risk for assault and harm (Shinoda-Tagawa et al. 2004; Burgess and Phillips 2006).

A study of resident-to-resident violence used a population-based cohort of community-residing older persons placed in long-term care facilities, and the results showed that 89 percent of incidents requiring law enforcement involvement were simple or aggravated assaults (Lachs et al. 2007). An analysis of perpetrators of these incidents showed that 62 percent were involved in one incident, 19 percent were involved in two incidents, and another 19 percent were involved in three or more incidents. Half of the persons involved had dementia. Qualitative analyses of the incidents suggested five typologies: (1) unprovoked assaults, in which a resident who had dementia struck another resident; (2) space invasion, in which a resident entered another resident's room; (3) assaults involving two men with a history of aggression; (4) competition for resources, involving escalating arguments leading to an assault; and (5) an aggressive response by a resident after a history of long-standing difficulties.

Sexual Abuse

Residents who sexually assault other residents are a challenge for long-term care staff. These individuals may be cognitively impaired or may have criminal offender backgrounds. Many health care professionals have not been trained to recognize and respond to suspected sexual abuse, and at the moment there are little empirical data to create training programs and clinical practice guidelines.

A growing body of research is beginning to clarify the prevalence and clinical characteristics of sexual offenses by nursing home residents. A study of substantiated cases of sexual abuse in home and long-term care settings from Virginia APS records over a three-year period revealed that most victims had some cognitive impairment, were female, and lived in a nursing home (Teaster et al. 2000). The most frequent perpetrators were other residents, followed by staff members. Teaster and Roberto (2004) examined verified cases of sexual abuse of female nursing home residents collected over a 5-year period by Virginia APS workers. Perpetrators were all male, mostly over age 70, and the victims largely women with functional and cognitive limitations who were age 80 or older. Nursing home residents accounted for 90 percent of the perpetrators.

Detection, investigation, and response to sexual abuse of residents-by-residents has complex clinical, legal, ethical, and practical challenges in long-term care settings, given the functional and cognitive impairments of victims and perpetrators. Although reports of alleged and confirmed sexual abuse of residents-by-residents may be relatively rare compared to other violent acts, the prevalence is likely under-reported. Furthermore, risk assessment and intervention policies and practices must be incorporated into the spectrum of violent resident behaviors.

Responsibilities of Physicians and Staff

Physicians and other clinical staff members can and should play a significant role in identifying, intervening, and preventing mistreatment in long-term care settings because they see residents on a regular basis for health care and monitoring. State laws require physicians to examine patients for admission to nursing homes and assisted living facilities. After admission, each nursing home resident must be followed by an attending physician or by a physician's assistant, nurse practitioner, or clinical nurse specialist supervised by a physician. Evaluations must be done every three months or when there is a change in the resident's condition.

The physician can monitor the possibility of abuse or neglect in several ways: participation in resident care plan meetings with other staff; evaluating the need for medications, including psychotropic medications, nutritional supplements, and other health care interventions and procedures; and checking reports, including monthly pharmacist reviews of medications and reports of substandard care by an appropriate state agency.

Legal Consequences of Elder Abuse

Elder mistreatment has been successfully prosecuted in both criminal and civil courts (Heisler 2000), but a 2001 national survey of prosecutors unfortunately showed that only 42 percent of prosecutors had ever handled elder abuse and neglect cases. Persons and corporations have been found criminally liable in home and long-term care settings, but many times abuse goes ignored and unrecognized.

Litigation of elder mistreatment cases in both civil and criminal arenas is beset by a number of intrinsic problems (Heisler and Steigel 2004). Evidence may rely on persons who have impaired cognitive and communication abilities, and direct first-hand testimony is hard to find. Home and community service providers and health care professionals may be hesitant about participating in legal proceedings. Because court proceedings may be prolonged for long periods of time, victims and witnesses become unavailable for many reasons, including deterioration and death, disenchantment, or staff turnover. Many victims are intensely afraid of losing misperceived love or economic security from abusive caregivers, and when perpetrators are members of the victim's family, the prospect of alienating relatives can be intimidating. The existence of these practical obstructions and the low fee potential often diminishes the interest of attorneys to take on these cases. Furthermore, the significantly reduced government support for legal service and advocacy programs has curtailed the availability of legal resources and representation.

In addition to criminal liability for abuse, exploitation, and neglect under state elder abuse statutes, physical abuse may be classified as assault or battery, and financial exploitation can meet state definitions of theft, extortion, embezzlement, fraud, or other crimes. Civil rights protection has been used to establish a case of neglect, giving federal protection to patients. However, problems with evidence, court procedures, and lack of resources in many prosecutors' offices across the country obstruct active enforcement. Financial exploitation by caregivers can be difficult to prove because it is not a single overt theft but rather a subtle and sinister crime that occurs over time.

Even when prosecutions are successful, these cases are expensive, time-consuming, frustrating, and demanding. Even in the most horrifying circumstances, the outcomes may be disheartening, as the following case illustrates:

The victim, TG, was a 91-year-old white female who had a history of schizophrenia and had been bedridden off and on for eight years. There were three abusers: MG, the 69-year-old daughter, who was the primary caregiver; DG, the 54-year-old son; and SG, the 54-year-old daughter-in-law. The daughter lived with TG in the first floor of a two-story townhouse. MG had retired from a position in the federal government to be a caregiver for her mother. DG lived upstairs with his wife, SG, and he was the principal of a local high school. His wife occasionally helped out with the caregiving.

The family called EMS and law enforcement personnel to assist with an apparent natural death. The decedent was found lying supine in a hospital bed in the bedroom, and various sick room items (e.g., adult diapers, lotions) were on the dresser and tables. The decedent appeared emaciated; her eyes were sunken with open fixed pupils, and her mouth was open without teeth. She was covered up to the neck by a blanket and was lying on an egg crate mattress. There was a strong smell of feces and urine, a common occurrence with natural death.

The law enforcement officer met with the family to express condolences and interview them about the decedent. The family reported a sketchy medical history: TG had fallen about 20 years ago and had had surgery, after which time she became morbidly obese. After a crash diet 10 years later, causing a 100-pound weight loss, TG's symptoms of schizophrenia became worse, and she was bedridden. A review of medical records later confirmed a limited number of physician visits.

A local funeral home was called, but while the EMS were preparing the body for removal, they found pads and clothes covered with urine and feces under the body as well as several large bedsores. Body fluids, urine, and other liquid substances had seeped through the victim's diaper, into the egg crate padding, and then into the mattress. A dark black fungus had started to grow. The bedroom was cold, and a number of deodorizing sheets were hanging from the walls. The coroner's office was called, and the body was taken to the funeral home for further examination, including photographs.

Law enforcement officers interviewed DG, who indicated that he left the caregiving to his sister and wife. Occasionally, he would help turn his mother and expressed surprise at the mention of bedsores. DG indicated that hospice had brought them a bed several years ago, but they had not needed their help.

The coroner's inspection of the body revealed a dark fluid with the consistency of coffee grounds draining from the mouth. The decedent's flesh had the consistency of biscuit dough, and it appeared that she had been malnourished and dehydrated. TG had dirty fingernails and toenails. The toenails were approximately 1½ inches long, and they were bent over and to the side. This appeared to be the result of the constant pressure of bed sheets that pressed her feet into the edge of the bed. There was packed fecal matter from her back and pubic area down her thighs. TG had several decubiti, the largest of which was 3–4 inches in diameter at the surface. It was located at the base of the spine and the bone was visible. A large number of bobby pins were found under and on the body. At least 10 were embedded in her bedsores as well as other parts of the body.

TG's body did not appear to have been washed for a long time. Analyses indicated that the foul smelling clothes, egg crate, and mattress had been rotting for several months. After the body was cleaned for autopsy, the decubiti were much larger, the exposed spine was deteriorating, rotting flesh was found under the armpit and breasts, and fecal matter had to be removed from the vaginal canal and cavity. Analyses of tissue and bone sections from the spine verified the presence of infection from the decubiti that likely led to sepsis, causing her death. The lack of proper personal care and hygiene created conditions for the infection to develop, and the lack of regular and proper medical attention allowed infected areas to become worse.

After the investigation by the coroner and law enforcement, the decedent's daughter, son, and daughter-in-law were all arrested and charged under the state statute with a neglect violation of the Omnibus Adult Protection Act. During a bench trial, the entire community rallied around the family and tied yellow ribbons around trees to show their support. Town meetings were held to protest the police interference. Editorials in local papers also supported the family and criticized the intrusion of government and law enforcement in the lives of good people in the community.

MG, DG, and SG were all found guilty and sentenced to 3 months' probation (case material, Randy Thomas).

This case raises many questions about possible points of primary, secondary, and tertiary prevention and appropriate punishment:

• At the level of primary prevention, the victim's physician(s) could have checked on her at regular intervals and could have recommended home and community-based services. Others who had regular contact (e.g., mail delivery personnel, gas meter readers) could have been trained in Gatekeeper Programs to recognize warning signs, and neighbors could have talked with the family about getting in-home help.
• A secondary prevention response assumes that this case was recognized. Many questions are unanswered. What if the patient had been forced to leave the home and was relocated to a nursing home? If the family caregivers were prosecuted, what might have happened to the patient?
• Tertiary responses target the question of how the abuse could have been prevented. The family members could have been trained to care for the patient appropriately and also required to participate in counseling. They could also have been prosecuted and convicted of several crimes.
• Finally, the community that rallied behind the principal and his family could have been better informed about the issues of neglect and the responsibilities of caregivers.

Principles of Managing Elder Mistreatment

1. Every health care setting should have a protocol for elder mistreatment screening and intervention.

2. Clinicians should know the reporting requirements for their respective states.

3. Clinicians should screen for the presence and severity of cognitive impairment when investigating a suspicion of elder abuse or neglect.

4. The clinician's responsibility is not to prove that elder mistreatment has occurred, but rather to document a high index of suspicion.

The detection of elder abuse and neglect is clearly a complicated challenge. The magnitude of the public health problem and the potential for injury and death for vulnerable older persons make assessment/intervention protocols a critical component of health care.

18

Violent Deaths

Violent deaths—suicide and homicide-suicide—are an emerging public health challenge worldwide. This chapter reviews the epidemiology of violent deaths, risk factors and warning signs, intervention and prevention strategies, the impact on surviving family members, and traumatic grief interventions.

Approximately 50,000 Americans die a violent death each year; about 30,000 are suicides, and about 20,000 are homicides. Although the Centers for Disease Control and Prevention does not keep statistics on homicide-suicide as they do for suicide and homicide deaths, the best estimates are that 1,500–2,000 homicide-suicide deaths occur each year in the United States (D Cohen 2002). The 2002 World Health Organization (WHO) report on world violence and health (www5.who.int/violence_injury_prevention/main.cfm?p=0000000117) estimated that 1.6 million people met premature and violent deaths in 2000. At least 815,000 people killed themselves, making suicide the thirteenth most common cause of death; and persons age 60 or older were most likely to commit suicide. Although 520,000 persons were murdered and 310,000 died in wars, suicides accounted for as many deaths as homicide and war combined. Global suicide statistics can be retrieved from WHO sources (www.who.int/health_topics/suicide/en/).

Suicide

Suicide is a tragedy at any age, leaving an average of six family members or intimates to deal with the aftermath. U.S. suicide statistics can be found at the website of the American Association of Suicidology (www.suicidology.org). Based on the more than 738,000 suicides that have occurred in the United States from 1976 through 2000, there are at least 4.4 million

American lives touched by the self-inflicted death of a loved one—or 1 in 62 Americans in 2000. Given the estimate that one person commits suicide every 18 minutes, there are 80 new suicides and 320 new co-victims or survivors each day.

It is well established that the highest suicide rates occur in the population age 65 or older and increase dramatically with advancing age (http://mentalhealth.samhsa.gov/suicideprevention/). This reflects the sharp rise in rates for older men, particularly older white men, who commit more than 80 percent of all suicides. The high rates in the older population have been a consistent finding in the United States since the 1930s. WHO surveys report the same for most of the developed countries in the world since the 1950s (www5.who.int/mental_health/download.cfm?id=0000000382). Increasing suicide rates with advancing age are observed in countries with high life expectancies (Shah 2009).

Older persons show a greater degree of premeditation and lethality of intent than younger persons. Older adults are less likely to attempt suicide, with an average of four attempts for every completed suicide compared to 100–200 attempts for every completed suicide in younger age groups (www.suicidology.org). More than 70 percent of older suicides involve firearms, compared to 57 percent for the general population. Careful planning, increased vulnerability, decreased reserve capacity to recover, and relative social isolation contribute to increased lethality in aged people. Older persons are less likely to be discovered after a suicide attempt, and they are less communicative about their ideation than younger persons.

Predicting suicide rates is a challenge, given the many changing demographic, economic, social, political, and generational forces that will affect society in the future. Suicide rates in the baby boom generation, those 76 million persons born between 1946 and 1959, are higher than suicide rates in previous generations, but it is not known whether this trend will continue as the boomers age (Conwell 2009; Sudak 2010). Furthermore, if this sequential birth cohort effect continues for the Generation X and Generation Y groups, suicide rates may continue to increase.

Risk Factors and Risk Markers

Suicide is associated with many different risk factors that are in turn associated with other forms of psychological dysfunction not specific to suicide alone (Maris et al. 2000). The influence of specific risk factors may change over the lifespan, and the effects may have a cumulative effect. There are also protective factors that prevent the occurrence of some risk factors, diminish the effects of others, increase resistance, or block the causal sequence of effects leading to suicide.

Risk factors for late-life suicide include the following (Conwell et al. 2002; Duberstein et al. 2005; Loebel 2005; Mann et al. 2005):

- Advancing age
- Male gender
- Caucasian race
- Depression and other psychopathology
- History of one or more suicide attempts
- Family history of suicide
- Alcohol use / dependency
- Poor physical health
- Use of multiple medications
- Health changes
- Not being married
- Socially disconnected from others
- Multiple losses
- Firearm(s) in the home
- Cultural factors, such as shame and embarrassment over events in the family
- Recent media attention on a suicide

The coexistence of depression with physical impairments differentiates older from younger populations at risk for suicide. Risk may be elevated in persons who have cancer or mul-

tiple debilitating conditions compared to other illnesses (Kendal 2007). There is no clear evidence of increased rates in persons who have dementia (Haw et al. 2009; Purandare et al. 2009), but cognitive impairment is a modest risk factor for suicide ideation (Draper et al. 1998).

Most of our understanding of late-life suicide is based on analyses of information from national vital statistics data and psychological autopsy studies in which data are collected from informants. Suicide occurs with a low prevalence compared to heart disease, stroke, and cancer, the top three causes of mortality, and this makes it difficult to analyze the interactions between various risk factors in prospective studies. In what may be the only community-based prospective study to date, a total of 14,456 older subjects were enrolled in the Established Populations for Epidemiological Studies of the Elderly, and 21 persons committed suicide over a 10-year period (Turvey et al. 2002). Depression, perceived health status, poor sleep, and absence of a confidante predicted suicide. These four variables predicted overall mortality as well, diminishing the will to live even in the absence of suicidal thoughts and behaviors.

Assessing Risk and Treating Suicidal Behavior

Not all suicides can be prevented, but a careful and thorough assessment of risk factors is essential, especially in primary care settings (Tadros and Salib 2007; Conwell and Thompson 2008; Conwell 2009). Most older patients who commit suicide have had a longstanding relationship with a primary care physician and have seen the doctor shortly before the suicide (Luoma et la. 2002; Schulberg et al. 2004). However, they are unlikely to communicate suicidal thoughts. As many as 45 percent of patients visited their physician within a month of killing themselves. Seventy-five percent had contact with their primary care physician within a year of their suicide, and there was pattern of contacting more than one physician during that year (Deisenhammer et al. 2007).

Detection and treatment of depression

and suicidality in managed care settings is a challenge because of the use of primary care physicians and fiscal care protocols for mental health evaluation and treatment. Suicide prevention rests on a thorough evaluation of suicide potential and imminent risk because among older persons the first suicide attempt is more likely to be successful and therefore to be the last. Bharucha (2001) argued that clinicians in managed care settings must clearly document objective indicators of risk, advocate for the mental health care of suicidal patients, make referrals to psychiatrists, and be aggressive in appeals when care is denied.

Several education and training resources are referenced on the American Association of Suicidology's website (www.suicidology.org). Recognizing and Responding to Suicide Risk: Essential Skills for Clinicians (RRSR) is an advanced, interactive training based on core competencies that mental health professionals need to effectively assess and manage suicide risk (www.suicidology.org/c/document_library/ get_file?folderId=233&name=DLFE-33.pdf). Recognizing and Responding to Suicide Risk: Essential Skills in Primary Care (RRSR-PC) is a one-hour training program for physicians, nurses/nurse practitioners, and physicians assistants that provides information to enable them to integrate suicide risk assessments into office visits, formulate relative risk, and work with patients to create treatment plans (www .suicidology.org/c/document_library/get_file/ folderId=233&name=DLFE-163.pdf). The Suicide Prevention Resource Center provides a suicide prevention toolkit for rural primary care (www.sprc.org/pctoolkit/index.asp).

Several basic areas need to be considered in the process of assessing risk and dealing with suicidal behavior (Maris et al. 2000): identifying the problem, exploring the problem, addressing high risk environmental factors, addressing high risk behavioral situations, focusing on problem-solving, and committing to an action plan.

The first step is to define the presence, nature, and characteristics of the suicidal thoughts and behaviors. If suicidal ideation is present, it is necessary to assess the content,

such as ambivalence, psychological pain, hopelessness, helplessness. Determination of intent requires an evaluation of the method being considered and its lethality, whether the individual has the knowledge and skills to commit suicide, and the availability of psychosocial supports or protective resources that can be mobilized. Questions should be asked about whether the individual has a suicide plan, and if so, details of the plan as well as whether the individual has made any previous suicide attempts or tried to harm themselves (e.g., self-mutilation).

The next phase is to explore the antecedents of the circumstances, including key problems that may have triggered the emotional crisis. Questions should be asked to clarify each event or issue surrounding key problems. As the context of the situation becomes clearer, the person should be asked to focus on specific issues associated with the problem situation. This process not only provides information about what is contributing to the suicidality, but it also provides the opportunity to focus on concrete issues and thus to diminish the sense of overwhelming emotional distress.

There are several ways to begin to intervene and try to reduce the dangerousness of the situation associated with high-risk environmental and behavioral factors, for example, removing lethal items or convincing the individual to do so by giving them to family members and communicating with the patient's family or significant others to reduce isolation while maintaining contact with the patient. The clinician should pay careful attention to the person's affect as well as to the content of the answers to questions, validate the emotional pain but emphasize the importance of tolerating negative emotions, and try to generate hopefulness and reasons for living. Short-term somatic treatment, such as not consuming alcohol or sleep medications, might be considered.

Specific actions to take during the problem-solving phase include:

- Emphatically instructing the person not to commit suicide

- Focusing the person on alternatives to help improve the situation and those who are available to help
- Confronting the person about the outcome of his or her actions
- Giving advice and making direct suggestions about how to change the person's circumstances
- Clarifying and reinforcing more adaptive solutions
- Identifying how to deal with factors that interfere with a productive plan of action

Committing to an action plan includes several components:

- Reassessing the potential for suicide
- Anticipating and being prepared for a recurrence of the crisis response
- Considering prescribing psychotropic medication but assuring the availability of a 24/7 support system, because suicidal risk may increase in the initial phase of antidepressant medication
- Recommending or considering hospitalization
- Considering involuntary commitment when necessary

Factors Associated with the Risk of Imminent Suicide

Direct indications of imminent risk include suicidal ideation, suicide threats, suicide plans or preparations, history of a suicide attempt in the last year, and the availability of a gun, poison, or plan to use a car in a closed garage. Indirect indices include recent losses or disruptions, depressive affect, indifference or dissatisfaction with therapy, presence of hopelessness and anger or both, increased anxiety, a recent medical care visit, indirect references to death, and giving things away.

Circumstances associated with suicide in the next several hours or days include:

- Major depression with severe agitation, insomnia, helplessness and hopelessness, severe anhedonia
- Consumption of alcohol
- Suicide note written or in progress

- Specific plans to commit suicide
- Methods available or easily obtained
- Specific precautions about not wanting to be discovered
- Giving house keys to a friend or lawyer just in case
- Checking insurance policy re: suicide
- Insinuating to a spouse or others about going away

Considering or Recommending Psychiatric Hospitalization

Several considerations for hospitalization include the following circumstances: the suicidal person is not responding to outpatient therapy, and depression is severe or anxiety disabling; the person is in an overwhelming crisis and at serious risk to harm him- or herself or others; this is a first-time psychosis, and the person has little support and expresses suicidal ideation. Hospitalization is recommended in the following situations: the patient is in a psychotic state, threatening suicide, and identifies specific means; the risk of suicide outweighs the risk of an inappropriate hospitalization; suicide threats are escalating, the patient is drinking alcohol, using illicit drugs, or taking psychotropic medications and has a history of serious drug overdose.

Suicide Pacts

Suicide pacts are rare in all age groups, accounting for less than 0.05 percent of all suicides (Brown and Barraclough 1997; Hunt et al. 2009). Suicide pacts in the older population, characterized by explicit mutual intent of the persons involved, are not spousal homicide-suicides, but both types of linked dyadic deaths share similar risk factors. Older couples often go to great lengths to plan a deliberate death, and the older man usually uses a gun to kill his wife before killing himself. The method of death for the case described below may be unusual in the United States, but the antecedent circumstances—incapacitating illness, depression and hopelessness, and a suicide note or written documentation of intent—are not.

The day MS, age 85, and ES, age 80, planned to die was New Year's Eve 2003. They had complained to a maintenance man at their condominium that the screens in their bedroom blocked the ocean breeze. He removed them, and several hours later the couple committed suicide together.

The results of the medical examiner's investigation indicated that MS and ES had crawled across their bedroom floor to the window and fell 17 floors to their death. Both relied on walkers to get around their one-bedroom condominium. ES appeared to have helped her husband, who was weak and frail due to emphysema, by pushing him out the window first before she followed. A note with the name of their attorney and estate information was taped to the telephone, and ES had a card in her blouse pocket with emergency contact information.

The Ss had been married 42 years when they died. They had no children and ran a resort together as well as traveling around the world. In their retirement years, the Ss spent most of their time together but also went out with friends. M played poker several times a week with friends in the condominium, and E volunteered at a local hospital. The couple's only niece and their neighbors, who saw the Ss frequently, were shocked by the couple's death, and even in retrospect, saw no signs that the couple were planning to commit suicide together.

This case illustrates many of the characteristics of the victims and circumstances of suicide pacts. Most couples have been married a long time and have enjoyed what appears to have been a successful marriage. However, disabling chronic or terminal illness accompanied by depression and other late-life stressors intervene and begin to limit their control and independence. The decision to commit suicide together is made reflectively, and typically the event is carefully planned. Often the double suicide occurs on a date significant for the couple or at a time shortly after one or both experience a significant deterioration in health.

Antecedents of Suicide: The Psychological Autopsy

It is usually easy to understand the many factors and circumstances leading to suicide in retrospect after a psychological autopsy, a method developed by Edwin Schneidman (1994), to clarify the nature of equivocal deaths. The psychological autopsy is a comprehensive retrospective investigation of the intentions, lethality, and motivations of the victim to be dead (Cavanagh et al. 2003; Knoll 2008). Information is obtained by interviewing individuals who had a close relationship with the deceased and knew his or her background, character, behavior, personality, and concurrent stressful life events. Clinicians should gather the following data:

- Details of death, including mode of death and physical evidence at the death scene
- Clues to or communication of suicidal intent
- Life history, including education, marital/dyadic relationships, family, work, military, and social activities
- Personality and lifestyle
- Medical history
- History of prior suicide ideation or attempts, family history of suicide
- Legal history and current circumstances, if any
- Financial history and current status
- Recent contacts with medical, legal, financial, or other professionals or agencies
- Recent life stressors or changes in health, lifestyle, relationships, economic or legal status
- Assessment of intent and lethality

Preventing Suicide: A National Agenda

The urgency of preventing suicide is underscored by several national reports. In 1999, the Surgeon General issued a groundbreaking report, *The Surgeon General's Call to Action to Prevent Suicide* (USPHS 1999), and in 2001 the Office of the Surgeon General followed up with the *National Strategy for Suicide Prevention*, which specified goals and recommendations for action, including the importance of reducing suicide mortality in the aged (USPHS 2001). In 2002, two reports were issued: the Centers for Disease Control published *Suicide Prevention Now: Linking Research to Practice* (CDC 2001), and the Institute of Medicine published *Reducing Suicide: A National Imperative* (IOM 2002). These documents are critical roadmaps for a challenging future in which older people, at the highest risk for suicide, are the fastest-growing segment of the population (Conwell and Pearson 2000; Pearson 2006).

Homicide-Suicide

Homicide-suicides, also referred to as murder-suicides in the public domain, are tragedies in which a perpetrator, usually a man, kills one or more victims, usually a wife or intimate, and then commits suicide within minutes or hours, but no later than 24 hours later. The most common homicide-suicide in all age groups involves spouses or intimates, but homicide-suicides may also involve infants and children, entire families, or multiple victims in the workplace or school (Marzuk et al. 1992; Cohen et al. 1998; Bossarte et al. 2006; Salari 2007; Eliason 2009; Liem et al. 2009).

Until recently, it was believed that homicide-suicides occurred most frequently in the young, usually involving a jealous, angry man who would kill a wife or girlfriend when he believed the relationship was threatened with dissolution. Homicide-suicides in older people were considered to be suicide pacts, mercy killings, or altruistic homicide-suicides in which both partners were old and sick (McIntosh et al. 1994). However, a body of research since the 1990s has dispelled these myths (Cohen et al. 1998; Malphurs and Cohen 2005):

• Homicide-suicide rates are higher in the population age 55 or older compared to the population age 54 or younger, although numerically more homicide-suicides occur in the latter because the population is larger.
• Homicide-suicides are not suicide pacts or altruistic acts.
• Older men are perpetrators 90–95 percent of the time.

• Victims, including spouses and intimates, are not willing or knowing participants.

Homicide-suicides are rare compared to both homicides and suicides, but they are an emerging public health issue, especially in the population age 55 or older. It is estimated that they account for 1,500–2,500 deaths each year in the United States, similar to the number of deaths due to meningitis, viral hepatitis, or pulmonary tuberculosis (Marzuk et al. 1992). At least 20 percent of homicide-suicides across the United States involve older persons, with 300–500 deaths annually.

Although many papers have been published about homicide-suicides since 1900, it was not until 1995 that rates and clinical patterns were empirically studied in older persons (Cohen 1995; Cohen et al. 1998). The few papers that mentioned older perpetrators or victims reported only the number of events and sometimes health status. The available taxonomy systems, which classify homicide-suicides by age, relationship, and presumed motivation, all assumed homogeneity of motives by the perpetrators (Marzuk et al. 1992; Hanzlick and Koponen 1994; Berman 1996).

The prevalence rates for homicide-suicide have consistently averaged 0.2 to 0.3 per 100,000 over the years throughout the world, although rates vary according to geographic areas. The relative stability of homicide-suicide rates has been interpreted to reflect that the amount of psychopathology in the population remains about the same. However, the variation in homicide-suicide rates across cities, metropolitan areas, counties, and countries probably reflects differences in age demography, suicide and homicide rates, and other factors, including culture.

The characteristics of perpetrators and victims and the frequency distribution of various homicide-suicide subgroups are similar in old and young age groups (Cohen et al. 2003):

• 90 percent of old and young perpetrators are male.
• 78 percent of older victims and 72 percent of younger victims are women.

- Most homicide-suicides were spousal/consortial (72 percent of old and 74 percent of young).
- Familial homicide-suicides accounted for 10 percent of older homicide-suicides and 8 percent of younger homicide-suicides.
- Children were victims in both old and young, 5 percent and 6 percent respectively.
- Extrafamilial homicides accounted for 10 percent of all homicide-suicides in old and young.
- Mass murders or workplace killings accounted for 2 percent of all homicide-suicides in old and young.
- 85 percent of older perpetrators and 87 percent of younger perpetrators used firearms.

Clinical Patterns of Spousal Homicide-Suicide

The motivations for spousal homicide-suicide are complex. Although some investigators have argued that these are extended suicidal processes in which relationships have been loving, empirical data are lacking. Depression and other forms of psychopathology in the perpetrator play an important role as well as relationship variables such as a strong attachment to the victim, marital and family conflict, caregiving burden, a pending separation such as a move to a long-term care residence, and other life event stressors (Malphurs and Cohen 2005).

There are at least three types of spousal/consortial homicide-suicide: dependent-protective, symbiotic, and aggressive (Cohen 2000). A common feature of all three is the perpetrator's perception of separation as an unacceptable threat to the integrity of the relationship.

Half of all spousal/consortial homicide-suicides are the dependent-protective subtype. The husband-perpetrator, usually two to four years older than his wife, may or may not have a serious illness. In most circumstances, however, he is caring for a wife who is chronically ill. There is evidence of serious depression—including helplessness, hopelessness, and vital exhaustion—which in most circumstances has gone undetected and untreated despite frequent medical care contacts. Most of these men have seen a physician within a few weeks of committing the homicide-suicide.

Dependent-protective homicide-suicides are not impulsive acts. The men who commit these acts have usually thought about or planned the act for months or sometimes more than a year. Although illness, age, depression, and other life stressors may be predisposing factors, a real or perceived decline in the perpetrator's physical health and discussions about, or a pending move to, a nursing home or assisted-living residence are precipitating factors.

Caregiving responsibilities over time appear to cause significant strain and depression in perpetrators of a dependent-protective homicide-suicide (Malphurs and Cohen 2005). These men are consistently described by surviving family and friends as having dominant or controlling personalities. Thus, depression and helplessness, coupled with a perceived inability to manage the situation, to make the wife better, or to protect her appear to be significant risk factors for homicide-suicide.

Available data indicate that many older women who are killed may not be knowing or willing participants. Most wives are shot in their sleep or in the back of the head or chest. It appears that most homicide-suicides involving older spouses and consorts are the result of unilateral decisions by men with controlling personalities with no evidence from surviving informants that the homicide victim had spoken about wanting to be dead or to be killed.

The symbiotic subtype accounts for 20 percent of older homicide-suicides. In these cases, the male perpetrator tends to be a few years older than the victim, and both the husband and wife are sick. There is no suicide note signed by either party, and there is no evidence that this was a pact. However, neighbors and/or family members have reported that both persons had talked about wanting to die or being better off dead.

One-third of older homicide-suicides are the aggressive subtype, in which there is a history of verbal and/or physical conflict and/or domestic violence. The male perpetrators are usually 9 to 10 years older than their victims. Neither the perpetrator nor victim has a physical illness. What usually triggers the homicide-suicide is the victim talking or making plans about separation, divorce, or moving out of the home. The homicide is usually a surprise, is usually violent, and often the victim is shot or stabbed multiple times.

Intervention and Prevention

Because older perpetrators have usually thought about the act for a long time, there is a window of opportunity for the prevention of a homicide-suicide. Clinicians should assess the risk for homicide-suicide in all older patients when the following factors exist: (1) the patient has been married for a long time, and one or both members of the couple have real or perceived health problems; (2) there is evidence or reports of domestic conflict, discord, violence, the existence of a restraining order, or a pending separation or divorce; and/or (3) there is a history of ideation about suicide, homicide, or violence.

In the case of dependent-protective and symbiotic homicide-suicides, the older couple has been married a long time; they appear to be interdependent on each other; and the husband has a dominant, commanding, or controlling personality. The wife is usually sick, frail, and chronically or terminally ill. The husband is usually the primary caregiver (even when others give some assistance) and is depressed. Results from a recent case control study of older married men who committed suicide and those who committed a homicide-suicide show that the men who committed suicide were care recipients in contrast to the homicide-suicide perpetrators, who were caregivers (Malphurs and Cohen 2005).

Because the male is usually the perpetrator and a caregiver, it is essential to query the wife, if possible, during medical care contacts and to evaluate the husband for depression and other psychiatric problems. Assessment can be complicated because the potential victim rather than the potential perpetrator may be the patient, and the perpetrator may resist an evaluation.

Clinicians should consider administering brief depression screening instruments (chapter 3) to both parties while couples are sitting in the waiting room. If possible they should meet with the wife alone and inquire about changes in the husband's behavior such as increased anxiety and agitation, giving possessions away, talk of feeling helpless or hopeless or of being too exhausted to go on, crying, and/or difficulty sleeping or sleeping too much. Has the couple has been fighting? Have there been discussions about divorce, a history of estrangement, or threats to harm her?

Ask whether there are guns and ammunition in the house or whether the husband is considering buying them. Inquire whether the husband has given a house key to a neighbor, friend, or attorney. Talk with adult children and other caregivers such as home-health aides about any threats. It is not uncommon for the perpetrator to tell children or close relatives, "There is something I must do." Although adult children may suspect suicide, a homicide-suicide is usually not part of the equation for them.

Women rarely commit a homicide-suicide, but the wish to kill a spouse and themselves is not uncommon. Although women caregivers have a greater prevalence of depression, most older women have had little experience with guns, the most common method for a homicide-suicide, and their approach to caregiving is less task-focused than men and more emotion-focused. When older husbands or wives express homicidal and suicidal ideation or talk about a specific method to kill themselves and their spouse, it is essential to take the threat seriously.

There are several situations in which the danger of homicide-suicide is especially high: the period before and after a move to a long-term care residence; circumstances during which an individual is spending days at the hospital bedside of a terminally ill spouse or in which the spouse is about to be discharged from the hospital to a nursing home, hospice, or home; and situations in which a person has been spending most of their waking hours for months or more with a spouse who is institutionalized. It is important for staff members in health care facilities to be aware that these are high-risk periods and to talk with the patient, spouse-caregiver, and other family members about it. In many cases, men have told one or more adult children of their intentions, and the children were too embarrassed to tell anyone.

The strong evidence of undetected and untreated depression in almost all perpetrators of homicide-suicides and the existence of domestic violence in one-third of older homicide-suicides emphasize the importance of careful interviews when one or both spouses are in the acute or long-term care system. Interventions should include intensive treatment of depression and other psychiatric problems when appropriate, removal of guns or other lethal weapons, social support for spouses and families in caregiving situations, and appropriate interventions to deal with marital conflict—especially when the woman is a potential victim of aggressive, lethal behavior.

Intervention is complicated and should be done on a case-by-case basis. Separating the perpetrator and victim and arranging for respite care are usually appropriate to diffuse the tension, protect the victim, and help the caregiver. A careful clinical plan is essential, however, because separation is often the trigger for violence. Finally, clinical staff and family members as well as individuals who have continuing contact with older people—clergy, senior center staff, home health care staff, and others—should be educated about warning signs and trained to ask questions and seek appropriate help. The Department of Justice maintains a website with resources for homicide-suicides associated with domestic violence (www.ojp.usdoj.gov/nij/topics/crime/intimate-partner-violence/murder-suicide.htm).

The Impact of Violent Deaths on the Family and Community

Sudden, messy, and violent deaths have a significant, devastating impact on family members and family relationships as well as on the communities where they occur. It is common for family members, whom Spungen (1998) refers to as co-victims, to be hurt, angry, grief-stricken, and almost emotionally paralyzed; they are at risk of developing depressive and anxiety disorders. The suddenness of the violence, the public nature of these tragedies, and the inability to fathom how this could happen often irrevocably transforms the family.

After a violent death(s), family members have many natural reactions, and some are likely to last a long time:

- Persistent thoughts about the deceased
- Visualization of the bodies and the crime scene
- Strong desires for things to be the way they were before
- Mixed feelings of anxiety, anger, sadness, and numbness
- Withdrawal from others
- Memory problems and difficulty thinking
- Sleep disturbances
- Shame and embarrassment
- Self-blame and guilt
- A desire for help but an inability to ask for it
- Inability to talk about feelings and what happened

A violent death may provoke every conceivable human emotion: shock, numbness, anger, fear, anxiety, guilt, shame, and pain. It is natural for survivors to be angry with the perpetrator. Many say they can perhaps understand that a father or grandfather would kill himself, but they believe that it is unacceptable to kill a wife, sister, or other relative. Some family members describe the anger as so intense and uncontrollable that it scares them, because they have never felt this way before. Anger toward the perpetrator can be intense and last a long time. Some family members report that their anger is confusing; it is a combination of anger toward the deceased, anger coupled with guilt because they should have seen it coming, and anger combined with shame that this happened in the family. Some family members fight, often blaming each other for not seeing the signs or not recognizing the depression. This is common among siblings as well as adult children of the deceased. Feelings of anger and rage are normal. Co-victims frequently vent their anger on people around them—family, friends, law enforcement officers, and professionals working with the family. Anger is an emotional response to block painful emotions, and getting angry is a way to get rid of the tension, anxiety, guilt, hurt, and frustration.

The grief can be overwhelming. Shock, sadness, and confusion may last for weeks, months, or longer. It is not uncommon for co-victims to cry uncontrollably, to become irritable or angry and even scream and rage, to feel helpless and hopeless, and to withdraw from others. The immediate grief is only the beginning of the experience, and family members often experience a roller coaster of emotions, sometimes a year and often more after the incident has occurred.

Family members will often benefit from counseling, psychotherapy, family therapy, and support groups. Questions every co-victim asks are, "Why did this happen?" or "Why did this happen to me?" or "Why did Dad kill Mom?" or "What could I have done to prevent it?" There are usually no certain answers to these questions. Even when the deceased perpetrator and victim have had a history of arguments and domestic violence, these same questions arise. With two or more parties deceased, family members often obsess about circumstances leading to the violent death or blame one another for not being aware of the pending violence. Clinicians need to be aware of the impact of these traumatic events and keep in mind that a suicide is a risk factor for further suicides in family members. Judicious monitoring and intervention, if necessary, is indicated.

Guilt and shame are also common emotions. Guilt, like anger, is a normal reaction. Self-blame can be adaptive in the early phases of grief because it allows the individual to make some sense of what happened, but if it goes on too long, it interferes with mourning. Even the most competent and resourceful individuals can be devastated by violence and suddenness of these occurrences. It is not a sign of personal weakness to feel these emotions, to be incapacitated by them, and to reach out for help. In these circumstances, clinicians have several responsibilities:

• Being supportive and listening carefully
• Urging family members to seek psychological help
• Assessing short-term problems, such as employment leave, and financial and legal issues
• Assessing long-term risks such as depressive and anxiety disorders
• Referring family members to appropriate resources and professionals

The journey from co-victim to survivor is a long and difficult one as those left behind struggle to rebuild their lives. Mental health professionals have a powerful role to help individuals heal themselves—forgive the perpetrator, forgive themselves, make sense of the chaos and violence, and find meaning and pleasure in the future.

19

Disasters and Terrorism

Major disasters, mass violence, and terrorism have affected communities throughout the United States and abroad, but disaster research programs began to evolve only after World War II, partly as a response to the consequences of the bombings in Japan. An extensive literature documents the emotional and behavioral after-effects of natural disasters and human-caused disasters, but comparatively little is known about the psychological impact of terrorist attacks and mass casualty attacks (Bonger et al. 2006). Documentation of effective mental health interventions in response to all forms of disasters, mass violence, and terrorism is limited, but consensus about best practices is beginning to emerge (Ritchie et al. 2004; BD Stein et al. 2004; Everly et al. 2008; Patterson 2009).

Contemporary concerns about people's vulnerability to disasters and terrorism are leading to concerted efforts to prepare and intervene. Resources include, but are not limited to, a SAMHSA training manual (DHSS 2004a), a WHO report (Van Ommeren et al. 2005), and consensus recommendations developed by the National Voluntary Organizations Active in Disaster (Everly et al. 2008) for the continuum of specialized mental health services. SAMHSA maintains a Disaster Technical Assistance Center (http://mentalhealth .samhsa.gov/dtac/dialogue/Issue4_09.asp). Several reviews provide useful clinical and ethical guidelines for physicians (Fetter 2005; Braga et al. 2008). The American Association of Geriatric Psychiatry maintains a listing of Internet disaster relief resources for professionals (www.aagpgpa.org/prof/disaster.asp).

Many environmental, psychosocial, cultural, economic, and health variables mediate the impact of disasters and terrorism on all age groups (Norris et al. 2002a, b). Older people

are likely to be more vulnerable than younger adults to physical and interpersonal consequences, including displacement from their home, injury or death of family members, and loss of access to medical, pharmacy, and community services (Fernandez et al. 2002; Sanders et al. 2003; L Brown et al. 2006). The available information suggests that mental health interventions may be particularly important for older adults who are socially isolated, frail, chronically ill, or cognitively impaired. However, the greater population of older persons may be more resilient than the general population because of a lifetime of experiences in dealing with psychological trauma (L Brown et al. 2006; Cohen and Kallimanis-King 2010).

Improving the preparedness of, and developing a prompt emergency response for, this population should be a priority in disaster plans (Sakauye et al. 2009). Two major reports published by the Institute of Medicine gave almost no consideration to older adults (IOM 2003a, 2005). However, following the devastation caused by Hurricane Katrina in 2005, the American Association of Geriatric Psychiatry (AAGP) convened a Disaster Preparedness Task Force (Sakauye et al. 2009). During Katrina, 74 percent of the deaths were people age 60 or older, and half were age 75 or older. More than 56 percent (5,846) of the people who went to the New Orleans Astrodome were age 65 or older (Dyer et al. 2008). After the storm, the mortality rate for older people was higher than that for younger age groups. The impact of Katrina also significantly increased rates of mental health problems and suicidality, reported to be more than 60 percent above the levels of previous years. The AAGP's position statement emphasized the vulnerability of frail and cognitively older persons and recommended disaster preparedness services and research priorities to meet the needs of older Americans.

This chapter (1) reviews what is known about the psychological and behavioral consequences of disasters and terrorism on older adults; (2) identifies the challenges of responding to the needs of older persons and their families in the community; (3) examines the special vulnerabilities of long-term care residents; (4) describes strategies to assess the vulnerabilities and mental health risks of various older populations; and (5) provides an overview of interventions.

There are several valuable web-based resources: emergency and disaster preparedness for special populations, including older adults, maintained by the National Institutes of Health National Library of Medicine (http://sis.nlm.nih .gov/outreach/specialpopulationsanddisasters .html); and a disaster mental health and human services training manual maintained by SAMHSA's National Mental Health Information Center (http://mentalhealth.samhsa.gov/ publications/allpubs/ADM90-538/tmsection3 .asp). A consortium of Geriatric Education Centers created curricula and training for bioterrorism and emergency preparedness in aging (BTEPA) and made recommendations for clinical practice, policy, and research (Johnson et al. 2006).

The Psychological Impact of Disasters and Terrorism

Age is one of many risk factors that mediate the severity of adverse consequences associated with disasters (Norris et al. 2002a, 2002b; Ferraro 2003; Deeg et al. 2005). Children are the most vulnerable to severe mental health problems, and middle-aged persons, 40–60 years, sustain more adverse effects than individuals age 60 or older, who are more resilient.

Terrorist attacks are similar in many characteristics to natural and human-caused disasters. These traumatic events occur suddenly and unexpectedly, and while the magnitude of the violence adversely affects a defined population, repercussions are often widespread. Such attacks disturb or destroy human lives and families as well as social structures and dynamics, threatening the integrity of organizations and the functioning of communities and larger geographic areas, even those not directly affected (Fullerton et al. 2003; IOM 2003a). Every aspect of community life may be affected, which in turn disrupts individuals' support systems. Homes, worksites, hospitals, long-term care facilities, educational institutions, and emergency responder operations may have been destroyed, and large numbers of people may be injured, sick, or dead.

The immediate consequences of a terrorist attack cause many powerful emotional reactions in adults of all ages: shock and disbelief, apprehension about future attacks, anxiety, anger, and the need to reconnect with family, pets, neighbors, and friends. Most healthy older persons will cope with the immediate emergencies, but there are populations at high risk for negative consequences: persons who are socially isolated, frail, chronically ill, or cognitively impaired or who have a history of psychiatric illness or exposure to an extreme and prolonged traumatic stressor. Older persons who require medications as well as other medical procedures and devices may also be vulnerable.

An empirical analysis of 177 articles describing 130 different samples, made up of 60,000 persons who experienced 80 different events, reviewed the range, magnitude, and duration of effects of natural disasters and mass violence (Norris et al. 2002a). Victims/survivors of natural disasters, technological disasters, and mass violence experienced a high prevalence of psychiatric disorders, physical health problems, disrupted psychosocial functioning, and diminished resilience.

Psychiatric distress and disorders are more prominent after human-caused than natural disasters, especially when there is widespread damage and a high prevalence of injury and death (Norris et al. 2001). In general, disasters caused by malicious human intent are more disturbing than either human-made or natural disasters (Norris et al. 2001; Beaton and Murphy 2002). In these circumstances, there may be a greater need for mental health services to prevent serious and pervasive mental health problems.

Several factors mediate the likelihood and severity of negative psychological outcomes, including post-traumatic stress disorder (PTSD) (Creamer and Parslow 2008). Individuals who perceive being at risk for death or injury and those who are temporally or geographically close to the event are at higher risk for adverse consequences. Personal injury and physical harm, exposure to dead or mutilated bodies, and the violent, sudden death of family, friends, or co-workers are potent mediators of both acute traumatic stress disorder and PTSD. Although the type and severity of catastrophic disasters influence psychological outcomes, the premorbid existence of psychiatric symptoms is the best overall predictor of long-term maladaptive psychosocial functioning (Knight et al. 2000).

The Resilience of Older Persons

Resilience refers to the process of adapting successfully to stressful circumstances such as illness(s), difficult life experiences, misfortunes, and traumatic events (Rutter 1987). Resilience involves a dynamic biopsychosocial interaction of attitudes, attributions, cognitions, behaviors, and physiologic responsivity that mediate effective coping with adversity. Although resilient individuals are not immune to emotional distress, they are flexible, able to modify their thinking and behavior under stress, and can return to their prior level of functioning relatively quickly.

Older adults have an extensive background of life experiences that influences their vulnerability or resilience following exposure to traumas. Resilient older adults have several characteristics: optimism about the future, a sense of personal mastery, the ability to use cognitive and behavioral rather than emotional strategies to cope, and an ability to find some deeper meaning in the experience (APA 2002a). These qualities allow older individuals to minimize the negative influences of the stress by proactive thoughts, feelings, and actions.

Although older adults tend to be resilient in the face of life challenges, including disasters, some older adults, such as Holocaust survivors, former prisoners of war, and persons exposed to interpersonal violence or abuse as children or adults, may be particularly vulnerable (Green et al. 2000; Port et al. 2001, 2002; Bleich et al. 2005). Exposure to extreme, prolonged stress may result in permanent developmental effects that increase vulnerability to future traumatic events throughout the lifespan.

The Impact of 9/11 on Older People

An estimated 6,300 residents age 65 or older lived within several blocks of the World Trade Center, site of the terrorist attacks of September 11, 2001, and at least 18,000 lived in neighborhoods close by which were also affected by the attacks (Salerno and Nagy 2002). Police barricades blocked these neighborhoods for several weeks after the attack, contributing to many problems in providing emergency assistance to older residents, including inadequately coordinated community services, the absence of a system to identify and locate older adults, and the lack of mechanisms to convey pertinent information. Emergency organizations such as the Federal Emergency Management Agency (FEMA) and the American Red Cross were not prepared to assist older and disabled people living near Ground Zero. For more than a week after the attacks, large numbers of racially diverse older people were still unidentified and neglected in their homes (Chen et al. 2003; Strug et al. 2003; Chung 2004).

Breakdowns in communication, the most immediate problem, significantly affected older people. Telephone and television cables were destroyed as the towers fell. Few older people had cell phones, available phone lines were jammed, the electricity was out, and televisions, nonbattery radios, and computers could not be used. Mail and newspaper delivery were discontinued, making it difficult for many older people to find out what was happening as well as to contact family, friends, and health care providers.

Isolation was another serious issue. Most of the older population lived alone or with an older spouse, and those who were ill, frail, or cognitively impaired remained isolated in their homes. They were located only after relief workers and volunteers canvassed the neighborhoods door to door in the second week after the attacks. Immediate responders were overwhelmed, and access avenues such as bridges, tunnels, and airports were closed. Many Manhattan agencies that provided home and community-based services did not have disaster plans for their older clients or staff, and personnel could not get through police barricades or telephone their clients. It was several weeks before agencies were able to obtain the necessary permits to be in these areas, but many staff members were hesitant or afraid to enter what could have been a contaminated area.

Consequently, many older persons were found with little or no food and water, and others needed medications and emergency medical care. Older adults who were not affiliated with a community service agency or registered with the county for special needs shelters were at risk for not receiving services from emergency providers. Many had resisted pre-enrolling in programs designed to identify vulnerable adults, fearing they might be forced to move from their home to a long-term care facility.

Various city agencies held meetings shortly after the events of 9/11, resulting in a report that described shortcomings in the existing emergency response system and presented a disaster response plan to meet the needs of older residents more effectively (O'Brien 2003). Two important conclusions emerged: (1) community-dwelling older adults, frail and homebound persons, and older adults living in long-term care facilities had distinctively different needs; and (2) current emergency response plans did not adequately address those differences. The special disaster considerations for long-term care facilities and home health agencies included the level of care and assistance needed by patients or residents, medical resources and equipment required to provide care, and the ability of residents to assist themselves or others during a disaster.

Older adults have significant difficulties recovering after a disaster (Brennan et al. 2004).

Water, food, medications, and a safe place to live are the initial priorities, followed by mental health interventions and financial assistance, but many older adults may not be in a position to benefit from these interventions. Their ability to cope is mitigated by many factors, including feelings of stigma about receiving help, fears of losing entitlements, and cultural and literacy barriers. Some older adults may be reluctant to accept assistance from governmental agencies or may find completion of the paperwork required to receive aid daunting. Some may be more willing to receive assistance from the Salvation Army, Red Cross, or church groups than from governmental agencies. Penner (2003) recommended that mental health crisis workers be knowledgeable about existing service providers and provide older adults with assistance in identifying organizations to help with disaster response and recovery.

In an ideal world, home health aides would continue to provide daily care during disaster evacuations and accompany frail older adults to temporary or long-term shelters. However, the probability of service interruptions to the homebound is high. A survey of New York City public health nurses attending an emergency preparedness program revealed that 90 percent of the attendees reported at least one barrier (i.e., family responsibilities, transportation problems, and personal health issues) to their ability to report for duty in the event of an emergency (Qureshi et al. 2002).

Priorities in the Assessment of Older Adults

A sudden, threatening, traumatic event induces fear, helplessness, and vulnerability in everyone affected, but when an older person already feels susceptible because of impaired health, mobility, or sensory and cognitive abilities, the feelings of powerlessness and helplessness can be overwhelming. Unexpected evacuations from nursing homes, assisted living facilities, senior living communities, or trailer parks or moves from one facility to another can be frightening experiences causing disorientation, confusion, and anxiety. Cognitive and sensory impairments usually make it harder for older persons to understand evacuation instructions and emergency assistance information, cope with a chaotic environment, and respond to emergency workers and friends who want to assist them (Massey 1997). Social support is often mobilized when an older person's life or health is threatened after a natural disaster, but assistance is less available when property is damaged or destroyed, electricity or telephone communication is lost, or daily routines are disrupted (Kaniasty and Norris 1993).

The deaths of children or grandchildren in disaster situations are among the most difficult situations for older persons not only because of the unexpected, violent death of a loved one but also because a sense of the continuity of the family, including traditions and legacies, is lost. Family support and contact with older relatives may decrease in the immediate aftermath of a tragedy as everyone in the family and community is consumed with the struggle to deal with immediate losses, injuries, and deaths. When family support is less available, it is common for older persons, especially those who have health problems, to fear being moved into an institution, which causes them to withhold concerns, difficulties, and emotional reactions.

The psychological effects of severe violence and mass trauma have not been well studied in the older population (Cook et al. 2001). Older persons who are geographically distant from the attack appear to recover faster than younger adults, but the recovery rate for persons in affected areas will vary, depending on the many circumstances discussed previously. Although older adults may not meet the full diagnostic criteria for PTSD or other anxiety disorders, they may manifest clinical symptoms that interfere with biopsychosocial functioning (subthreshold PTSD). The literature suggests that a small group of older persons will develop full-blown PTSD, but the prevalence of more widespread subsyndromal PTSD could be a serious consequence of mass disasters.

The few studies that have examined the prevalence of PTSD in older adults suggest that often it is not identified or is incorrectly diagnosed (Davidson 2001; Port et al. 2001). Some researchers have hypothesized that older adults are not diagnosed because they do not consider their post-trauma difficulties abnormal since friends and family are experiencing similar problems. Furthermore, because PTSD often co-occurs with other illnesses, clinicians may misdiagnose symptoms as alcoholism, depression, or anxiety disorders.

Assessment of Risk

The clinical challenge is to distinguish between normal and abnormal reactions to terrorism and disasters. Older adults should be screened to identify risk factors for developing PTSD. Some factors that increase an individual's risk, such as a history of significant traumatic stressors or a psychiatric history, cannot be altered; whereas other factors, such as loss of resources and social support, can be modified by interventions. Given the high prevalence of psychiatric comorbidity, assessment for depression and other psychiatric symptoms and disorders is necessary.

Clinicians should include the following areas in risk assessment:

- Extent of preparedness for terrorism or disaster (e.g., food, water, medications, radio, information, shelter)
- Health status and frailty
- Disability
- Mobility
- Cultural background
- Previous exposure to serious trauma
- Religious beliefs
- Proximity of family members
- Injury or death of family members from the violence
- Availability of other social supports
- Exposure to weather, extreme fatigue
- Exposure to toxic contamination

- Living situation
- Availability of transportation and communication

Older adults rarely access mental health services after a disaster (L Brown et al. 2006). Following 9/11, the visits of patients already in therapy increased dramatically, but there was no significant increase in mental health visits by adults, young or old, who were not previously receiving mental health care, despite the availability of free services (Boscarino et al. 2004). Older adults usually look to religious leaders, family member and friends, or their personal physician to deal with emotional distress.

Intervention Strategies
Primary Exposure

Crisis intervention services are effective in delivering emergency mental health care to individuals and groups. Clinicians should allow people to talk when ready, validate their emotional reactions, avoid diagnostic language, and communicate person to person rather than expert to victim. The American Psychological Association (2002) suggests several levels of intervention for older persons, including building resilience with psychosocial and behavioral support, therapeutic interventions for persons who have psychopathology, and using older persons as resources in the community to cope with community needs and restore normalcy. The timely delivery of appropriate treatment is imperative following the acute crisis phase to lessen the risks for acute stress disorder, PTSD, and other forms of anxiety and depressive disorders. Although older persons are at low risk for mental health problems, those who do develop serious psychiatric distress may go unrecognized, untreated, or inadequately treated after a terrorist attack.

Older people themselves can do many things to build their resilience and increase their preparedness for disaster or terrorism. These include, but are not limited to, education about normal reactions to disaster, maintaining routines as much as possible, focusing on self-care, engaging in pleasurable activities, staying connected to family and friends, talking with others about feelings, writing a journal or diary, reaching out for help if needed, prioritizing problems, developing a concrete plan of what needs to be done, volunteering, and examining personal strengths and finding personal meaning in the experience. All of these straightforward strategies are essential to dealing with the immediate and short-term aftermath of mass disaster.

Secondary Exposure

The events of 9/11 caused horror and emotional distress in most television viewers, and research targeting the impact of media broadcasting and print stories on traumatic stress in individuals not present at the actual event revealed a dose-response effect: those who watched the most television coverage reported higher levels of distress, and people who lost friends or family were the most vulnerable (Ahern et al. 2002). Older adults in both community and institutional settings were more likely to watch television coverage for extended periods of time. Because the magnitude of the attack was so catastrophic and horrifying, it elicited strong reactions that increased retention of information, even in persons who had dementia (Budson et al. 2004).

A study investigating memory and emotions among older adults regarding the events of 9/11 showed that patients who had dementia were more likely to remember personal information (e.g., how they heard the news) than factual information (e.g., details of the attack) compared to those who had mild cognitive impairment or to those who were cognitively intact. They did not differ in the level of emotional intensity (i.e., sadness, anger fear, frustration, confusion, and shock) to the terrorist attacks (Budson et al. 2004).

Challenge for the Future

A number of catastrophic events have increased concerns about the vulnerabilities of older adults. A series of named hurricanes, the tsunami in Southeast Asia, tornados in the Midwest, and heightened fears of terrorist attacks in the United States and abroad have raised concerns about susceptibility and the need for response planning and preparation for disasters and terrorism. The disastrous aftermath of Hurricane Katrina demonstrated the inadequacy of preparations and responses by all branches of city, state, and federal governments as well as the heightened vulnerability of older people, who had the highest casualty rate of any age group (Dyer et al. 2008). This finding of heightened vulnerability, also reported in other studies of disasters, is likely a function of impaired mobility and sensory impairments that contribute to heightened risk (Fernandez et al. 2002).

Nursing home residents are at very high risk in a disaster. Before a series of major hurricanes in the Gulf Coast since 2004, few long-term care administrators knew about the emergency support functions within their states. Decision-making criteria were absent for resident evacuation, and communication systems were usually compromised. The relocation and tracking of residents was not planned, and many frail and cognitively impaired nursing home residents were lost because there was no patient identification system. Preparedness guides were conspicuous by their absence.

In advance of the 2006 hurricane season, planning for preparation, response, and recovery were accelerated. Federal officials from the Center for Medicare and Medicaid Services, Department of Health and Human Services, Department of Homeland Security, Department of Defense, and Federal Emergency Management Agency, as well as representatives from foundations, professional organizations, health care institutions, and state agencies focused on strengthening the infrastructure of long-term care facilities to minimize stressful evacuations and improve policies and procedures for resident safety. These policies included a management structure and process for long-term care services, creation of decision-making rules for facilities similar to those of hospitals, planning for effective communica-

tion systems in the likelihood of a breakdown in services, and tracking residents, especially those who are frail or cognitively impaired.

Several measures have been developed to identify and manage vulnerable older populations. The Seniors Without Family Team (SWIFT) triage was developed by a Houston team working in the Texas astrodome with about 20,000 Katrina evacuees who were older, frail, and in poor health (Dyer et al. 2008). The Impact of Event Scale—Revised (IEC-R) is a self-report questionnaire to screen for PTSD following a traumatic event. It is reported to discriminate between traumatized and nontraumatized groups along different dimensions of stressors (Christiansen and Marren 2009).

The challenge to mental health professionals and trained volunteers is to find a balance in responding to the special needs of vulnerable populations and supporting the resiliency of others in affected communities. Responding professionals need to be trained to understand that older adults who have mental health problems are responsive to psychotherapies, group therapies, counseling, and psychotropic medications when necessary (APA 2002). Older adults appear to be more willing to accept help on many levels from families or in familiar settings, including senior centers and religious institutions. However, older persons may be especially reluctant, ashamed, or embarrassed to admit and discuss mental health problems, given the mass devastation, injury, and deaths in the aftermath of disaster.

Education to decrease misattribution of somatic symptoms and increase acceptance of mental health treatment is essential. Effective screening measures need to be validated with older adult populations so that those at risk for psychopathology after a disaster can be quickly and accurately identified. Programs to reduce the stigma and enhance the attractiveness of mental health interventions need to be developed. Following acts of terrorism, intervention should focus on building a recovery environment that restores social supports and normalcy.

Although exposure to traumatic stressors can be hazardous to an individual's psychological well-being, times of crisis may lead to personal growth. Gerald Caplan, the founder of modern crisis intervention, argued that crisis is a necessary precursor to growth (Caplan 1961). The coping process, a time when an individual strives for equilibrium or stability in response to a stressor, provides a venue for achieving either a higher or a lower level of functioning than the pre-crisis state and creates a foundation for future development (Brown et al. 2003). This appears to support the data on older persons exposed to mass violence and disasters, who largely show greater resilience and adaptation than middle-aged and younger adults.

The older population is an underused community resource to assist with everything that must be done to help victims and their families, restore normal routines, deliver basic necessities of life, provide child care, and canvas communities (L Brown et al. 2006). Older adults have significant generative roles and responsibilities to assist children and other adults cope with short-term and long-term effects. Indeed, those who have grown older show us by their very existence that there are many ways to survive pain and injury, disease and disability, death, economic loss, war and hatred, as well as every known natural and human-made disaster. Older people are more than role models and teachers for survival; they are also symbols that we shall prevail.

20

End-of-Life Care

More than 80 percent of deaths in the United States occur among persons age 65 or older (Cassel and Foley 1999). Many chronic diseases (e.g., cancer, vascular and pulmonary diseases, and cardiac, renal, and hepatic failure) routinely progress to a point where they cause death. About 90 percent of Medicare beneficiaries die with one or more of these conditions, and many experience emotional and physical pain, which are treatable or preventable with appropriate palliative care. Unfortunately, people who have chronic illness, including the dementias, too often receive less-than-optimal care at the end of life (Mast et al. 2004; Sachs et al. 2004; Chatterjee 2008).

Advances in medical sciences, clinical care, and public health have progressively altered the nature and course of dying. Over the past century, longevity has increased in developed countries, shifting most deaths into later life. Technologies, medications, and clinical procedures are now available to prolong survival, and these interventions can be applied to save lives as well as prolong or postpone dying. As a result, we are now confronted with new and complex ethical dilemmas about end-of-life choices. Increasingly, patients and families are in the position of choosing procedures to sustain or limit terminal care, and cultural issues are potent mediators of choices along with personal preferences and clinical practices (Frank et al. 2008). Although most Americans want to die at home, at least 85 percent die in hospitals and nursing homes, and of this group, 70 percent have chosen to refuse or withhold some forms of life-sustaining intervention (Ahmad and O'Mahoney 2005; Kaufman 2005).

Because many people who are dying are likely to lose the capacity to make decisions about their end-of-life care as they near death,

clinicians should make every effort for them to state their care preferences in advance while they are able to do so. Preferences about future medical treatment may be described in general terms, or specific procedures may be identified as acceptable or unacceptable. There are several ways that individuals declare their wishes: specific physician instructions (e.g., "Do Not Resuscitate") that are placed in their medical files; living wills, documents that detail their requests or prohibit specific interventions; oral statements about care preferences to family members or health care providers; or the appointment of a health care proxy or equivalent (e.g., durable medical power of attorney). The efficacy of these directives may vary depending on the circumstances and availability during a medical emergency.

Clinicians should bring up advance care directives with patients as early as possible and explain specific health care choices. The American Bar Association Commission on Aging website (www.abanet.org/aging/) maintains a listing of downloadable advance care directive forms and information from state bar associations for each state. Because a patient may be in denial or anxious and fearful after a diagnosis and avoid the topic, it is important for the clinician to give her or him time to think about decisions that may lie ahead, to ask questions about what happens with different procedures, and to discuss the benefits and liabilities of various interventions. These topics are best handled in several conversations to help individuals identify their values and preferences, which should be documented in the patient's chart. Discussions regarding funeral/burial plans as well as other arrangements, including organ donation and postmortem examinations, may also be timely. These conversations can help patients and family members deal with denial as well as prevent future conflict about postmortem arrangements.

Clinicians have the responsibility to advise patients and family members about their options and the need to obtain information and resources for putting financial and legal matters in order. Serious illnesses affect more than a person's health. The American Bar Association published a report commissioned by the National Hospice and Palliative Care Organization (NHPCO), *The Legal Guide for the Seriously Ill,* which is an informative resource not only for patients and families but also for health care professionals, service providers, faith-based organizations, and others who work with seriously ill populations (www.caringinfo.org/UserFiles/File/PDFs/ AdvanceCarePlanningLegalIssues/Legal_ Guide_for_Seriously_Ill.pdf).

This chapter reviews the nature of palliative and hospice care, palliative care guidelines, and clinical roles across the continuum of end-of-life care. The evaluation and treatment of individuals and strategies for dealing with pain, depression, suicidality, anxiety, and delirium are also examined, as are guidelines for having discussions with patients and families. One of the more significant decisions to be made concerns the strategy of palliative care. Cultural and religious issues that affect attitudes, beliefs, and practices, as well as the application of individual and family therapies are described. In the final section, advance care planning, withholding life-sustaining treatment, and the controversial issues of terminal sedation, assisted suicide, and euthanasia are discussed, as is end-of-life care for individuals who have dementia.

Palliative Care

The National Hospice and Palliative Care Organization Standards of Practice for Hospice Programs defines palliative care as treatment that enhances comfort and improves the quality of an individual's life during the last phase of life (NHPCO 2007: www.nhpco.org/i4a/ pages/index.cfm?pageid=5308). The test of palliative care lies in the agreement among the individual, physician(s), primary caregiver, and the hospice team that the expected outcome is relief from distressing symptoms, the easing of pain, and/or enhancing the quality of life.

Palliative care is a philosophy of caring without reference to a specific life expectancy, and it includes a number of core assessments and interventions (Ferris et al. 2004; Ferrell et al. 2005; Emanuel and Librach 2007). Palliative care not only includes attending to individuals who are close to death but also refers to a process of ongoing discussions about personal wishes concerning end-of-life care. Ideally, individuals should talk about choices before a serious condition develops as well as early in the course of a grave or life-threatening illness. The dialogue should continue as a patient's circumstances, desires, and wishes change or new care options become available (Larson and Tobin 2000).

Palliative care is suitable for people who have any number of conditions, including cancer, AIDS, congestive heart failure, chronic obstructive pulmonary disease, end-stage organ disease, dementia, and other degenerative diseases. However, the trajectory of change associated with each of the various disease conditions influences the frequency and content of these discussions. For example, the deterioration is usually slow in persons who have Alzheimer disease, amyotrophic lateral sclerosis, motor neuron disease, and some cancers. The clinical course may fluctuate with acute medical crises associated with pulmonary or cardiovascular disease, any one of which might cause death or lead to a partial or full return to functional effectiveness.

Palliative care is also the conceptual basis of hospice care programs, many of which focus on care during the last six months of life (Cassel and Foley 1999; International Association for Hospice and Palliative Care: www.hospicecare .com/manual/principles-main.html). Hospice uses a comprehensive team approach to provide integrated clinical care, pain management, and psychological and religious/spiritual support according to an individual's preferences. The hospice team usually consists of the patient's physician; the hospice physician;

nurses; home health aides; psychologists; social workers; speech, physical, and occupational therapists as needed; clergy or other spiritual counselors; and trained volunteers. Culturally appropriate supportive services, including translators, are also available. Hospice care can be provided at home or at freestanding hospice centers, hospitals, nursing homes, and assisted living facilities. Services are covered under Medicare, Medicaid, most private insurance plans, HMOs, and other managed care organizations. However, there is significant variability in the use of hospice in medical centers well known for their good-quality care of chronic illness (Wennberg et al. 2004) as well as in the use of hospice by minority populations (Washington et al. 2008).

Hospice care was added to Medicare in 1983 for persons in the community who have terminal illness to provide an alternative to curative care at the end of life, to improve the experience of dying, and to reduce costs (Enck 2009). Hospice care was extended to nursing home residents in 1989, and the growth of hospice programs in long-term care settings has been considerable. Most nursing homes contract with hospice agencies, and 87 percent of nursing homes have one or more contracts (Stevenson and Branson 2009). One in five Medicare hospice patients lives in a nursing home (Office of Inspector General 2007). Huskamp and associates (2009) argued that Medicare palliative care coverage needs to be altered based on residents' documented needs rather than physician certification of six-month prognosis, and residents should be allowed to choose care that supports quality of life rather than waive the right to curative treatments.

Hospice programs in the twenty-first century differ from those that evolved in England in the 1960s under the leadership of Dame Cicely Saunders, who opened the first hospice, St. Christopher's, in 1967 (www.stchristophers.org.uk; Clark 2001). The first U.S. hospice, based on the St. Christopher's model, opened as the Connecticut hospice in 1974 (Lack 1978). From its inception, hospice was predominantly a volunteer movement offering palliative care rather than aggressive medical

approaches to postpone death. Some hospice programs have become medicalized and institutionalized, with patients being put on ventilators or feeding tubes, having pacemakers implanted, and receiving blood transfusions, chemotherapy, and cardiopulmonary resuscitation (Syme and Bruce 2009; Field 2010). This transformation of hospice, referred to as open access, means that patients can continue a range of disease-focused treatments financed by Medicare hospice benefits. The open access movement emerged when younger patients who had HIV/AIDS began to enroll in hospice but were unwilling to forgo some aggressive medical treatment, hoping for a breakthrough cure.

The decision to use hospice care is beneficial for most people, because hospice maximizes the interactions between the person who is dying and family members. Programs may be based in institutions, but they are run as quasi-independent clinical operations with nursing aides and physicians trained in palliative care. In recent years, home-based hospice, in which nurses visit daily, has become increasingly popular. Under both arrangements, family members are free to visit and interact with the patient without the restrictions of the usual hospital or nursing home rules.

Clinical Guidelines for Palliative Care

The National Consensus Project for Quality Palliative Care, a consortium of five major palliative care organizations in the United States, established Clinical Practice Guidelines in an effort to maximize good-quality care across the continuum of health care in the United States (NCP 2009). This collaborative initiative evolved out of recommendations of several major publications: several Institute of Medicine reports (Field and Cassel 1999; Field and Behrman 2003); a report by the American Association of Colleges of Nursing (2002); and a report generated by the National Hospice Workgroup, the Hastings Center, and the National Hospice and Palliative Care Organization (Jennings et al. 2003).

The National Consensus Project identified eleven core elements supporting tenets described in the World Health Organization of Palliative Care:

1. Patient populations should include people of all ages who have been diagnosed with a debilitating chronic or life-threatening disease or injury.

2. Care plans should be determined by the goals, values, and preferences of patients and family members, with decision-making assistance from health care professionals.

3. Care begins with diagnosis and continues with regular contact until either the patient's condition improves or the patient dies. Care also includes grief support for the individual and bereavement support for the family.

4. Care is a comprehensive ongoing process of clinical assessment, diagnosis, care planning, interventions, and follow-up.

5. Care is provided by an interdisciplinary team.

6. Care targets the prevention and relief of pain and suffering.

7. Clinicians' effective communication skills are essential for good-quality care.

8. Care is based on specific knowledge and skills and evidence-based standards, when available.

9. Care should be integrated throughout the continuum of health care.

10. Health care teams should ensure equitable access to palliative care.

11. Care services should be evaluated regularly to ensure that the highest-quality care is being provided.

Cultural background usually has profound influences on the ways individuals experience illness, participate in end-of-life decision-making, experience and express grief, participate in palliative care, and follow customs and rituals surrounding dying and death (Krakawer et al. 2002; Crawley 2005; Bosma et al. 2009). Palliative care programs should have procedures to evaluate and document cultural influences that affect the way patients and family members view illness and death, and these beliefs and practices should be integrated into the interdisciplinary team's care plans. Communication is essential, and interpreter services, including signing, should be accessible as needed. Finally, it is essential to accommodate the patient's personal preferences, including language, diet, religious and cultural rituals, and, where desired, the involvement of alternative care practitioners (e.g., healers, shamans).

Making Palliative Care Part of Disease Management Guidelines

The American Hospice Foundation Palliative Care Guidelines Group developed a template for integrating palliative knowledge, skills, and services into existing guidelines for life-threatening diseases (Emanuel and Librach 2007). The template is a guide for developing patterns of palliative practice and not the result of evidence-based data. The group identified core practices that should help clinicians decide to perform a full evaluation of palliative care needs: discussion of the prognosis and impact of the illness on the patient; an assessment of the patient's medical and psychosocial status, spiritual values and needs, family caregivers, and living arrangements; setting goals and revising them as the illness progresses; and family grief and bereavement support and care.

Clinical Roles of Mental Health Professionals

Geriatric mental health professionals have many opportunities to deal with end-of-life issues with patients and family members. The American Psychological Association report on end-of-life care identified five arenas where this can take place: (1) before individuals get sick; (2) during and after diseases are diagnosed and treatments begin; (3) when individuals have a high probability of succumbing to disease because of genetic risk or exposure to a lethal substance; (4) during advanced phases of disease and the process of dying; and (5) after the death of the patient, supporting family and intimates (Haley et al. 2003; www .apa.org/topics/death/end-of-life.aspx).

Before Major Illness Strikes

Older people who are able to invest time and energy in decisions about future end-of-life issues have a greater feeling of control about their lives. Expressing these wishes is important, especially for those who are chronically and seriously ill. Only 15–25 percent of the general population has a living will, although the prevalence is much higher for older adults (Kahana et al. 2004). That number is growing as a result of federal regulations requiring these documents during hospitalizations and surgery.

During and after Diagnosis

The period during which individuals are being diagnosed is often an emotional roller-coaster because of the patient's and family's fears and uncertainty. At this point clinicians can help people understand the diagnosis and how the illness may affect them. In addition to information, people usually need support and guidance to make sense of the diagnosis and prognosis, appreciate their options, and learn and practice effective coping strategies. Home and community-based services, psychosocial supports, and opportunities to communicate treatment preferences to their medical providers and family are essential when possible. This process needs to be tailored to the person's medical and psychological sophistication, family and social supports, personality, cultural background, and gender.

When People Are at Genetic Risk or Are Exposed to Risk

Palliative care specialists regard education and discussions about advance disease planning as important when individuals and family members may be at risk for a life-threatening illness (e.g., HIV/AIDS, breast cancer, Huntington disease). If a person has a significant family history for a life-threatening condition, referral for genetic counseling may be advisable. Likewise, if an individual has engaged in risky sexual behavior or has been exposed to toxic substances, testing and/or referral to a specialist are important. Other interventions may include providing information about the disease, including symptoms to anticipate, and being available for follow-up.

During More Advanced Disease States

As serious illnesses progress to more advanced stages with increasing debilitation and discomfort, care plans may need to shift from cure-oriented therapies to managing the disease and symptoms. This is frequently a period of difficult adjustment for patients, family members, and significant others, including clinicians, who may see this as a defeat and react accordingly, even to the point of withdrawal. Fortunately, a great deal can be done to provide support, including behavioral and psychosocial interventions as well as religious and spiritual support, to help patients and others cope with anticipatory grief and emotional distress. As symptoms increase and become more debilitating, pain control and the detection and treatment of depression, anxiety, and delirium become critical aspects of care. The clinician should anticipate increasing support for those close to the patient.

Emanuel and Emanuel's (1998) framework for "a good death" identifies six dimensions of patients' experiences for intervention: (1) physical symptoms; (2) psychological and cognitive symptoms; (3) social relationships and support; (4) economic and caregiving needs; (5) hopes and expectations; and (6) religious, spiritual, and existential beliefs. Unfortunately, many of these needs, all of which can be dealt with successfully, are frequently unmet. Estimates are that 20–70 percent of patients who are dying experience inadequate pain relief, more than 33 percent are depressed, and 35 percent have unmet emotional needs (Bradley et al. 2000).

Families caring for dying relatives are at risk for mental health problems, disruption of work/life, and even increased mortality (Boerner and Schultz 2009). Spouses caring for patients in hospice who have lung cancer report an average of more than 120 caregiving hours per week. Haley and colleagues (2001, 2003) found that spouses caring for terminally ill patients who had lung cancer or dementia showed rates of depression about three times higher than observed in non-caregiving populations. Hospice care is associated with greater caregiver satisfaction with end-of-life care, lower anxiety while caregiving, and lower depression after the patient has died (Abernethy et al. 2009).

Talking with Patients and Family Members

Effective communication and a positive relationship are essential for achieving beneficial outcomes from the beginning of a serious or life-threatening illness through the final stages of dying. The clinician should begin the initial discussion with open-ended queries to clarify the individual's personal values and priorities, personality style, and perspectives on family, illness, pain and suffering, and medical treatments, as well as dying and death in a culturally sensitive manner. It is critical to communicate at least four important messages empathically and clearly: (1) understanding of the patient's values, beliefs, and needs; (2) respect for the patient's wishes; (3) commitment to be available and supportive; and (4) commitment not to abandon the patient or family.

There are many challenges in the ongoing dialogue with patients and their families: delivering bad news, preparing individuals for the course of illness and possible changes in symptoms, assisting with decision-making about care options, dealing with ambiguity, and answering questions and titrating information in a way that is honest, supportive, and compassionate (Parker et al. 2007; Brunnhuber et al. 2008).

Delivering Bad News

As the patient's condition deteriorates and complications develop, the clinician needs to give the patient and family members relevant facts in ways that maintain or enhance the therapeutic alliance and partnership (Ammann and Baumgartner 2005; Thistlethwaite 2009). When the information to be communicated is unequivocally serious, making a statement up

front that there is bad news and asking the patient whether she or he wants to talk at that time is a way to assess the person's preparedness to talk. When the health information is less dire but not definitive, such as test results, a neutral question is appropriate, such as "I have the results of the last blood tests. Would you like to talk about them now?"

Clinical Course of Symptoms

Throughout the course of the illness, the clinician must evaluate the patient's symptoms and personal needs to develop therapeutic and palliative care plans. The severity and nature of any pain, physical and emotional symptoms, and changes in functional status should be monitored regularly. However, there are a number of barriers to this process. Patients may not admit to certain symptoms because they do not believe that these can be treated. They may be afraid that revealing symptoms will be signs of serious problems and lead to more "bad news." Building an alliance with older adults is important not only to be supportive but also to create a trusting environment in which to elicit symptoms and the subjective experience of the illness. The clinician may need to involve family members, fictive kin, and other knowledgeable informants, when available, to assess symptoms and symptom history in dying persons who have dementia or delirium.

Mental health professionals may need to play the role of intermediary between the physician(s) providing the medical/surgical management and the patient/family, especially in hospital settings. Some treating physicians may view discussions about the patient's clinical state as relieving their feelings of carrying an uncomfortable burden, whereas other physicians may see the mental health professional as interfering. Being available to the patient and family is optimal for care, whereas communicating with attending clinicians is an obligation. Fortunately, rejection of assistance from mental health professionals is rare, but as much as possible the mental health clinician must accommodate the needs of the patient and family.

Decision-making

Patients and family members face many decisions, including:

• Decisions about starting and continuing treatments that may slow the disease process and extend life but also have a high probability of causing pain and discomfort
• Decisions about whether to challenge a physician's judgment that the patient is dying, to seek a second opinion, and to continue or start other disease-focused interventions
• Decisions about emergency procedures (e.g., mechanical ventilation, cardiopulmonary resuscitation)
• Decisions to enter hospice care

Clinicians are responsible for initiating discussions about advanced disease planning. Although they need to be sensitive and supportive, they must also be direct. Patients and families are entitled to timely information that is accurate and comprehensible in order to examine competing options and reach decisions consistent with the patient's values and preferences.

When clinicians share information, they must consider the individual's right to privacy. Some patients may insist on withholding dire information to protect others (e.g., spouse, children). In most instances, clinicians should encourage patients to be open with family members on the premise that open communication facilitates support and quality of personal and family life. In all instances, however, clinical staff members are bound by the patient's wishes.

The context that clinicians use to deliver information, their choice of words, tone of voice, attitude, and time allotted to be with the patient, all affect the therapeutic liaison. When patients are deliberating over interventions to prolong their death rather than life, they may elect palliative care instead of life-extending care, provided they can accurately understand the prognosis or appreciate the low probability of recovery (Lyness 2007). Whatever the clinician's personal beliefs, it is the patient who

must decide, and the clinician must take care not to generate feelings of pressure or guilt in patients who do not wish to act according to advice. The clinician serves as a consultant and educator, not a salesperson for a particular end-of-life pathway.

Terminality

Most deaths in older persons are expected; only 10 percent occur suddenly, usually the result of a heart attack or stroke. Although the nature of the patient's medical condition, medications, and other factors influence what happens as an expected death approaches, general changes in the patient include (Nuland 1994; Kafetz 2002):

• Decreased interest and activity
• Diminished communication
• Reduced desire to eat and drink
• Periods of delirium
• Decreasing body temperature
• Falling blood pressure
• Decreased circulation to the extremities
• Breathing changes from a normal rate and rhythm to a pattern of several rapid exchanges of air followed by a period of no breathing
• Changing skin color
• Lapsing into a coma lasting minutes to hours to days before death occurs

Several scales are useful to predict the likelihood of death (Knaus et al. 1985), and patient management categories based on ICD-10 diagnostic codes can predict mortality with greater than 80 percent accuracy. The Acute Physiological and Chronic Health Evaluation (APACHE) index is a hospital-based scale used to chart twelve physiological variables (e.g., blood pressure, heart rate, age, state of alertness) in severely ill patients in the first twenty-four hours after admission (Knaus et al. 1985, 1991; Muckart et al. 2005). The higher the patient's score, the higher the probability of death and the need for decision-making concerning terminality.

Dealing with Ambiguity

Patients and families frequently ask, "How long will I live?" or may make statements such as "I'm going to live to see my daughter get married next summer." There are several reasonable responses to these situations. With regard to the question of longevity, the clinician must acknowledge that it is usually not possible to predict how long an individual person will live, but the clinician will always be there to help the patient. When individuals protest that they want to outlive the odds to participate in a celebration or benchmark event, an empathic response should emphasize that the exact course of illness is uncertain, but the team will be available and supportive.

Family Conflict at the End of Life

Anger is common in conflicts over end-of-life care in the absence of clear guidelines, especially when relationships have been strained or estranged. A history of conflict, communication problems, and family members' attempts to exert control can pit individuals against each other about whether to treat a catastrophic illness aggressively or discontinue life-sustaining measures. In the light of these intense passions, it is amazing how rarely these conflicts are argued in the courts.

Rejected parents, rival siblings, or adult children who disappointed parental expectations bring a great deal of emotional baggage to the bedside as well as their cultural, religious, and ethical beliefs. When families are hostile or cannot reconcile differences, the death of a loved one often eliminates the possibility for reconciliation and understanding. This emphasizes how critical it is to obtain a clear oral, and preferably written, statement of the patient's wishes at a time when he or she is not clinically depressed or compromised in decision-making capacity. Having a nonfamily member witness written advance directives and sharing these preferences widely among family members and health professionals can be very helpful.

Direct Treatment of Pain

Pain is probably the most feared symptom of people who are dying. The International Association for the Study of Pain (IASP; www.iasp-pain.org/AM/Template.cfm?Section=Home) defines pain as "a complex, unpleasant sensory and emotional experience associated with actual or potential tissue damage or expressed in terms of such damage." However, for the purposes of clinical treatment, "Pain is what the patient says it is." Between 70 and 90 percent of patients who have advanced cancer experience significant pain, but almost all could have relief with proper treatment. Pain goes undetected and untreated in patients who have many other serious conditions, and it is particularly neglected among nursing home resident, of whom 40–80 percent are in significant pain (Shega et al. 2007; Zwakhalen et al. 2006).

The clinical goal is to eliminate pain or reduce it as much as possible. This is usually achievable, although some individuals will protest any interventions to treat their discomfort, even when it is intense. Careful probing is necessary to identify whether this results from fears of taking medications, depression, or religious and cultural values prohibiting the use of pain treatments.

Current regulations of the Joint Commission on Accreditation of Health Care Organizations (JCAHO) specify that hospitals and health care facilities must evaluate, monitor, and manage pain in all patients or risk losing accreditation (Sandlin 2000). The guidelines and tools for assessment and management are available at the JCAHO website (www.jcaho.org). In addition to blood pressure, pulse rate, respiratory rate, and temperature, pain has been designated as the fifth vital sign.

Because pain is subjective, the best way to find out about it is to ask the patient to rate the pain on a scale of 0 to 10 (0, none, up to 10, excruciating) and then to describe the nature of the pain (e.g., stinging, burning, throbbing). Observer ratings are not reliable, and clinicians and family members usually underestimate or do not understand the intensity of a person's pain. Patients may not act as if they are in severe pain but rather complain about somatic problems or be depressed, agitated, or irritable. Unfortunately, clinicians may dismiss some patients as complainers or whiners who are not in serious distress, when their pain is real. Persons who have dementia or communication impairment are especially difficult to evaluate. At least twelve observational pain assessment tools are being developed for cognitively impaired persons (Zwakhalen et al. 2006); among the most useful are the Pain Assessment Checklist for Seniors with Limited Ability to Communicate (PACSLAC) and the Assessment of Discomfort in Dementia (ADD) Protocol (Kovach et al. 1999, 2002).

Analgesic drugs are usually the first-line treatment for pain (American Geriatrics Society 2002b; American Pain Society 2003). The World Health Organization three-step analgesic ladder (1990) provides a framework for the treatment of mild, moderate, and severe pain and emphasizes that older patients need careful monitoring (Barakzoy and Moss 2006). Step 1 targets mild pain for which acetaminophen and nonsteroidal anti-inflammatory drugs are appropriate. Step 2 focuses on moderate pain for which opioids are given, usually in conjunction with a step 1 drug. For step 3, severe pain, opioids such as morphine are the treatment of choice. The route of administration depends on the drug, the patient's ability to swallow or absorb an oral dose, and the appropriateness of other routes for treating patients (e.g., nasogastric or direct enteral access, permanent intravenous ports, subcutaneous morphine drip).

Treatment of pain may also include interventions for specific diseases, even when these therapies are not expected to improve survival or minimize the progression of the illness (e.g., antianginal drugs for angina pain, corticoids or nonsteroidal anti-inflammatory medications to minimize pain associated with inflammation and edema). When patients have severe bone pain from metastatic cancer, opioids may be effective, but other causes of bone cancer make treatment challenging (Goblirsch et al. 2006). Tricyclic antidepressants often provide relief for

patients who have neuropathic pain syndromes that do not respond to opioids (Dworkin et al. 2007; Pergolizzi et al. 2008).

Patients may not tolerate the side effects of analgesic medications such as opioids, which frequently cause nausea, constipation, drowsiness, or psychiatric symptoms (McNichol 2003; Swegle and Logemann 2006). The clinician may need to try prescribing different opioids to maximize pain relief and minimize side effects or to prescribe opioids with other analgesics, which may reduce the opioid dosage yet offer adequate pain control. Other medications, such as laxatives to prevent constipation or stimulants (e.g., methylphenidate) to reduce sedation, may counteract the side effects of opioids.

Nonpharmacological interventions may relieve pain, although efficacy varies, depending on the patient's condition and the therapeutic modality (Menefee and Monti 2005; Morrison and Morrison 2006). These interventions can be invasive (e.g., anesthesia or surgery) or noninvasive (e.g., physical rehabilitation, transcutaneous electrical nerve stimulation, or acupuncture) as well as psychiatric (e.g., cognitive/interpersonal therapies, meditation, guided imagery, or relaxation techniques). Music, massage, and aromatherapy are other nontraditional approaches to the management of pain.

Emotional and Spiritual Issues Associated with Dying

People who are dying face many personal issues that contribute to what has been described as spiritual pain—intense, diffuse cognitive and emotional pain (Stanworth 2003). Spiritual pain affects a person's desire to continue living in the context of perceived and real losses, and it is mediated by the individual's personality, life experiences, supportive relationships, personal beliefs and values, and religiosity or spirituality (Chochinov and Cann 2005; Chochinov 2006; Balboni et al. 2007). The experience of a life-threatening illness has been described as a loss of self in many dimensions:

- Feelings of not being a whole person
- Physical unattractiveness
- Inability to participate in a sexual relationship
- Not having "normal" interactions with others
- Inability to tolerate stress of any kind
- Diminished pleasurable activities

Each patient will emphasize a personal agenda, and the clinician will serve the individual's best interests by listening and observing him or her carefully and offering to bring in an appropriate spiritual counselor. Sensitive, compassionate discussions about these personal changes, existential issues, and lifestyle alterations may be a strong antidote to the meaninglessness associated with spiritual pain and reactive depression.

Mental Health Issues with People Who Are Dying

Depression

The estimated prevalence of depressive disorders and clinically relevant symptoms reported in populations of dying patients ranges from 15 to 60 percent (Lander et al. 2000; Wasteson et al. 2009). Diagnosis is often difficult because many of the disease symptoms may be similar to those of depression (e.g., cachexia, anorexia, weight loss, weakness, fatigue, insomnia, anhedonia, poor concentration, pain, or psychomotor disturbances). Dy and associates (2008) describe evidence-based guidelines for managing cancer fatigue, anorexia, depression, and dyspnea. The standard of care in working with dying patients is to diagnose and treat the underlying depression when emotional symptoms are present with the somatic manifestations, regardless of cause (Block 2005). However, defining ideational symptoms (e.g., hopelessness, helplessness, thoughts of death) is difficult when death is pending.

Antidepressant therapy is effective, but only a few empirical studies have been conducted among dying patients (Cochrane Library 2010). However, there are guidelines for recognizing and treating depression in dying patients (Lyness 2007):

1. Self-report depression measures described in earlier chapters are useful screening instruments, but so is a brief psychiatric interview.

2. Not diagnosing and treating depression leads to a desire for a hastened death, excess functional disability, and decreased quality of life.

3. Effective treatment of pain or other uncomfortable physical symptoms can improve depressive symptoms and functional effectiveness.

4. At this time, there are no controlled trials of medications or psychosocial treatments. However, dying patients have a good probability of responding to standard antidepressant treatments, although response rates may be more variable than in healthy populations.

5. Psychostimulants may relieve anergia, anhedonia, and abulia when patients do not manifest a major depressive syndrome or when patients have a short life expectancy and rapid relief of symptoms is desirable.

6. Clinicians should assess patients for suicidality. The most common reasons for wanting to commit suicide include the level of pain, fears of greater pain in the future, fears of being dependent and a burden, fears of dying alone, loss of dignity, fears of disfigurement, and a desire to be with previously deceased loved ones.

Anxiety

Although prevalence data are lacking, anxiety is common and may contribute to a desire for a hastened death to end a tortured existence (Lyness 2007). Anxiety may manifest alone, in conjunction with depression, or secondary to the occurrence and/or treatment of medical conditions. Anxiety usually presents as a generalized anxiety pattern, although panic attacks or acute stress disorder may also occur (chapter 11).

Controlled trials of anxiety drugs are lacking in terminally ill patients (Roth and Massie 2007), although there are a number of effective approaches to treating and managing anxiety (Miovic and Block 2007). When rapid control of symptoms is desirable in the context of acute distress or nearness to death, the clinician can prescribe benzodiazepines or antipsychotic medications, sometimes in conjunction with opioids or other sedatives (Jackson and Lipman 2010). Opioids may be especially effective when dyspnea occurs from cardiac or pulmonary disease. When the patient is not imminently dying, appropriate antidepressant medications, particularly SSRIs, may be valuable to treat generalized anxiety or panic-pattern symptoms or if the anxiety occurs with significant depressive symptoms. Cognitive-behavioral and supportive therapies may be useful for patients who have sufficient time, cognitive capacity, and motivation for treatment (Hirai et al. 2003). Group treatment and spiritual or pastoral counseling are significant components of a comprehensive approach to palliative care for many patients, and the clinician should offer them.

Delirium

People who are dying may manifest delirium resulting from central nervous system disturbances secondary to the terminal disease or reactions to certain medications, such as narcotics (Breitbart and Strout 2000). Prevalence rates vary widely, from 8 to 85 percent, depending on age, severity of illness, and stage of the disease (Michaud et al. 2004). The evaluation may be difficult because of the complex biopsychosocial issues dying patients face, but treatment is frequently successful. Patient/family decisions to adhere to a strict palliative strategy may preclude a work-up for underlying causes, despite significant emotional distress from the symptoms (Morita et al. 2004). Furthermore, the causes may not be remediable or may lead to a dilemma if the delirium results from the palliative use of opioids or glucocorticoids.

The recommended strategy is to carefully reconsider the risks and benefits of all medications with central nervous system side effects and consider the tradeoffs of the beneficial effects for the patient's comfort with the possible risk of delirium (Breitbart and Alici 2008). Symptoms such as agitation, psychosis, and emotional lability often respond to antipsychotic medications, which may have sedative properties in patients who are terminally ill.

Supportive Psychotherapy and Family Therapy

Psychotherapy and family therapy are valuable for life review, to enable patients to identify goals for the remaining time, to resolve conflicts and personal relationships, and to leave a legacy (Cohen and Block 2004; Ando et al. 2007; Allen et al. 2008). Family members and patients need support during the dying process (Andershed 2006; Ohlén et al. 2007), and clinicians need to be culturally competent about these needs (Wong and Chan 2007). Help for the family may include education and grief support, referral to home and community-based services, and therapies to improve communication, problem-solving, and caregiving behaviors (Erikson et al. 2006). The clinician should make a serious attempt to reconcile troublesome family differences, but family conflicts over clinical decisions may not be resolvable when the party legally empowered to act is at odds with others.

End-of-Life Issues
Patient's Capacity

People who are dying may not be able to make decisions about their clinical care for many reasons, including severe cognitive impairment, delirium, fluctuating consciousness, coma, and other conditions that affect communication and competency. The clinician may need to evaluate the patient's capacity with regard to specific decisions or actions (chapter 16): a patient's understanding of the facts of the condition and the options; an appreciation of the significance of these facts; and the patient's ability to make a reasonable choice based on a logical consideration of the situation consistent with her or his personal and cultural values.

Withholding/Terminating Life-Sustaining Treatment

Patients and families may be confronted with decisions about initiating certain interventions (e.g., mechanical ventilation, cardiopulmonary resuscitation, or artificial administration of fluids and nutrition) or discontinuing these treatments after they have begun. Clinicians can facilitate decision-making by describing the nature of such interventions, the probability that each will lead to a consequential recovery, and, if implemented, whether the effect will be short term or more long lasting. This type of information can help the patient and family think about what contributes to a quality of life consistent with their values. However, some people have religious or cultural values that will make them adamant about not using any life-sustaining treatments. In these situations, bringing in a pastoral counselor or culturally appropriate and acceptable professional to talk with everyone may help identify possible options.

Clinicians and ethicists have different positions about whether there is an ethical distinction between terminating treatment and not initiating treatment when patients are terminally ill (Meisel et al. 2000). Because it is common for people to believe that the cessation of treatment "causes" death, the social impact of withdrawing treatment often has a greater emotional influence. It may also have legal implications. Some states differentiate between withholding treatment (e.g., life support technology) and nutritional interventions (e.g., IV, feeding tube).

Clinicians may explain to family members that withholding or terminating these interventions allows the disease to take its natural course toward death as opposed to continuing treatments that postpone death and prolong suffering. Withholding artificial hydration and nutrition usually contributes to a more comfortable death with gradual loss of consciousness, and the available evidence indicates that tube feeding does not lengthen or improve the quality of life for people who are dying (American Academy of Hospice and Palliative Medicine: www.aahpm.org/positions/nutrition .html; Schultz 2009). Educating patients and family members about these issues is essential, because many believe that this constitutes a painful process of starving the patient to death or having the patient endure the experience of intense thirst.

Terminal Sedation

Although palliative care eliminates or diminishes physical suffering for most people who are dying, a small group remains uncomfortable despite the best clinical efforts. For some clinicians, patients, and family members, terminal sedation (i.e., the use of medications to cause the patient to become unconscious and allow the patient to die from the underlying disease condition) is an acceptable option to living with unbearable pain and suffering (Cowan and Walsh 2001). The sedative dose is insufficient to cause death, but the patient is unable to communicate. Medications commonly used include benzodiazepines, opioids, and anesthetics.

The current literature indicates significant variability in conclusions about the prevalence of use of terminal sedation, the effects, the decision-making process, fluid and food intake, and life-shortening effects (Good 2006; Claessens et al. 2008). The position of the American Medical Association can be found at www.ama-assn.org/ama1/pub/upload/ mm/369/ceja_5a08.pdf, and the position of the American College of Physicians can be found at www.acponline.org/running_practice/ ethics/. Terminal sedation should be used as a last resort after thorough conversations with the patient and family. The process of talking about it is usually comforting, and actual implementation is less frequent; therefore, the clinician should bring up terminal sedation as an option for consideration earlier in the illness rather than at the last possible moment. The patient and family need to be educated that this is not euthanasia. The purpose is to reduce pain and suffering, not to accelerate death.

Physician-Assisted Suicide and Euthanasia

Physician-assisted suicide (PAS) is defined as allowing a person to die by using medications or a device a physician provides for that explicit purpose. This differs from euthanasia, which is physician-controlled purposeful termination of life by active means, usually by a lethal dose of a sedating medication administered by the physician or a designated person such as a nurse (Quill et al. 2008). Most clinicians and ethicists agree that PAS and euthanasia are different from the reduction of more or less useless aggressive therapies and of medications to control pain or suffering, because the explicit goal and dosage of the latter are appropriate to reduce suffering rather than to cause death. This distinction, known as the doctrine of double effect, has been accepted as a component of proper palliative care. However, other clinicians and ethicists argue that this distinction does not adequately address the intentionality of hastening a patient's death as opposed to allowing a patient to die a "natural death" from the disease.

Euthanasia and PAS continue to be controversial issues, with concerns ranging from the individual's right to choose when to die to the availability of safeguards to protect vulnerable populations (Loewy 2004; Quill et al. 2008). About 10 percent of patients consider PAS, but only about 1 percent request it (Bascom and Tolle 2002). Empirical data about the circumstances and characteristics of patients who successfully sought PAS and euthanasia as well as physician practices in these situations have been difficult to ascertain in the United States because it is illegal in most states. Oregon legalized PAS in 1997, Washington State legalized it in 2008, and Montana legalized it in 2009 (Cassity 2009). These laws specify criteria for allowing terminally ill patients to receive prescriptions with lethal dosages from physicians for the purpose of ending their lives. The Netherlands legalized PAS and voluntary euthanasia in 2002, but Dutch courts have permitted them since 1984. Belgium legalized euthanasia in 2002 but does not specify the method. Switzerland has permitted PAS and non-physician-assisted suicide since 1941.

Euthanasia is illegal in all 50 states. Although sometimes used interchangeably, the terms *euthanasia* and *PAS* describe distinctly different types of assisted death. As legally defined in Oregon and Washington, PAS refers to death caused by ingesting a lethal dose of medication obtained by prescription from a physician for the purpose of ending life, but it is permitted only after a second opinion about the patient's terminality and after a determination of competency and the absence of depression. In contrast, euthanasia refers to death that occurs from direct intervention with lethal intent.

Special Considerations in End-of-Life Care for Dementia

Clinicians face many significant issues in the course of palliative care for individuals who have dementia, including the burden of family decision-making when a cognitively impaired patient has not made her or his wishes known; special guidelines for palliative dementia care; defining end-stage dementia and eligibility for hospice care; the patient's risk for severe/lethal violence; and caregiver education about dying and end-of-life care (Blasi et al. 2002; Volicer et al. 2003; Kim et al. 2005).

There are unique challenges when people who have dementia are dying (Volicer 2005; Chatterjee 2008). They are clinically and psychosocially vulnerable and dependent on others to make decisions on their behalf. Many individuals and family members have not discussed preferences for end-of-life care options, and family members may disagree about the right time to let go, especially in the late stages. It is common for family members who have the primary burden of caring to feel death wishes accompanied by guilt, especially when the advanced or final stages are protracted and the patient becomes fearful and agitated. Dementia is painful for everyone, and a common reaction is to deny, run away, or attempt to eliminate the cause of the pain. As a result, some caregivers distance themselves or think about ways to kill the person rather than see him or her suffer (chapter 18). These thoughts and feelings, coupled with depression and the intense distress of caregiving, can even lead to a premature, violent death.

Discussions about death and dying involving people who have dementia are especially distressing to families (Hurley and Volicer 2002) and involve much ambivalence and the potential of intrafamily conflict. Social isolation of patients and caregivers is a widespread phenomenon and prevents important discussions about end-of-life preferences and final arrangements. Psychological distress becomes more intense when patients are deteriorating into the terminal phase, a process family members have described as a "living funeral."

Approximately 1.8 million people in the United States are in the final stages of Alzheimer disease or related dementias. Although good-quality palliative care can be provided at home when supplemented by hospice (Volicer et al. 2003), end-of-life issues are uncharted territory for physicians and other health professionals, and despite the interest in providing adequate palliative care, little is known about effective strategies (Hurley and Volicer 2002; Sampson et al. 2005). Most physicians do not get to know the personal and family history of their terminally ill patients, knowledge that could be used to mediate a dignified death as well as comfort grieving families. Often, in the absence of DNR or other instructions, medical practice is to ignore dementia and continue with clinically indicated procedures for medical co-morbidities instead of finding ways to make patients more comfortable (Morrison and Morrison 2006). Physicians who do not know their patients seldom discuss dying and palliative care, or they communicate poorly, leaving patients and caregivers with little or no support at this stressful time.

Consensus is emerging for the care of patients who have advanced progressive dementia, recognizing that patients and families have special needs (Hurley et al. 1995; NHPCO 2008), but evidence-based practice guidelines are needed (Hancock et al. 2006). An advisory group convened by the U.S. Department of Veterans Affairs and the Alzheimer's Association drafted recommendations that enhanced general recommendations for standards of care at the end of life (Cassel and Foley 1999).

Although a number of studies have documented significant inadequacies in caring for people who have terminal illness (Shega et al. 2004; Harris 2007; Lorenz et al. 2008), people who have dementia are particularly at high risk across the continuum of care for many reasons. Almost 75 percent of all people who have dementia die in nursing homes and assisted living residences, where most staff members are not trained to deal with terminal care (Volicer 2005). Unfortunately, few people who have dementia are admitted to hospice, but when they are admitted, the care is beneficial (Mitchell et al. 2007). Of the estimated 540,000 terminally ill Americans admitted to hospice, less than 3 percent have a primary diagnosis of dementia (Hanrahan and Luchins 1995). Pain management, one of the central tenets of hospice care, can be particularly difficult with people who have dementia and cannot communicate how and what they feel.

A significant obstacle for people who provide hospice and long-term care for patients who have dementia is the difficulty in predicting six-month survival, a Medicare and Medicaid requirement for hospice reimbursement (Schonwetter et al. 2003; McCarty and Volicer 2009). With increasing federal regulation and fear of denial of payment, some hospices have been hesitant to admit patients who have dementia. The National Hospice and Palliative Care Organization first developed dementia guidelines in 1996 and later published medical guidelines for determining prognosis in advanced dementia that successfully target six-month survival in 85 percent of patients (NHPCO 2007). Specific indicators are quantified regarding the severity of co-morbid conditions, the rate of physical deterioration, difficulty with swallowing and feeding, and recurrent infections despite antibiotics.

A number of innovative hospice adaptations have been created and evaluated to overcome some of the barriers to good-quality dementia palliative care in home and long-term care settings (Stevenson and Bramson 2009). The Jacob Perlow Hospice, Beth Israel Medical Center, in New York City, developed a full-service hospice program targeting patients who had advanced-stage dementia and met specific end-stage criteria, the most important being eating and swallowing problems, recent weight loss, incontinence, and recurring infections (Brenner 2000). The model program resulted in 70 percent of patients dying comfortably at home, compared to 17 percent in the hospice inpatient residence and 13 percent in nursing homes.

Investigators at the University of Chicago and the Hospice of Michigan created a two-pronged hospice approach known as PEACE—the Palliative Excellence in Alzheimer's Care Efforts (Sachs et al. 2004; Shega et al. 2004). The PEACE project integrated palliative care into the primary care of people who had dementia from the time of diagnosis at a geriatric outpatient clinic through the course of illness and death. Preliminary results showed high ratings of the quality of care at enrollment and greater satisfaction over time: mean pain ratings averaged little or no pain, but family stress remained high. More than 60 percent of PEACE patients died at home, and less than 20 percent died in the hospital.

Karlawish and associates (1999) advocated expanding the clinician's role beyond explaining medical circumstances to actively guiding dialogue to facilitate decision-making when patients were too cognitively impaired to participate. Narratives about other patients and families were used to clarify the values of the patient, family caregivers, and professionals mediating terminal care. The meaning of suffering is highly subjective, and understanding the experience of persons who have late-stage dementia is extraordinarily difficult. Families benefit from guided support because they have to live with themselves after the patient has died.

The latest research findings indicate that stomach tubes, which have been used increasingly over the past fifteen years, are not medically or ethically justified to feed patients (Cervo et al. 2006; Chernoff 2006; Gillick and Volandis 2008). Feeding tubes not only can cause diarrhea, bloating, infections, and other health problems, but they also are not effective in reducing the risk of pneumonia or choking. Perhaps the best approach for clinicians to pursue with families who want a feeding tube is to acknowledge the symbolism of nutrition and search for another way to meet their needs (Gillick and Volandis 2008). Educating staff members about end-of-life care and nutrition

management and establishing interdisciplinary palliative care teams are useful approaches to deal with these issues (Monteleoni and Clark 2004).

Interacting with the Family after a Death

The death of the patient marks the beginning of a changed life for survivors. Clinicians need to be sensitive to the family's needs with the call after the patient dies, to recognize the comprehensive impact of bereavement, to be alert to the signs of health and social complications in the grieving process, and to be prepared to help more severely distressed survivors cope with their loss (Chochinov and Cann 2005; Chochinov 2006; LoboPrabhu et al. 2008). Grieving is an appropriate reaction to loss, and clinicians should take care to allow for a reasonable period of grief and mourning. Many cultures and religions have rituals and supports for the recently bereaved.

Individuals show many different types of grief, and those who suppress grief or fail to move beyond grief and adjust to new circumstances are at risk for serious problems (chapter 10). Although most people cope effectively, bereavement has been associated with serious neuroendocrine disturbances and sleep disruption, generalized anxiety or panic syndrome, depression, and increased mortality (Clayton 2007).

The palliative care team should evaluate family members' reactions to the circumstances of the death to determine who may be at risk for negative outcomes associated with protracted and intense grief. Chronic and unremitting grief is typically associated with sudden, unexpected, or traumatic death; untimely loss, such as the death of a child or young person; and the closeness of the relationship (Kaltman and Bonanno 2003; Schum et al. 2005; Gillies et al. 2006). Serious conflict or estrangement from the decedent before the illness may create a significant barrier to coping and adapting to death (Worden 2008).

Identifying bereaved persons at risk is the first step to help survivors adapt to the short-term and long-term challenges of loss (Worden 2008). Immediately after death has occurred, for example, the family and intimate friends may benefit from being coached in symptom management, using techniques such as relaxation skills, thought stopping, and a review of the meaning of the death (Neimeyer 2000). Over time, however, survivors may need more psychological assistance to find personal ways to deal with the loss (Jacobs and Prigerson 2000).

Attempting to rebuild a world of meaning that has been challenged by the death of a loved one is a core process in grieving (Neimeyer et al. 2006). Many bereaved people find new and powerful meanings in their losses, experiencing what is referred to as "post-traumatic growth" with or without professional help (Calhoun and Tedeschi 2001). Grief is a normal process, and rapid interventions, including medications, may not be advisable. If the grief is prolonged and unremitting after six weeks with the emergence of serious depressive symptoms, more aggressive involvement may be needed (Jacobs and Prigerson 2000; Neimeyer et al. 2006).

Future Challenges to Approaching Death

There are several end-of-life care curricula for various professionals, including:

- Physicians: The American Medical Association's Project to Educate Physicians in End-of-Life Care (www.epec.net)
- Hospice/Palliative Care Training for Physicians: The UNIPAC Book Series (www .liebertpub.com/publication.aspx?pub_id=119)

- Nurses: The End-of-Life Nursing Education Consortium Project (www.aacn.nche.edu/elnec)
- Psychologists: American Psychological Association Working Group on Assisted Suicide and End-of-Life Decisions (www.apa.org/pi/aids/programs/eol/index.aspx)
- Across Professions: End-of-Life/Palliative Education Resource Center (www.eperc.mcw .edu)
- Interprofessional Fellowship in Palliative Care (www.va.gov/oaa/fellowships/palliative.asp)
- Support Workers: Palliative Care for Support Workers (www.chpca.net/initiatives/train_the_trainer.htm)

Geriatric mental health professionals can do a great deal for patients across the continuum of palliative care: risk reduction in high-risk patients, therapies to modify the disease process, therapies to relieve pain and/or improve quality of life, preparation for the end of life, care in the last hours, and bereavement care. However, as the field of palliative care has emerged, empirical research is relatively sparse and limited primarily to populations of patients who have cancer or HIV/AIDS. A major research effort is needed to clarify how biological, psychological, and psychosocial factors mediate the dying process. Clinical trials are also needed to test the feasibility and efficacy of psychopharmacological and psychotherapeutic interventions to relieve pain and suffering as well as maximize comfort and quality of life. These challenges focus on improving the quality of end-of-life care and support for surviving loved ones.

21

Geriatric Mental Health Policies

Mental health problems are a global public health priority: they are the single greatest cause of health disability in all age groups. The President's New Freedom Commission on Mental Health (2003: www.mentalhealthcommission.gov) highlighted data from the World Health Organization (2001: www.who.int/whr/2001/en/) ranking mental health problems among the top three causes of disability in the United States, Canada, and Western Europe. Mental illnesses ranked highest (24 percent), followed by alcohol and drug abuse (12 percent) and Alzheimer disease and other dementias (7 percent). The U.S. Surgeon General's Report on Mental Health (USDHHS 1999a) emphasized the prevalence and severity of mental health problems, including those of older adults, and the need for action at all levels of government and nongovernmental agencies.

The magnitude of the unmet need for mental health care in the older population continues to be high (Jeste et al. 1999; Karlin and Duffy 2004). At least two-thirds of older adults who have a mental disorder do not receive needed services, and although older adults are becoming more willing to seek mental health care than in the past, the outcome is disturbing (Borson et al. 2001; Bartels et al. 2003). Only 48 percent of older persons who received psychiatric help were considered to have received minimally adequate care, and of the great majority who received mental health care in the general medical sector, only 12.7 percent received adequate care. Because the majority of Americans, particularly older Americans, use general physicians as de facto mental health care providers, these data reflect the inadequacy of the current patterns of practice.

Many factors in the provider and health care system contribute to the inadequacy of geri-atric mental health care across the continuum of acute and long-term care settings. On the provider side, these factors include negative attitudes about older adults and therapeutic nihilism; lack of knowledge about needs, functionality, diagnosis, and effective treatments; and poor referral rates from primary practice clinicians to mental health specialists. Systemic factors in the organization and financing of health care that create barriers include the lack of available, accessible mental health services; a historical lack of parity between mental health care reimbursement and that for other medical disorders; limited reimbursement in long-term care settings; limited coverage under private insurance and managed care programs; and perceptions by third-party payers that mental health care is open-ended, leading to high costs.

This chapter reviews the history of public policies that have affected the mental health of older adults in the United States, presents major geriatric mental health policy issues for the near future, and examines policy challenges within the context of broader social and health policies affecting our aging society. For several reasons, mental health policy targeting older people cannot be understood in isolation from social, economic, health, and welfare concerns. Aging is a developmental process in which biopsychosocial and environmental factors interact at multiple levels to influence health or disease and functional effectiveness or disability across the lifespan (chapter 2). The emergence of illness, including mental illness, in later life usually reflects the consequences of genetics, accumulated trauma, health and lifestyle behaviors, environmental factors, personal losses, and a variety of stressors.

Mental health policies are inextricably intertwined with broader health, social, and human services policies. Physical health and mental health are intimately interrelated (Weiss et al. 2009), and it is estimated that at least 50 percent of all diseases are affected by behavioral factors (e.g., poor nutrition and exercise patterns, substance abuse, lack of adherence to prescribed medication). Aging is also a sociopolitical experience that affects every person, family, and community as well as every component of a society's infrastructure. Thus, a healthy society must develop policies that create and sustain mental and physical health, vitality, economic security, and meaningful involvement of people of all ages.

Historical Review of the Impact of Public Policy on Geriatric Mental Health

Five White House Conferences on Aging in the United States, spanning fifty years, have stimulated a number of major national policies and programs that have had a direct or indirect impact on geriatric mental health care (www .whcoa.gov/about/history.asp). Several national conferences held earlier laid the groundwork for the first designated White House Conference on Aging in 1961. For instance, in 1950 President Truman directed the Federal Security Administration to hold a national conference on aging to evaluate the shifting age demography.

Health care was the major focus of the 1961 White House Conference on Aging, which catalyzed legislation establishing Medicare and Medicaid, ultimately signed into law in 1965 under President Johnson (Tibbitts 1960). However, long-term care was largely ignored, and reimbursement for mental health care was restricted relative to that for other acute health care services. Inpatient psychiatric care and psychological testing were covered, but only $250 was allowed annually for outpatient services, and there was a higher co-payment than for other medical conditions. The Older Americans Act, creating the Federal Administration on Aging, a body to be advisory to the Secretary of Health and Human Services, was also passed in 1965.

The focus of the 1971 White House Confer-

ence on Aging, held under the auspices of President Nixon's administration, was economic security, but several recommendations centered on research and training (WHCOA 1971). The National Institute on Aging was established in 1974, and the National Institute of Mental Health created the Center for the Study of Mental Health and Aging. The executive and legislative branches implemented the majority of the recommendations from the 1971 White House Conference on Aging. Major developments included a national nutrition program for older people and the creation of the Federal Council on Aging and the Senate Special Committee on Aging.

The 1981 White House Conference on Aging was planned under President Carter and implemented under President Reagan (Cowell 1981; Heppler 1981). Social Security and long-term care were major areas of concentration, and as a result of recommendations, the federal Omnibus Budget Reconciliation Act was passed in 1987. This legislation mandated that mental health services be provided in long-term care facilities to include staff education and assessments of quality of life. The 1981 conference also produced other mental health recommendations that were implemented over the years. The $250 cap on outpatient mental health services under Medicare Part B was increased first to $400, then to $1,000, and finally was repealed under the Omnibus Budget Reconciliation Act of 1989. Medicare was also modified to permit reimbursement for certain services provided by psychologists and clinical social workers. However, at that time, parity between health care and mental health care was not achieved, with mental health care services reimbursed at 50 percent in contrast to 80 percent for other medical care. Not until 2008 was parity achieved, in part with the passage of the Mental Health Parity Act, which mandated insurance parity for companies of fifty or more employees beginning in 2010.

During the 1980s federal legislation expanded reimbursement for home health care, occupational therapy, and certain therapeutic interventions in long-term care institutions. An interagency task force on Alzheimer disease was organized, and federal funds were increased for mental health and dementia research as well as for the creation of clinical research centers for geriatric mental health. Geriatric mental health awards were developed to provide opportunities for scientists to obtain specialty training in geriatric mental health research. The Department of Veterans Affairs (VA) created a panel to discuss the VA's future health care system, the single largest health system in the country. Recommendations included having better integration of mental health care with health care and more clinical geriatric research and demonstration programs for older populations.

The 1995 White House Conference on Aging, convened under President Clinton, was originally planned to occur in 1991 under President George H. W. Bush (Blancato 1994). This conference focused on supporting and reforming existing social and health programs—Medicare, Medicaid, and the Older Americans Act. Few new initiatives were endorsed, but a substantial oral commitment was made to support the field of geriatric mental health and to target future national policy focused on an aging population, not just aged persons.

At least four major developments occurred in the 1990s. Funding for research on Alzheimer disease grew substantially. In 1991 representatives of several organizations formed the National Coalition on Mental Health and Aging, whose mission was to be a vigorous advocate for policy reform. Another milestone event was the 1999 Surgeon General's report on mental health. Finally, the 1999 Olmstead decision of the U.S. Supreme Court established that "the institutionalization of persons who have disabilities, including those with mental illnesses, who could live in the community given appropriate resources, is a form of discrimination that violates the Americans with Disabilities Act."

The 2005 White House Conference on Aging, convened under President George W. Bush, identified fifty resolutions targeting present and future aging issues; and the need to improve the recognition, detection, and treatment of mental illness, particularly depression, emerged as one of the top ten priorities. Mental health issues were also addressed in other resolutions regarding Medicare and Medicaid, geriatric manpower, and long-term care reform (www.whcoa.gov/about/history.asp). The success or failure of the policy efforts of the 2005 White House Conference remain to be seen as 76 million baby boomers enter later life and the proportion of older Americans continues to grow (Kennedy 2006).

The Mental Health Parity Act of 2008, mentioned earlier, was a major advance in mental health policy reform. However, although it mandates insurance parity for larger companies, significant variation still exists for smaller companies. The legislation, which did not prevent insurance companies from denying mental health coverage for certain conditions, was reversed by the Health Care and Education Reconciliation Act of 2010.

An Integrated Framework for Mental Health and Social Policy

Future mental health care policies need to maintain a focus on recognizing the multiple interactive factors that support mental health and maximize the functioning, well-being, and quality of life of the individual. These goals should not be pursued in a vacuum, and we have identified core thematic components of a conceptual framework to integrate mental health, health, and social policies, expressed in the acronym SAFE HAVENS:

- *Security*
- *Alternatives*
- *Functionality*
- *Engagement*
- *Health*
- *Ability*
- *Value*
- *Environment*
- *New Information*
- *Simplicity*

SAFE HAVENS embodies three different meanings that underscore principal themes for comprehensive geriatric policy reform. First, SAFE HAVENS refers to what should be a time of life to feel secure and enjoy the rewards of decades of productivity as the individual grows older. Second, SAFE HAVENS refers to the potential of later life as a time for those who so choose to retool themselves to take on new roles and remain actively engaged in family and community life. Finally, SAFE HAVENS is a reminder that policies negatively affecting the independence and functioning of older persons have the potential to adversely affect mental health through a process of increasing marginalization and eventual decline and dependency.

Security

Financial, physical, and emotional security are the foundation for successful aging and mental health, and the policy issues encompass the nature and financing of pensions, Social Security, Medicare, and health care benefits. Although social policies are economically based, they should be driven by beliefs in the value of older people. Successive generations of older people have achieved a great deal, contributing to the well-being of their families and communities, and they have earned honor and respect for these contributions. Older adults also deserve opportunities and support to continue to learn and contribute in meaningful ways.

The case for providing an adequate support system stems not only from the moral principles of earned rewards for generativity but also from the perspective that programs that benefit older people also help their families and the community. Social Security and Medicare are not simply entitlement programs but also family-oriented programs. Social Security was originally conceived to save families from economic hardship because parents and older relatives were living longer, and the provision of pensions for older adults who could afford to retire opened up jobs for younger persons entering the labor force. Likewise,

Medicare was intended to assist families with the costs of acute health care for aging relatives. However, continued federal financing of these programs is an ongoing challenge in the light of the increasing number of older people, a declining proportion of workers to retirees, a declining workforce making contributions because of the economic recession, and other factors.

The older population may be increasing, but they embody successive cohorts of individuals who enter the period after age 65 with better health and increased vigor and vitality, capacity, and knowledge. Old chronological labels (e.g., age 45 as an older worker or mandated full retirement at age 65 or 70) are no longer appropriate. Retirement from previous occupational roles should not be regarded as the result of a decreased ability to contribute to the workplace or community. The simplistic concept of age-related disengagement from society must be discarded or at least substantially modified, given the continued productivity and vitality of a large population of older persons. A paradigm shift is needed in the way we perceive policy issues affecting an increasingly healthy and diversified older population, who should be regarded as potential assets. Later life should be recast as a period of potential to be fueled by investment rather than as a time of liability and uselessness.

Medicare, funded by tax revenues, is an age-specific example of a successful policy that provides health insurance for the older population as well as for blind and disabled populations. It has eased the burden of health care payments for millions of middle-aged Americans who would otherwise be paying for the care of parents, grandparents, and children. From its inception, Medicare has been a success. It has improved access to health care and, as a result, improved the health and quality of life for older persons. Medicare has also allowed middle-aged workers to support their children's growth and education as well as pay for housing, transportation, health care, and other expenses that might have been assigned to the health care costs of parents and grandparents.

Although Medicare has shortcomings, specifically with regard to restrictions in long-term care, rising costs, and fraudulent abuse of the program, the fundamental principle of investment in health care financing remains sound.

Economic security is a lynchpin for policy concerns, but economic insecurity is becoming a growing concern of many Americans, given the publicized future shortfall in Social Security financing as well as the unfunded liability of an increasing number of corporate pension plans. The solvency of Social Security, now a pay-as-we-go program, is dependent on the ratio of workers to retirees, level of taxation, and other factors. Current projections indicate that over time there will be a shortfall of available funds for the growing population of retirees who, in turn, are supported by fewer workers paying into the program. At the same time, income from private pension programs is being significantly challenged as major corporations are defaulting or scaling down employee pensions to maintain profits or, in some instances, solvency. Thus, older persons, even those who had done everything possible to save for retirement, are experiencing anxiety associated with possible financial insecurity.

There are several options to reform Social Security and protect pension funds (American Academy of Actuaries 2007; Shelton 2008; Turner 2009). These include postponing retirement age, raising the earnings cap, and establishing parallel federal investment programs. Increasing the retirement age by two or three years and/or increasing the level of taxable employee earnings from $90,000 to a higher cap (e.g., $125,000) would significantly resolve economic disparities of cash inflow versus outflow in the short term. Creating a parallel supplemental federal security investment program to enhance individual retirement protection through low-risk personal/investment savings accounts in addition to Social Security also has merit, although fluctuations in the equity and bond markets can cause havoc with such accounts. Indeed, in one sense, these are already possible through IRAs and other savings plans, but, unfortunately, for many individuals the yield is small or these plans are not affordable or are even risky using current earnings.

First and foremost, Social Security needs to be depolarized. Reform needs to be empowered by active public education and citizen involvement in identifying options as well as a bipartisan review of national pension reform (e.g., a multipartisan commission to hold public hearings, analyze the alternatives, and develop recommendations for protecting the long-term solvency of the Social Security Administration and public and private plans).

Alternatives

Older people are increasingly characterized by heterogeneity with respect to all biological, psychological, behavioral, and social variables. As improved public health measures have led to increasing life expectancy and as advances in the biomedical sciences, coupled with economic improvements have contributed to a healthier, more active population, successive generations of older people have become even more diversified.

It is inappropriate, therefore, to create policies based on inaccurate notions that all older people are sick and dependent, lose cognitive abilities, or are less capable in the workplace. Policy reform needs to focus on increasing opportunities for older people to participate in meaningful ways, rather than promoting barriers that force individuals to retire and become marginalized. The ability to make meaningful choices and perceive alternatives in later life enhances mental well-being, and policy formulation must recognize this need.

Functionality

The assessment of functionality addresses opportunities to enhance lifestyle through rehabilitation and improved assistive devices. Not only is a program of investment in these approaches worthwhile, but also we should rethink the role of product design and move from concepts of barrier freedom to environmental enhancement.

Functionality is also the outcome of incorporating health promotion and risk prevention behaviors into personal lifestyles. Education about health maintenance strategies as well as establishing new behaviors, such as physical and cognitive exercise, enhances functional capacity. The Americans with Disabilities Act (www.ada.gov/pubs/ada.htm) has led to the clear appreciation that the ability to do the job trumps any limitation in other aspects of a person's life.

The need for broad educational opportunities for adults of all ages is a serious issue for those stakeholders who must assess the current policy value of limiting educational resources to the young. While early education is essential, educational opportunities throughout life and into old age are now equally necessary. The alternative is to risk obsolescence and enforced marginalization of an otherwise experienced segment of the population. Many years may have elapsed since older people completed formal education, but that does not make them less valuable or useful. Given the tools to retrain for workplace roles, older adults can be productive members of the workforce.

Functionality is a core concept in geriatric health and mental health care (chapter 3), and indeed caring for individuals who have functional impairment is often more challenging than curing a disease. The clinicians' role is to optimize function by a variety of approaches, integrating behavioral, social, technological, and pharmacological strategies to maximize performance and minimize acute crises.

Engagement

Engagement has many different meanings: to participate in work or an occupation; to collaborate with others to accomplish mutual goals; to begin or carry on an activity; to enter into a committed relationship with someone; to deal with other persons or activities for a long time. This refers to many aspects of a successful aging society: supporting older people to work or volunteer; encouraging functional roles in the family and community; helping older persons remain active in physical and social activities that provide personal pleasure and a sense of meaningful participation; appreciating the value of intimate relationships and friendships in later life; developing policies

that will continue to engage the growing aging population.

Many older people find meaning in family, parenting, and grandparenting relationships as well as in work and volunteer roles in the community. However, there are more broad-based concerns in the development of policies that encourage engagement. With life expectancy continuing to increase, what is the "shelf life" of an individual? What mechanisms are needed to outfit older people to maximize independence and interdependence as well as to encourage successful aging within a social structure? What stakeholders, public and private, have responsibilities to develop and implement policy changes?

Health

There are at least four arenas to be considered in developing health and mental health policy for an aging population: Is help available, accessible, affordable, and appropriate?

Availability in this context refers to the existence of effective clinical tools for the diagnosis, treatment, management, rehabilitation, and prevention of diseases and injuries. Accessibility and affordability are closely related: accessibility refers to the ease of obtaining care, and affordability refers to the ability to pay for care. The ability to find good-quality health and mental health care that is affordable, is accessible, and deals with the comprehensive functional needs of older persons remains a challenge in the United States. To work toward these objectives, we need to transform the nature of our health care delivery system and financing.

Relatively independent generalist and specialist physicians deliver most of the health care in this country, despite the recognition that the availability of nonmedical supportive services can decrease the burden of health care management. Policies to encourage the coupling of health and supportive services and to increase the number of geriatric health care professionals, which is woefully insufficient at this time, are critical to improve accessible and affordable care. The latter was among the top ten recommendations of the 2005 White

House Conference on Aging and a 2008 IOM report.

Although mental health and physical health are interrelated, the systems of delivering and financing care are very different (Kessler et al. 2005; Unutzer et al. 2006). Mental health has a powerful impact on health care costs, in large measure because mental illnesses are so prevalent, are frequently undetected, and dramatically affect physical health and functional effectiveness (Mojtabai 2009). Studies repeatedly show that the cost of health care is significantly affected by mental health problems, and depression and anxiety disorders significantly increase the cost of a patient's general medical or surgical care (Katon et al. 2003).

A Veterans Administration Hospitals demonstration project, the Unified Psychogeriatric Biopsychosocial Evaluation and Treatment Program (UPBEAT), demonstrated significant savings by having all geriatric medical outpatients seen by mental health professionals and then treated as part of a comprehensive approach to geriatric medical and surgical care (Kominski et al. 2001; Oslin et al. 2004). Older patients receiving UPBEAT care spent 3.3 fewer days in the hospital, and although the cost of outpatient care was about $1,171 higher per patient, the inpatient costs were $3,027 lower.

Because an individual's health behaviors mediate the risks for different illnesses and therefore affect health care costs, health care reform needs to address reinforcement for appropriate health promotion and risk reduction health and mental health behaviors (e.g., compliance with prescribed treatment). A related policy challenge lies in the personal versus societal responsibility to pay for health care for those who smoke, fail to control their blood pressure by not adhering to medications or diet, refuse to exercise, abuse drugs, or refuse rehabilitation or counseling. Programs to reduce risk and promote health should be available and paid for when individuals who have such behavioral problems want help. Furthermore, incentives in the form of reduced out-of-pocket payments or better insurance rates should be more widely used for those who practice healthy lifestyles.

An overarching issue in health and mental health policy is a three-way partnership among patients, health care providers, and third-party payers to provide good-quality care, minimize medical errors, and contain costs. This includes not only a partnership for the provision and payment of acute medical care and long-term care services, but also preventative screening and interventions (e.g., cholesterol, blood pressure, malnutrition, obesity, bone density screening) as well as vaccinations for conditions such as pneumonia and influenza. In addition, health maintenance behavior programs need to be implemented for patients as well as family members, who are frequently critical partners in the treatment/management plans.

A number of other important policy issues need to be addressed:

• Reimbursement should be provided for essential services that play a crucial role in health but do not fit the simple fee-for-service model. Physician assistants or advanced registered nurse practitioners can be used to provide ongoing management for chronically ill patients, particularly in rural areas where physician manpower is limited.

• Computerized records of medical care need to be implemented to prevent duplication of tests, procedures, and prescriptions as well as to coordinate patient care because the current pattern of health care delivery involves multiple specialty physicians. This computerized medical database must protect patient confidentiality but be accessible by all treating physicians and other health care professionals caring for a patient.

• More health care and human services professionals should be trained in geriatric care.

• Family caregiver supports and services should be inclusive of children, adolescent, and adult caregivers.

• Health care and social services should be provided in the same location for patients and caregivers.

- Resident-centered care interventions are priorities to improve long-term care in assisted living and nursing home settings.

Ability

This domain focuses on maximizing the potential of older persons. Because the language used in policy communicates underlying values as well as specific content, policy statements need to emphasize the concept of ability. In the absence of serious health problems, older adults can remain actively engaged and be productive members of society. Predicting where an individual performs on the spectrum of functioning from ability to disability is not always easy unless specific performance criteria are specified. The standards for evaluating performance on tasks such as driving a car, flying an airplane, sitting as a judge, or performing in other workplace roles are very different, but performance criteria can be defined, measured, and evaluated.

Unfortunately, however, public as well as professional assumptions and negative biases toward older people often presume age-related declining abilities without testing them. As a consequence, policies emerge that affect the ability to perform various roles and responsibilities. Although some older adults have impairments, these should be addressed on a case-by-case basis. Individual performance criteria should be used instead of chronological age. Age-based mandatory retirement in the corporate sector as well as for state judges and other occupations, age-of-entry cut-offs for law enforcement and other public safety occupations, and the age-60 rule for retirement of commercial airline pilots are prime examples of occupational requirements that presume but do not evaluate job-related abilities.

Value

We need policies that acknowledge older people as individuals and as valuable contributors to society, rather than policies that reinforce a devaluation of older adults. Social and health policies need to be formulated to address issues that improve participation in meaningful pursuits, creativity, quality of life, and, ultimately, mental health. For example, the development of community programs to allow older persons to train and participate in voluntary work as well as paid employment should be a priority. Policies restricting the participation of older adults in the workplace need to be carefully justified.

Environment

Most older people prefer to remain at home, even when illness and frailty threaten mobility, self-care, safety, and independence. "Aging in place" is a widely accepted concept used to describe an overarching policy goal to enable older persons to remain in their homes as long as possible (Cutchin 2003). It usually refers to helping people stay at home and securing necessary services and assistance as their needs change. However, aging in place is more broadly described as enabling people to continuing to live in a familiar community of their choice unless it is necessary to relocate individuals to appropriate living environments for agreed-upon support and care.

Although many individual, family, social, and political factors affect the ability of the older population to age in place, financial circumstances probably have the greatest impact. Older people who rent apartments, houses, or trailers may not have the option to remain at home or in familiar communities when properties are sold for commercial development, and finding affordable, desirable housing may be difficult. Even those individuals who own their homes may face diminishing financial resources to pay the mortgage, taxes, maintenance, insurance, and other expenses necessary to remain at home.

Aging in place is seen as desirable, but state policies need to facilitate the ability of the older population to stay in their homes by providing accessible needed services. These policies should address the availability of home and community-based services; accessible health care; coordination among health and aging networks; transportation options, including public transportation; caregiver support services; affordable and available housing, including assisted living; and home repair services.

New Information

The rapid expansion of information and access to information in contemporary society is a challenge for all age groups, and those individuals who are not equipped to access information inevitably become less well-informed and less able to function. Policies that support educational and training programs, sustain cognitive capacities, and help older adults develop new skills to prevent obsolescence are critical. Public-private sector partnerships of many different stakeholders are needed to extend educational opportunities to the older population.

Evidence-based practice has become the standard in medicine, other clinical fields, and social programs. This approach recognizes the gulf between scientifically demonstrated information and traditional practice patterns, and it attempts to improve the quality of care by using results confirmed by multiple studies to inform clinicians and patients about empirical standards of care and available choices. Evidence-based practice involves systematically synthesizing scientific data to evaluate the outcomes of diagnostic and treatment clinical strategies. Standards of evidence-based practice are evolving for the treatment of older adults, but the research is limited at this time (Bartels et al. 2002b; van Citters and Bartels 2004; Bartels 2005; Bruce et al. 2005).

Simplicity

The many governmental and nongovernmental programs and services for older people and their caregivers are a confusing morass. The full range of available social and health programs for the older population needs to be integrated and seamless. Just as the problem of multiple physicians with poor communication among them adversely affects health care, so the existence of multiple private and governmental agencies becomes a barrier to good-quality care. Many of these agencies require different sets of qualifications for the populations served and rarely share information on records among professionals in these programs. Older people themselves may not communicate information to staff members across the many settings. The unfortunate consequence may be that if they are turned away in one setting, they may not be aware of other options for assistance.

The need for the orchestration and simplification of caring is among the most important and problematic challenges the clinical community faces. Mental health clinicians may need to become involved in the process of helping patients negotiate the system. Policy reform should include assurances of funding for multiagency collaboration and the availability of service managers to help patients and families find the right care.

Mental Health Policy Reform

The New Freedom Commission on Mental Health identified many barriers to mental health care for older persons: a fragmented system of delivering services, antiquated Medicare policies, the double stigma of age and mental illness, and the lack of adequate interventions to detect and treat geriatric mental health problems. Specific policies identified to combat these obstacles include:

- Guaranteed access to affordable, comprehensive mental health care with a range of services
- Achievement of parity (which occurred in 2008/2010)
- Elimination of exclusions based on pre-existing conditions
- Coordination of benefits for persons who are eligible for Medicare and/or Medicaid
- Provision of Medicaid waivers for home and community-based services to avoid premature admission to a nursing home
- Provision of culturally competent care
- Encouragement of research and implementation of evidence-based practices
- Integration of mental health care across the continuum of care

• Screening for co-morbid health conditions and developing appropriate treatment strategies

The economics of Medicare and Medicaid and the affordability of these programs are being challenged for many reasons:

• Population growth and the rapid aging of the population
• The increasing costs of equipment, goods, services, and personnel
• The increasing costs of prescription medications, many of which may be more effective but more costly
• The increasing costs of technological advances, coupled with rapid obsolescence
• The increasing role of the private sector

Medicare (www.kff.org/medicare/upload/1066-12.pdf) does not have a means test for personal finances, but Medicaid (www.kff.org/medicaid/upload/7235_03-2.pdf) was specifically designed with a means test to provide health care to individuals who are medically indigent. Medicaid operates as a state-federal partnership: each state establishes financial thresholds for Medicaid; the federal government approves the eligibility requirements; and both state and federal governments share the costs. Medicare restricts aspects of mental health and long-term care, but Medicaid typically does not. Medicaid controls fee schedules, and states have established formularies to limit the choice of drugs to control costs.

Because indigence is a requirement for Medicaid reimbursement, patterns of delivering long-term care emerged that remain today. Individuals in low socioeconomic strata who need to be admitted to long-term care facilities with Medicaid beds usually have a long wait because of state limitations in the number of long-term care beds as well as low reimbursement rates. Most long-term care residents are admitted as privately paying and then spend their personal or family resources until they become medically indigent and are eligible to apply for Medicaid. Some prospective residents are advised to "spend down" their assets in anticipation of admission to a long-term care facility. "Spending down" refers to the transfer of funds away from the control of the prospective long-term care resident so that a financial investigation of the patient's means one or two years later or more (depending on a state's regulations) will qualify the person as medically indigent. Resources may be transferred to children, who obtain total control of the parent's assets but no legal responsibility to pay for care, thus leaving the burden solely on Medicaid.

Medicare retained its primary focus on acute illnesses for forty years after it became operational in 1966, despite the increasing number of older Americans who have chronic illnesses (www.kff.org/medicare/medicaretimeline.cfm). The Medicare Prescription Drug Improvement and Modernization Act of 2003, also known as the Medicare Modernization Act (MMA), included several provisions to begin to reorient Medicare policy to focus on chronic diseases (www.cms.gov/PrescriptionDrugCovGenIn/01_Overview.asp; Ganz 2004; Anderson 2005). The Kaiser Family Foundation site (www.kff.org) provides updates regarding the impact of the 2010 Health Care and Education Reconciliation Act on Medicare. The 2010 bill eliminated the "doughnut hole," in which Medicare beneficiaries who do not have coverage have to pay the full cost of the drugs out of pocket, and had provisions to standardize coverage for Medicare beneficiaries enrolled in different drug plans (Jacobsen and Anderson 2010).

Section 721 of the Medicare Modernization Act created the Chronic Care Improvement (CCI) pilot program in 2004 to improve care for chronically ill patients covered by Medicare (Berenson 2004; Garrett 2005). CCI pilot program currently provides "patient-centered and physician-guided" services to Medicare recipients who have one or more of the following conditions: congestive heart failure, chronic obstructive pulmonary disease, and complex diabetes. Ten pilot projects have been initiated in different states to reduce the fragmentation of services and provide disease management for patients who have one or more of these chronic conditions. If the results of these pilots are successful, the CCI will be permanently included in Medicare.

Other provisions of the CCI address the role of physicians as case managers, the use of electronic records and computerized prescription writing, physician access to evidence-based medical protocols, and the development of a strategy to improve the quality of care and reduce the cost of chronic disease management (Anderson 2005). Costs are projected to increase initially as care is coordinated and health information is widely shared across providers. However, case management should improve health care outcomes as well as reduce the duplication of medications, tests, and hospitalizations, which in turn should lead to fewer errors and long-term savings.

Although the Medicare Modernization Act represents a significant improvement in health care for older adults, it does not include psychiatric disorders, which are common comorbid conditions for the targeted chronic illnesses. It also does not reimburse nonphysicians unless these professionals are directly responding to physician orders. Medicare modernization also needs to address a number of other significant issues: support for family caregivers, long-term care insurance (with the elimination of long-term care funding under Medicaid), strategies to minimize Medicare and Medicaid fraud, and strategies to reduce bureaucratic costs.

The availability of prescription medications has played a signal role in helping to improve health while at the same time contributing to a substantial increase in health care costs. Medicare Part D went into effect in 2006, also as a result of the 2003 Medicare Modernization Act. It was an effort to help all Medicare recipients, regardless of income, health status, or prescription drug usage, pay for prescription medications and reduce their out-of-pocket spending. At least 40 percent of older Americans reported not filling their prescriptions or cutting their doses because of the high costs of medications (Kaiser Family Foundation 2007; www.kff.org/rxdrugs/index.cfm). The average annual out-of-pocket prescription drug costs

in the Medicare population rose from $644 in 2000 to $999 in 2003, and costs are projected to increase to $2763 in 2013.

Medicaid recipients are automatically enrolled in a Medicare Part D program, but non-Medicaid recipients must sign up with one of more than 600 private insurance/ HMO plans with different costs, benefits, and convenience (e.g., pharmacies covered and availability of mail order option) on the theory that market forces will play a role in containing costs. However, the law protects the pricing practices of pharmaceutical companies by blocking price negotiations, thus fixing prices. The private HMOs and insurance companies involved in the Medicare Part D plans have implemented a number of cost-cutting strategies, including the development of formularies to limit the use of more expensive drugs in favor of older, less costly medications and generic formulations.

Nursing homes are required to assist residents to enroll in the most appropriate prescription drug plan. Residents may have a family member help them choose a plan or choose an agent in the long-term care facility, such as a registered nurse, to act as her or his designated representative.

Medicare Part D is a voluntary program available through stand-alone prescription drug plans or the Medicare Advantage Plan. Medicare recipients who do not have high drug costs may opt out of the program, but individuals will be penalized if they enrolled at a date later than November 2006 and do not have evidence of current enrollment in a private plan that provides at least the equivalent coverage of Medicare.

The Future of Mental Health Policy Reform

Although mental health care has advanced significantly since the 1950s, future mental health policy reform will not be successful unless it can be integrated into a broader health and social policy that addresses parity, access to integrated and culturally appropriate services, caregiver support services for youth and adults, and long-term care as well as a recognition that chronic illnesses require physician-guided disease management, including mental health care.

Policy changes rarely occur rapidly, but they inevitably come to fruition when there is a perceived need and a commitment to action by dedicated individuals who can mobilize sufficient public support to influence policy makers at the local, state, and federal level. Strong leadership will be needed to translate the health and mental health recommendations in reports from the Institute of Medicine, the Surgeon General, and the 2005 White House Conference on Aging into sound public policy. Improvements in mental health policy and care of older persons will occur if there is sustained informed leadership coupled with an educated, involved public.

A major advance in mental health care came with the passage and signing of the Mental Health Parity and Addiction Equity Act of 2008, a bill requiring parity in funding of mental health services and medical care by third-party payers nationwide, beginning in 2010. The resolution of this longstanding disparity applies to major mental illness, including chronically mentally ill patients and families who have been denied adequate coverage for care. The indirect effects of this legislation on manpower and resource development remain to be seen.

2010 Health Care Reform Bills

On March 23, 2010, President Obama signed into law the "Patient Protection and Affordable Care Act" (PL 111-148). A week later, on March 30, he signed the Health Care and Education Reconciliation Act of 2010, companion legislation that included amendments to the original act emerging from political compromises and commitments made to ensure its passage of the principal bill (PL 111-148).

These two pieces of legislation, fiercely opposed by the Republican legislators in both houses of Congress, comprised the fulfillment of the Democratic administration's stated commitments to the most significant health reform since Medicare and Medicaid. However, even after these bills passed into law, partisan

rancor continued, and numerous states (15 at this writing) with Republican attorneys general organized to file law suits in the federal courts, arguing that at least one provision of the law was unconstitutional (i.e., requiring people to obtain health insurance by the year 2014). These bills also became a rallying point for the 2010 congressional election, in which Republicans hoped to increase their presence in Congress and to amend or eliminate health care reform, presumably because of the image of federal intrusion ("big government") and the ("arguable") negative impact on the federal deficit. The future of this reform therefore may be affected in future elections.

While the major impetus of the law(s) was to reduce the large number of Americans without health insurance and to place controls on the ability of insurance companies to refuse to insure persons who have pre-existing conditions, mental and behavioral health issues were also included. Mental health and substance abuse as well as behavioral health care are to have parity with medical and surgical care under future insurance and be part of the basic benefits package. Psychotherapy under Medicare will continue the 5 percent payment restoration through 2010, and psychologists will have broadened practice parameters with interdisciplinary health programs and be allowed to provide care to chronically mentally ill people through state options. Wellness and illness prevention programs will be strengthened to include depression and elder abuse as well as the development of best practice initiatives by professional organizations.

The new laws also contained requirements for education and training as well as research. They stipulated funding for workforce development, such as loan repayment practice opportunities, including geriatric training. Research priorities included comparative effectiveness of interventions to enhance clinical treatment initiatives, long-term care services and support for those who have functional limitations, and family caregiver health and effectiveness.

The specific implementation of these new mandates is under development. The short-term impact on the older population, apart from a commitment to eliminate the famous "doughnut hole" under Medicare Part D, is not yet clear. The "doughnut hole" is that portion of drug costs which many on Medicare experience during mid-calendar year, depending on the specifics of the plan they have elected, because they are fully responsible for the costs of their medication during the period of no reimbursement. The result has been a serious economic burden for many even forcing some to be unable to fill their prescriptions. Although the change in Medicare Part D reimbursement is welcome, pharmaceutical companies need to be engaged in drug price controls as part of health care reform implementation.

Several other aspects of the legislation target Medicare and long-term care oversight. Tighter controls on Medicare expenditures to eliminate waste and fraud as well as programs to make care more efficient are promised, with anticipated billions of dollars in future savings. A Payment Advisory Board for medical reimbursement under Medicare and adjustments to Medicare Advantage plans is also proposed. Transparency of the ownership of long-term care facilities is also mandated and should be of considerable value to patient, families, and oversight agencies.

This legislation is a landmark step in broadening the provision of health care. Its impact over the next years will be the consequences of specific administrative decisions and the political climate consequent to its implementation. Clinicians and students should acquaint themselves with the specific state regulations and opportunities as well as the national initiatives that will affect clinical care, education, and clinical research.

Long-Term Care Policies

Health policy reform to enhance care in nursing homes and assisted living facilities continues to be national priority. The Nursing Home Reform Act of 1987, which established specific rights and guaranteed care and protection for residents, has still not been fully implemented (Castle 2001; Klauber and Wright 2001; Zhang and Grabowski 2004). The act was part of the Omnibus Budget Reconciliation Act of 1987,

and it was the result of a congressionally mandated study by the Institute of Medicine that found that nursing home residents were being abused, neglected, and receiving inadequate care (Mechanic and McAlpine 2000).

Recent takeover activity by large equity firms has led to substantially reduced quality of care and accountability in for-profit nursing homes, the largest sector of nursing homes in the country (Wells 2009). These takeovers have also had a major negative impact on the quality of life of residents and challenged family caregivers; the lack of transparency attendant to for-profit takeovers has led to the prominent public conclusion that "most people would rather die than go to a nursing home" (Wells 2009).

A policy focused on providing needed care must target patients, the potential for non-health-based noninstitutional care, family and companion caregivers, and the provision of medical and nursing care as adjunctive to social care, which would define a new strategy. Because nursing home residents have significant mental health problems, with few programs available apart from medication, such reformulation would be a policy milestone. Mental health policy for older people needs to be set in the context of programs that help those who are older but also younger families who provide care. This is the only way our country will retain its own moral integrity by helping people return to health or be cared for in the optimal way.

Meeting the Challenge of Caring

The health and mental health care system of the United States is a collection of practitioners, state and regional clinics, and for-profit and not-for-profit hospitals. These create a patchwork distribution of health and mental health care sites. This non-system is essentially a series of cottage industries rather than an integrated system of health, mental health, and human social services. An integrated continuum of care remains as an urgent health care agenda for the future. Perhaps, as suggested, the 2010 law reflects only the first step in an organized system for improving mental health, substance abuse, and behavioral care—or perhaps not.

A recurring theme throughout this volume is the significance of the ecological setting on all aspects of an individual's life. The genetic and epigenetic substrates cannot in themselves account for the health, mental health, and functional capacity of the individual, and the more impaired the person, the greater the saliency of her or his environment. Social and health policies as discussed in this chapter play a powerful role in the practice of patient care. In fact, whether the individual can be seen as a patient as well as the conditions under which care is provided and reimbursed are consequential for public and private policies. Although clinicians in training are often spared the details of compensation for services and the organizational challenges of caring for patients, clinicians need to be informed about and recognize the impact of community resources and financial factors that affect patient care and practice. Eternal vigilance is not only the price of freedom, it is also a requirement for the quality of patient care.

REFERENCES

Aalten P, Verhey FRJ, Boziki M, Bullock R, Byrne EJ, Camus V, Robert PH: Neuropsychiatric syndromes in dementia: Results from the European Alzheimer Disease Consortium: Part I. *Dementia and Geriatric Cognitive Disorders* 2007; 24: 457–63.

AARP: Issue Brief, Valuing the Invaluable: A New Look at the Economic Value of Family Caregiving. Washington DC: AARP, 2007.

Aarsland D, Sharp S, Ballard C: Psychiatric and behavioral symptoms in Alzheimer's disease and other dementias: Etiology and management. *Current Neurology and Neuroscience Reports* 2005; 5: 345–54.

Abernethy A, Burns C, Wheeler J, Currow D: Defining distinct caregiver subpopulations by intensity of end-of-life care provided. *Palliative Medicine* 2009; 23: 66–79.

Abraham PF, Shirley ER: New mnemonic for depressive symptoms. *American Journal of Psychiatry* 2006; 163: 329–30.

Abrams RC, Bromberg CE: Personality disorders in the elderly: A flagging field of inquiry. *International Journal of Geriatric Psychiatry* 2006; 21: 1013–17.

Adams SM, Miller KE, Zylstra RG: Pharmacologic management of adult depression. *American Family Physician* 2008; 77: 785–92.

Agronin ME: Somatoform disorders. In Blazer DG, Steffens DC, Busse EW (eds.), *The Textbook of Geriatric Psychiatry,* 3rd edition. Washington, DC: American Psychiatric Press, 2004, pp. 295–302.

Agronin ME, Maletta G: Personality disorders in late life: Understanding and overcoming the gap in research. *American Journal of Geriatric Psychiatry* 2000; 8: 4–18.

Aguzzi A, Heikenwalder M: Pathogenesis of prion diseases: Current status and future outlook. *Nature Reviews: Microbiology* 2006; 4: 765–75.

Ahern J, Galea S, Resnick H, Kilpatrick D, Bucuvalas M, Gold J: Television images and psychological symptoms after the September 11 terrorist attacks. *Psychiatry* 2002; 65: 289–300.

Ahmad S, O'Mahony MS: Where older people die: A retrospective population-based study. *Oxford Journal of Medicine* 2005; 98: 865–70.

Alagiakrishnan K, Blanchette P: Delirium. Retrieved from eMedicine from WebMD 2009, August 3.

http://emedicine.medscape.com/article/288890 -overview.

Alagiakrishnan K, Lim D, Brahim, A, Wong A, Wood A, Senthilselvan A, Chimich W, Kagan, L: Sexually inappropriate behavior in demented elderly people. *Postgraduate Medical Journal* 2005; 81: 463–66.

Alagiakrishnan K, Masaki K: Vascular dementia. Retrieved from eMedicine from WebMD, 2009. http://emedicine.medscape.com/article/292105 -overview.

Alatas E, Yagci AB: The effect of sildenafil citrate on uterine and clitoral arterial blood flow in postmenopausal women. *Medscape General Medicine* 2004; 6: 51.

Albert MS, Levkoff SE, Reilly C, Liptzin B, Pilgrim D, Cleary PD, Rowe JW: The delirium symptom interview: An interview for the detection of delirium symptoms in hospitalized patients. *Journal of Geriatric Psychiatry and Neurology* 1992; 5: 14–21.

Alexopoulos GS: Clinical and biological interactions in affective and cognitive geriatric syndromes. *Focus* 2004; 2: 236–38.

Alexopoulos GS: The vascular depression hypothesis: 10 years later. *Biological Psychiatry* 2006; 60: 1304–5.

Alexopoulos GS, Abrams RC, Young RC, Shamoian: Cornell scale for depression in dementia. *Biological Psychiatry* 1988; 23: 271–84.

Alexopoulos GS, Meyers BS, Young RC, Kalayam B, Kakuma T, Gabrielle M, Hull J: Executive dysfunction and long-term outcomes of geriatric depression. *Archives of General Psychiatry* 2000; 57: 285–90.

Alexopoulos GS, Katz IR, Reynolds CF, Carpenter D, Docherty JP: The expert consensus guideline series. Pharmacotherapy of depressive disorders in older patients. *Postgraduate Medical Journal* 2001; 1–86.

Alexopoulos GS, Raue P, Arean P: Problem-solving therapy versus supportive therapy in geriatric major depression with executive dysfunction. *American Journal of Geriatric Psychiatry* 2003; 11: 46–52.

Alexopoulos GS, Schultz SK, Lebowitz BD: Late-life depression: A model for medical classification. *Biological Psychiatry* 2005a; 58: 283–89.

Alexopoulos GS, Katz IR, Bruce ML, Heo M, Have TT, Raue P, Reynolds CF: Remission in depressed

263

geriatric primary care patients: A report from the PROSPECT study. *American Journal of Psychiatry* 2005b; 162: 718-24.

Alexopoulos GS, Jeste DV, Chung H, Carpenter D, Ross R, Docherty JP: The expert The expert consensus guideline series. Treatment of dementia and its behavioral disturbances: Introduction: methods, commentary, and summary. *Journal of Psychiatric Practice* 2007; 13: 207-16.

Alexopoulos GS, Murphy CF, Gunning-Dixon FM, Latoussakis V, Kanellopoulos D, Klimstra S, Hoptman MJ: Microstructural white matter abnormalities and remission of geriatric depression. *American Journal of Psychiatry* 2008; 165: 238-44.

Alexopoulos GS, Kelly Jr. RE: Research advances in geriatric depression. *World Psychiatry* 2009; 8: 140-49.

Algase DL, Moore DH, Vandeweerd C, Gavin-Dreschnack DJ: Mapping the maze of terms and definitions in dementia-related wandering. *Aging and Mental Health* 2007; 11: 686-98.

consensus guideline series. Treatment of dementia and its behavioral disturbances: Introduction: methods, commentary, and summary. *Journal of Psychiatric Practice* 2007; 13: 207-16.

Allegri RF, Glaser FB, Taragano FE, Buschke H: Mild cognitive impairment: Believe it or not? *International Review of Psychiatry* 2008; 20: 357-63.

Allen JP, Wilson VB: *Assessing Alcohol Problems: A Guide for Clinicians and Researchers,* 2nd edition. Washington, DC: National Institute on Alcohol Abuse and Alcoholism, 2004.

Allen RP, Piccietti D, Hening WA, Trenkwalder C, Walters AS, Montplaisi J: Restless legs syndrome: Diagnostic criteria, special considerations, and epidemiology: A report from the restless legs syndrome diagnosis and epidemiology workshop at the National Institutes of Health. *Sleep Medicine* 2003; 4: 101-19.

Allen RS, Hilgeman MM, Ege MA, Shuster Jr JL, Burgio LD: Legacy activities as interventions approaching the end of life. *Journal of Palliative Medicine* 2008; 11: 1029-38.

Alliance for Aging Research: *Ageism: How Healthcare Fails the Elderly.* Washington, DC: Alliance for Aging Research, 2003.

Almeida OP, Fenner S: Bipolar disorder: Similarities and differences between patients with illness onset before and after 65 years of age. *International Psychogeriatrics* 2002; 14: 311-22.

Alzheimer A: Uber eigenartige Krankheitsfalle des spateren Alters. *Zeitschrift fur die gesamie Neurologie und Psychiatrie* 1911; 4: 356-85.

Alzheimer's Association: 2009 Alzheimer's disease facts and figures. *Alzheimer's and Dementia* 2009; 5: 234-70.

American Academy of Actuaries. Social Security Reform Options. 2007.

American Association of Clinical Endocrinologists: Medical guidelines for clinical practice for the evaluation and treatment of male sexual dysfunction: A couple's problem. *Update: Endocrine Practice* 2003; 9: 77-95.

American Association of Colleges of Nursing: *Peaceful Death: Recommended Competencies and Curricular Guidelines for End-of-Life Nursing Care.* Washington, DC: American Association of Colleges of Nursing, 1999.

American Bar Association Commission on Law and Aging, American Psychological Association: *Assessment of Older Adults with Diminished Capacity: A Handbook for Psychologists.* Washington, DC: ABA, APA, 2008a.

American Bar Association Commission on Law and Aging, American Psychological Association: *Assessment of Older Adults with Diminished Capacity: A Handbook for Lawyers.* Washington, DC: ABA, APA, 2008b.

American Bar Association Commission on Law and Aging, American Psychological Association: *Judicial Determination of Capacity of Older Adults in Guardianship Proceedings.* Washington, DC: ABA, APA, 2008c.

American Dietetic Association (ADA): Position of the American Dietetic Association: Nutrition intervention in the treatment of anorexia nervosa, bulimia nervosa, and other eating disorders. *Journal of the American Dietetic Association* 2006; 106: 2073-82.

American Geriatrics Society (AGA), Geriatrics Interdisciplinary Advisory Group: *Interdisciplinary Care for Older Adults with Complex Needs.* New York: AGA, 2002a.

American Geriatrics Society, Panel on Chronic Pain in Older Persons: The management of persistent pain in older persons: AGS panel on persistent pain in older persons. *Journal of the American Geriatrics Society* 2002b; 6: 205-24.

American Medical Association: *Diagnostic and Treatment Guidelines on Elder Abuse and Neglect.* Chicago: American Medical Association, 1992.

American Pain Society: *Principles of Analgesic Use in the Treatment of Acute Pain and Cancer Pain,* 5th edition. Glenview, IL: American Pain Society, 2003.

American Psychiatric Association: *Diagnostic and Statistical Manual of Mental Disorders,* 4th edition—text revision (IV-TR). Washington, DC: American Psychiatric Association Press, 2000.

American Psychiatric Association: *The Practice of Electroconvulsive Therapy: Recommendations for Treatment, Training, and Privileging.* Washington, DC: American Psychiatric Association, 2001.

American Psychiatric Association: *Fostering Resilience*

in *Response to Terrorism: For Psychologists Working with Older Adults.* Washington, DC: American Psychiatric Association, 2002a.

American Psychiatric Association: *Practice Guidelines for Treating Patients with Eating Disorders,* revised. Washington, DC: American Psychiatric Association, 2002b.

American Psychiatric Association: *Practice Guidelines for the Treatment of Patients with Alzheimer's Disease and Other Dementias.* Washington, DC: American Psychiatric Association, 2007.

American Psychiatric Association: *Practice Guideline for the Treatment of Patients with Obsessive-Compulsive Disorder.* Washington, DC: American Psychiatric Association, 2007.

American Psychiatric Association: *Practice Guideline for the Treatment of Patients with Panic Disorder.* Washington, DC: American Psychiatric Association, 2009.

American Psychological Association: Ethical principles of psychologists and code of conduct. *American Psychologist* 2002; 1–16.

American Psychological Association: *Guidelines for Psychological Practice with Older Adults.* Washington, DC: American Psychological Association, 2003.

American Psychological Association: Guidelines for psychological practice with older adults. *American Psychologist* 2004; 59: 236–60.

American Psychological Association, Committee on Aging: *Multicultural Competency in Geropsychology.* Washington, DC: American Psychological Association, 2009.

Amici S, Gorno-Tempini ML, Ogar JM, Dronkers NF, Miller BL: An overview of primary progressive aphasia and its variants. *Behavioral Neurology* 2006; 17: 77–87.

Ammann RA, Baumgarnter L: Bad news in oncology: Which are the right words? *Supportive Care in Cancer* 2005; 13: 275–76.

Ancoli-Israel S: Sleep apnea in older adults: Is it real and should age be the determining factor in the treatment decision matrix? *Sleep Medicine Reviews* 2007; 11: 83–85.

Ancoli-Israel S: Sleep and its disorders in aging populations. *Sleep Medicine* 2009; 10: 7–11.

Ancoli-Israel S, Ayalon L: Diagnosis and treatment of sleep disorders in older adults. *Focus* 2009; 7:98–105.

Ancoli-Israel S, Cooke JR: Prevalence and comorbidity of insomnia and effect on functioning in elderly populations. *Journal of the American Geriatric Society* 2005; 53: 264–71.

Andershed B: Relatives in end-of-life care—part 1: A systematic review of the literature the five last years, January 1999–February 2004. *Journal of Clinical Nursing* 2006; 15: 1158–69.

Anderson GF: Medicare and chronic conditions. *New England Journal of Medicine* 2005; 353: 305–9.

Ando M, Tsuda A, Morita T: Life reviews on the spiritual well-being of terminally ill cancer patients. *Supportive Care in Cancer* 2007; 15: 225–31.

Andrew MK, Freter SH, Rockwood K: Prevalence and outcomes of delirium in community and non-acute care settings in people without dementia: A report from the Canadian Study of Health and Aging. *BMC Medicine* 2006; 4.

Antinori A, Cingolani A, Lorenzini P, Giancola ML, Uccella I, Bossolasco S, De Luca A: Clinical epidemiology and survival of progressive multifocal leukoencephalopathy in the era of highly active antiretroviral therapy: Data from the Italian Registry Investigative Neuro AIDS (IRINA). *Journal of NeuroVirology* 2003; 9: 47–53.

Antonini A, De Notaris R, Benti R, De Gaspari D, Pezzoli G: Perfusion ECD/SPECT in the characterization of cognitive deficits in Parkinson's disease. *Journal of the Neurological Sciences* 2001; 22: 45–46.

Appelbaum PS: Involving decisionally impaired subjects in research: The need for legislation. *American Journal of Geriatric Psychiatry* 2002; 10: 120–24.

Appelbaum PS: Assessment of patients' competence to consent to treatment. *New England Journal of Medicine* 2007; 357: 1834–40.

Appelbaum PS, Bonnie RJ, Karlawish JH: The capacity to vote of persons with Alzheimer's disease. *American Journal of Psychiatry* 2005; 162: 2094–2100.

Appelbaum PS, Grisso T: *Assessing Competence to Consent to Treatment: A Guide for Physicians and Other Health Professionals.* New York: Oxford University Press, 1998.

Arean PA: Problem-solving therapy. *Psychiatric Annals* 2009; 39.

Arean PA, Ayalon L: Assessment and treatment of depressed older adults in primary care. *Clinical Psychology: Science and Practice* 2005; 12: 321–35.

Arean PA, Cook BL: Psychotherapy and combined psychotherapy/pharmacotherapy for late life depression. *Biological Psychiatry* 2002; 52: 293–303.

Arean P, Hegel M, Vannoy S, Fan MY, Unuzter J: Effectiveness of problem-solving therapy for older, primary care patients with depression: Results from the IMPACT project. *Gerontologist* 2008; 48: 311–23.

Arena J, Wallace M: Sexuality issues in aging: Nursing standard of practice protocol: Sexuality in older adults. 2008. Retrieved February 22, 2010, from Hartford Institute for Geriatric Nursing website: www.consultgerirn.org.

Arai AC, Kessler M: Pharmacology of ampakine

modulators: From AMPA receptors to synapses and behavior. *Current Drug Targets* 2007; 8: 583–602.

Arendash GW, Rezai-Zadeh K, Cao C, Mamcarz M, Dickson A, Schleif W, Runfeldt M, Lin X, Cracchiolo J, Shippy D, Raj A, Tan J, Potter H: O1-01-01: Caffeine: Evidence for protection against, treatment for, Alzheimer's disease by direct suppression of disease pathogenesis. *Alzheimer's and Dementia* 2007; 3: S166.

Arendash GW, Mori T, Cao C, Mamcarz M, Runfeldt M, Dickson A, Rezai-Zaldeh K, Tan J, Citron BA, Lin X, Echeverria V, Potter H: Caffeine reverses cognitive impairment and decreases brain amyloid-β levels in aged Alzheimer's disease mice. *Journal of Alzheimer's Disease* 2009; 17: 661–80.

Arkin S: Language-enriched exercise plus socialization slows cognitive decline in Alzheimer's disease. American Journal of Alzheimer's Disease and Other Dementias 2007; 22: 62–77.

Arneric SP, Holladay M, Williams M: Neural nicotinic receptors: A perspective on two decades of drug discovery research. *Biochemical Pharmacology* 2007; 74: 1092–1101.

Arno PS: The economic value of informal caregiving. Proceedings of the Care Coordination and Caregiving Forum, National Institutes of Health, Department of Veterans Affairs, Bethesda, MD, 2006.

Artero S, Petersen R, Touchon J, Ritchie K: Revised criteria for mild cognitive impairment: Validation within a longitudinal population study. *Dementia and Geriatric Cognitive Disorders* 2006; 22: 465–70.

Arvanitakis Z, Wilson RS, Bienias JL, Evans DA, Bennett DA: Diabetes mellitus and risk of Alzheimer disease and decline in cognitive function. *Archives of Neurology* 2004; 61: 661–66.

Asberg K: Assessment of daily living. In Copeland, Abou-Saleh, and Blazer (eds.), *Principles and Practice of Geriatric Psychiatry.* New York: John Wiley & Sons, 2002.

Atkinson RM: Alcohol use in later life: Scourge, solace, or safeguard of health? *American Journal of Geriatric Psychiatry* 2002; 10: 649–52.

Atkinson RM: Late onset problem drinking in older adults. *International Journal of Geriatric Psychiatry* 2004; 9: 321–26.

Aud MA: Dangerous wandering: Elopement of older adults with dementia from long-term care facilities. *American Journal of Alzheimer's Disease and Other Dementias* 2004; 19: 361–68.

Auld DS, Kornecook TJ, Bastianetto S, Quieion R: Alzheimer's disease and the basal forebrain cholinergic system: Relations to β-amyloid peptides, cognition, and treatment strategies. *Progress in Neurobiology* 2002; 68: 209–45.

Avis NE, Brockwell S, Randolph JF, Shen S, Cain VS, Ory M, Greendale GA: Longitudinal changes in sexual functioning as women transition through menopause: Results from the Study of Women's Health Across the Nation. *Menopause* 2009; 16: 442–52.

Ayers, CR, Sorrell JT, Thorp SR, Wetherell JL: Evidence-based psychological treatments for late-life anxiety. *Psychology and Aging* 2007; 22: 8–17.

Azad N, Power, B: Dementia in women: The role of hypertension and hypercholesterolemia. *Journal fur Hypertonie* 2008; 12: 17–21.

Aziz R, Lorberg B, Tampi RR: Treatments for late-life bipolar disorder. *American Journal of Geriatric Pharmacotherapy* 2006; 4: 347-64.

Babor TF, Higgins-Biddle JC, Saunders JB, Monteiro MG: *AUDIT: The Alcohol Use Disorders Identification Test: Guidelines for Use in Primary Care,* 2nd edition. Geneva: World Health Organization, Department of Mental Health and Substance Dependence, 2001.

Bachman D, Rabins P: "Sundowning" and other temporally associated agitation states in dementia patients. *Annual Review of Medicine* 2006; 57: 499–511.

Bacskai B, Frosch MP, Freeman SH, Raymond SB, Augustinack JC, Johnson KA, Irizarrry MC, Klunk WE, Mathis CA, Dekosky ST, Greenberg SM, Hyman BT, Growdon JH: Molecular imaging with Pittsburgh compound B confirmed at autopsy. *Archives of Neurology* 2007; 64: 431–34.

Baghai TC, Moller HJ: Electroconvulsive therapy and its different indications. *Dialogues in Clinical Neuroscience* 2008; 10: 105–17.

Balboni TA, Vanderwerker LC, Block SD, Paulk E, Lathan CS, Peteet JR, Prigerson HG: Religiousness and spiritual support among advanced cancer patients and associations with end-of-life treatment preferences and quality of life. *Journal of Clinical Oncology* 2007; 25: 555–60.

Baldessarini RJ, Tondo L, Hennen J, Viguera AC: Is lithium still worth using? An update of selected recent research. *Harvard Review of Psychiatry* 2002; 10: 59–75.

Ball K, Berch DB, Helmers KF, Jobe JB, Leveck MD, Marsiske M, Morris JN, Rebok GW, Smith DM, Tennstedt SL, Unverzagt FW, Willis SL: Effects of cognitive training interventions with older adults: A randomized controlled trial. *JAMA* 2002; 288: 2271–81.

Ballard C: Agitation and psychosis in dementia. *American Journal of Geriatric Psychiatry* 2007; 15: 913–17.

Ballard C, McKeith I, Burn D: The UPDRS scale as a means of identifying extrapyramidal signs in patients suffering from dementia with Lewy bodies. *Acta Neurologica Scandinavica* 1997; 96: 366–71.

Ballard CG, Margallo-Lana M, Fossey J, Reichelt K, Myint P, Potkins D, O'Brien J: A 1-year follow-up study of behavioral and psychological symptoms in dementia among people in care environments. *Journal of Clinical Psychiatry* 2001; 62: 631–36.

Baltes PB, Smith J: New frontiers in the future of aging: From successful aging of the young old to the dilemmas of the fourth age. *Gerontology* 2003; 49: 123–35.

Barakzoy AS, Moss AH: Efficacy of the World Health Organization analgesic ladder to treat pain in end-stage renal disease. *Journal of the American Society of Nephrology* 2006; 17: 3198–203.

Barch DM: Neuropsychological abnormalities in schizophrenia and major mood disorders: Similarities and differences. *Current Psychiatry Reports* 2009; 11: 313–19.

Barnett JH, Smoller JW: The genetics of bipolar disorder. *Neuroscience* 2009; 164: 331–43.

Barry D, Beital M: Cultural considerations in mental illness and healing. In S Loue and M Sajatovic (eds.), *Determinants of Minority Mental Health and Wellness.* New York: Springer, 2008.

Barry KL, Blow FC, Cullinane P, Gordon C, Welsh D: *The Effectiveness of Implementing a Brief Alcohol Intervention with Older Adults in Community Settings.* Washington, DC: National Council on Aging, Center for Healthy Aging, 2007. www.healthyagingprograms.com/resources/BI_StayingHealthyProject.pdf.

Barry PJ, Gallagher P, Ryan C: Inappropriate prescribing in geriatric patients. *Current Psychiatry Reports* 2008; 10: 37–43.

Bartels S: Quality, costs, and effectiveness of services for older adults with mental disorders: A selective overview of recent advances in geriatric mental health services research. *Current Opinion in Psychiatry* 2002; 15: 411–16.

Bartels SJ: Evidence-based geriatric psychiatry. *Psychiatric Clinics of North America* 2005; 28: xiii–xv.

Bartels SJ, Forester B, Miles KM, Joyce T: Mental health service use by elderly patients with bipolar disorder and unipolar major depression. *American Journal of Geriatric Psychiatry* 2000; 8: 160–66.

Bartels SJ, Coakley E, Oxman TE, Constantino G, Oslin D, Chen H, Sanchez HAB: Suicidal and death ideation in older primary care patients with depression, anxiety, and at-risk alcohol use. *American Journal of Geriatric Psychiatry* 2002a; 10: 417–27.

Bartels SJ, Dums AR, Oxman TE, Schneider LS, Areán PA, Alexopoulos GS, Jeste DV: Evidence-based practices in geriatric mental health care. *Psychiatric Services* 2002b; 53: 1419–31.

Bartels SJ, Dums AR, Oxman TE, Schneider LS, Areán PA, Alexopoulos GS, Jeste DV: Evidence-based practices in geriatric mental health care: An overview of systematic reviews and meta-analyses. *Psychiatric Clinics of North America* 2003; 26: 971–90.

Bartels SJ, Coakley EH, Zubritsky C, Ware JH, Miles KM, Areán PA, Hongtu C, Oslin DW, Llorente MD, Costantino G, Quijano L, McIntyre JS, Linkins KW, Oxman TE, Maxwell J, Levkoff SE: Improving access to geriatric mental health services: A randomized trial comparing treatment engagement with integrated versus enhanced referral care for depression, anxiety, and at-risk alcohol use. *American Journal of Psychiatry* 2004; 161: 1455–62.

Barth J, Schumacher M, Herrmann-Lingen C: Depression as a risk factor for mortality in patients with coronary heart disease: A meta-analysis. *Psychosomatic Medicine* 2004; 66: 802–13.

Bascom PB, Tolle SW: Responding to requests for physician-assisted suicide. *JAMA* 2002; 288: 91–98.

Bassiony MM, Steinberg MS, Warren A, Rosenblatt A, Bake AS, Lyketsos CG: Delusions and hallucinations in Alzheimer's disease: Prevalence and clinical correlates. *International Journal of Geriatric Psychiatry* 2000; 15: 99–107.

Bastos-Leite AJ, van der Flier WM, van Straaten ECW, Staekenborg SS, Scheltens P, Barkhof F: The contribution of medial temporal lobe atrophy and vascular pathology to cognitive impairment in vascular dementia. *Stroke* 2007; 38: 3128.

Bates D, Spell N, Cullen D: The Adverse Drug Events Prevention Study Group: The costs of adverse drug reactions in hospitalized patients. *JAMA* 1997; 277: 307–11.

Baum AE, Akula N, Cabanero M, Cardona I, Corona W, Klemens B, McMahon FJ: A genome-wide association study implicates diacylglycerol kinase eta (DGKH) and several other genes in the etiology of bipolar disorder. *Molecular Psychiatry* 2008; 13: 197–207.

Beaton R, Murphy S: Psychosocial responses to biological and chemical terrorist threats and events: Implications for the workplace. *Journal of the American Association of Occupational Health Nurses* 2002; 50: 182–89.

Beauchamp TL, Childress JF: *Principles of Biomedical Ethics,* 6th edition. New York: Oxford University Press, 2008.

Beck AT, Alford BA: *Depression Causes and Treatment,* 2nd edition. Philadelphia: University of Pennsylvania Press, 2009.

Becker A, Grinspoon S, Klibanski A, Herzog D: Current concepts: Eating disorders. *New England Journal of Medicine* 1999; 340: 1092–98.

Becker S: Global perspectives on children's unpaid

caregiving in the family. *Global Social Policy* 2007; 7: 23–50.

Behl C, Moosmann B: Serial review: Causes and consequences of oxidative stress in Alzheimer's disease. *Free Radical Biology and Medicine* 2002; 33: 182–91.

Bell DC, Richard AJ: The search for a caregiving motivation. *Psychological Inquiry* 2000; 11: 124–28.

Benedek DM, Friedman MJ, Zatzick D, Ursano RJ: Guideline watch (March 2009) practice guideline for the treatment of patients with acute stress disorder and posttraumatic stress disorder. *American Psychiatric Association Practice Guidelines* 2009; 1–12.

Bengtson V, Silverstein M, Putney N (eds.): *Handbook of Theories of Aging*. New York: Springer, 2009.

Benitez CIP, Smith K, Vasile RG, Rende R, Edelen MO, Keller MB: Use of benzodiazepines and selective serotonin reuptake inhibitors in middle-aged and older adults with anxiety disorders: A longitudinal and prospective study. *American Journal of Geriatric Psychiatry* 2008; 16: 5–13.

Benoit M, Brocker P, Clement JP, Cnockaert X, Hinault P, Nourashemi F, Pancrazi MP, Portet F, Robert P, Thomas P, Verny M: Behavioral and psychological symptoms in dementia: Description and management. *Revue Neurologique* 2005; 161: 357–66.

Berenson RA: Medicare disadvantaged and the search for the elusive "level playing field." *Health Affairs* 2004; W4: 572–85.

Berg K, Wood-Dauphinee S, Williams JI, Gayton D: Measuring balance in the elderly: Preliminary development of an instrument. *Physiotherapy Canada* 1989; 41: 304–11.

Berger A, Mychaskiw M, Dukes E, Edelsberg J, Oster G: Magnitude of potentially inappropriate prescribing in Germany among older patients with generalized anxiety disorder. *BMC Geriatrics* 2009; 9.

Bergman-Evans, B: Evidence-based guideline: Improving medication management for older adult clients. *Journal of Gerontological Nursing* 2006; 32: 6–14.

Berman AL: Dyadic death: A typology. *Suicide and Life-Threatening Behavior* 1996; 26: 342–50.

Berman K, Brodaty H: Tocopherol (vitamin E) in Alzheimer's disease and other neurodegenerative disorders. *CNS* 2004; 18: 807–25.

Berrios G, Freeman H: *Alzheimer and the Dementias*. London: Royal Society of Medicine Services, 1991.

Berry K, Barrowclough C: The needs of older adults with schizophrenia: Implications for psychological interventions. *Clinical Psychology Review* 2009; 29: 68–76.

Bertram L, Tanzi RE: The genetic epidemiology of neurodegenerative disease. *Journal of Clinical Investigation* 2005; 115: 1449–57.

Bertram L, Tanzi RE: Alzheimer disease: New light on an old CLU. *Nature Reviews Neurology* 2010; 6: 11–13.

Bharucha A: Suicide in the elderly. In Ellison J (ed.), *Treatment of Suicidal Patients in Managed Care*. Washington, DC: American Psychiatric Publishing, 2001.

Bhatt MH, Podder N, Chokroverty S: Sleep and neurodegenerative diseases. *Seminars in Neurology* 2005; 25: 39–51.

Bielak AAM: How can we not "lose it" if we still don't understand how to "use it"? Unanswered questions about the influence of activity participation on cognitive performance in older age—a mini-review. *Gerontology: Behavioral Science Section* 2009; 1–13.

Biessels GJ, Kappelle LJ: Increased risk of Alzheimer's disease in type II diabetes: Insulin resistance of the brain of insulin-induced amyloid pathology? *Biochemical Society Transactions* 2005; 33: 1041–44.

Black B, Muralee S, Tampi RR: Inappropriate sexual behaviors in dementia. *Journal of Geriatric Psychiatry and Neurology* 2005; 18: 155–62.

Black S, Iadecola C: Vascular cognitive impairment: Small vessels, big toll. *Stroke* 2009; 40: S38–39.

Blancato RB: The 1995 White House Conference on Aging. *Journal of Aging and Social Policy* 1994; 6: xiii–xvi.

Blanchard MR, Wattereus A, Mann AH: The nature of depression among older people in inner London, and the contact with primary care. *British Journal of Psychiatry* 1994; 164: 396–402.

Blashfield RK, Intoccia V: Growth of the literature on the topic of personality disorders. *American Journal of Psychiatry* 2000; 157: 472–73.

Blasi ZV, Hurley AC, Volicer L: End-of-life care in dementia: A review of problems, prospects, and solutions in practice. *Journal of the American Medical Directors Association* 2002; 3: 57–65.

Blasko I, Stamper-Kountchev MM, Robatscher P, Veerhuis R, Elkenboom P, Grubeck-Loebenstein B: How chronic inflammation can affect the brain and support the development of Alzheimer's disease in old age: The role of microglia and astrocytes. *Aging Cell* 2004; 169–76.

Blass DM, Rabins PV: Depression in frontotemporal dementia. *Psychosomatics* 2009; 50: 239–47.

Blazer D: Successful aging. *American Journal of Geriatric Psychiatry* 2006; 14: 2–5.

Blazer D, Hybels C, Pieper C: The association of depression and mortality in elderly patients. *Journal of Gerontology: Biological Sciences and Medical Sciences* 2001; 56: M505–9.

Blazer DG: The psychiatric interview of older adults. *Focus* 2004; 2: 224–35.

Blazer DG: Depression in late life: Review and commentary. *Focus* 2009; 7: 118–36.

Blazer DG, Steffens DC (eds.): *American Psychiatric Publishing Textbook of Geriatric Psychiatry*, 4th edition. Washington, DC: American Psychiatric Publishing, 2009.

Blazer DG, Wu LT: The epidemiology of at-risk and binge drinking among middle-aged and elderly community adults: National survey on drug use and health. *American Journal of Psychiatry* 2009; 166: 1162–69.

Bleich A, Gelkopf M, Melamed Y, Solomon Z: Emotional impact of exposure to terrorism among young-old and old-old Israeli citizens. *American Journal of Geriatric Psychiatry* 2005; 13: 705–12.

Blessed G, Tomlinson B, Roth M: The association between quantitative measures of dementia and of senile changes in the cerebral grey matter of elderly subjects. *British Journal of Psychiatry* 1968; 114: 797–811.

Blessed G, Tomlinson BE, Roth M: Blessed-Roth dementia scale (DS). *Psychopharmacology Bulletin* 1988; 24: 705–8.

Bliwise DL: Sleep disorders in Alzheimer's disease and other dementias. *Clinical Cornerstone* 2004; 6: S16–28.

Block SD: Assessing and managing depression in the terminally ill patient. *Focus* 2005; 3: 310–19.

Blow FC, Barry KL: Older patients with at-risk and problem drinking patterns: New developments in brief interventions. *Journal of Geriatric Psychiatry and Neurology* 2000; 13: 115–23.

Blow FC, Brower KJ, Schulenber JE, Demo-Dananberg LM, Young JL, Beresford TP: The Michigan Alcoholism Screening Test-Geriatric Version (MAST G): A new elderly-specific screening instrument. *Alcoholism: Clinical and Experimental Research* 1992; 16: 372.

Blow FC, Serras AM, Barry KL: Late-life depression and alcoholism. *Current Psychiatry Reports* 2007; 9: 14–19.

Blum B: The "IDEAL" protocol for undue influence: An introduction. *NCPJ Life and Times* 2003; 2, National College of Probate Judges.

Blum B: Forensic issues: Geriatric psychiatry. In Sadock B, Sadock V (eds.), *Kaplan and Sadock's Comprehensive Textbook of Psychiatry*, 8th edition. Baltimore: Lippincott, Williams and Wilkins, 2005.

Boerner K, Schulz R: Caregiving bereavement and complicated grief. *Bereavement Care* 2009; 28: 10–13.

Boettger S, Passik S, Breitbart W: Delirium superimposed on dementia versus delirium in the absence of dementia: Phenomenological differences. *Palliative and Supportive Care* 2009; 7: 495–500.

Boeve BF, Lang AE, Litvan I: Corticobasal degeneration and its relationship to progressive supranuclear palsy and frontotemporal dementia. *Annals of Neurology* 2003; 54: S15–19.

Bogner HR, Cary MS, Bruce ML, Reynolds CF, Mulsant B, Have TT, Alexopoulos GS: The role of medical comorbidity in outcome of major depression in primary care: The PROSPECT study. *American Journal of Geriatric Psychiatry* 2005; 13: 861–68.

Bogunovic OJ, Greenfield SF: Use of benzodiazepines among elderly patients. *Psychiatric Services* 2004; 55: 233–35.

Boldy D, Webb M, Horner B, Davey M, Kingsley B: *Elder abuse in Western Australia*. Perth, Western Australia: Curtin University of Technology, 2002.

Bonanno GA, Kaltman S: The varieties of grief experience. *Clinical Psychology Review* 2001; 21: 705–34.

Bonci CM, Bonci LJ, Granger LR, Johnson CL, Malina RM, Milne LW, Vanderbunt EM: National Athletic Trainers' Association position statement: Preventing, detecting, and managing disordered eating in athletes. *Journal of Athletic Training* 2008; 43: 80–108.

Bonger B, Brown L, Beutler L, Breckenridge J, Zimbardo, P (eds.): *Psychology of Terrorism*. New York: Oxford University Press, 2006.

Bonnie R, Wallace R (eds.): *Elder Abuse: Abuse, Neglect, and Exploitation in an Aging America*. Washington, DC: National Academies Press, 2002.

Bookwala J, Schulz R: A comparison of primary stressors, secondary stressors, and depressive symptoms between elderly caregiving husbands and wives: The caregiver health effects study. *Psychology and Aging* 2000; 15: 607–16.

Boothby LA, Doering PL: Acamprosate for the treatment of alcohol dependence. *Clinical Therapeutics* 2005; 27: 695–714.

Bootman J, Harrison D, Cox E: The health care costs of drug-related morbidity and mortality in nursing homes. *Archives of Internal Medicine* 1997; 157: 2089–96.

Borrayo EA, Goldwaser G, Vacha-Haase T, Hepburn KW: An inquiry into Latino caregivers' experience caring for older adults with Alzheimer's disease and related dementias. *Journal of Applied Gerontology* 2007; 26: 486–505.

Borson S, Bartels SJ, Colenda CC, Gottlieb GL, Meyers B: Geriatric mental health services research: Strategic plan for an aging population: Report of the health services work group of the American Association for Geriatric Psychiatry. *American Journal of Geriatric Psychiatry* 2001; 9: 191–204.

Borson S, Scalan JM, Watanabe J, Tu SP, Lessig M: Improving identification of cognitive impairment in primary care. *International Journal of Geriatric Psychiatry* 2006; 21: 349–55.

Boscarino JA, Adams RE, Figley CR: Mental health service use 1-year after the World Trade Center disaster: Implications for mental health care. *General Hospital Psychiatry* 2004; 26: 346–58.

Bosma H, Apland L, Kazanjian A: Cultural conceptualizations of hospice palliative care: More similarities than differences. *Palliative Medicine* 2009; 121–13.

Bossarte RM, Simon TR, Barker L: Characteristics of homicide followed by suicide incidents in multiple states, 2003–2004. *Injury Prevention* 2006; 12: ii33–38.

Bostock CV, Soiza RL, Whalley LJ: Genetic determinants of ageing processes and diseases in later life. *Maturitas* 2009; 62: 225–29.

Bourke A: Kin selection and the evolutionary theory of aging. *Annual Review of Ecology, Evolution, and Systematics* 2007; 38: 103–28.

Boyce N, Walker Z: Late-onset schizophrenia and very late-onset schizophrenia-like psychosis. *Psychiatry* 2008; 7: 463–66.

Braak H, Braak E: Argyrophilic grains: Characteristic pathology of cerebral cortex in cases of adult onset dementia without Alzheimer changes. *Neuroscience Letters* 1987; 76: 124–27.

Braak H, Del Tredici K, Rub U, de Vos RAI, Steur E, Braak E: Staging of brain pathology related to sporadic Parkinson's disease. *Neurobiological Aging* 2003; 24: 197–211.

Braak H, Rüb U, Steur J, Del Tredici K, de Vos RAI: Cognitive status correlates with neuropathologic stage in Parkinson disease. *Neurology* 2005; 64: 1404–10.

Bradley EH, Fried TR, Kasl SV, Idler E: Quality-of-life trajectories of elders in end of life. *Annual Review of Gerontology and Geriatrics* 2000; 20: 64–96.

Braga LL, Fiks JP, Mari JJ, Mello MF: The importance of the concepts of disaster, catastrophe, violence, trauma, and barbarism in defining posttraumatic stress disorder in clinical practice. *BMC Psychiatry* 2008; 8.

Braida D, Sala M: Epastigmine: Ten years of pharmacology, toxicology, pharmacokinetic, and clinical studies. *CNS Drug Reviews* 2006; 7: 369–86.

Bonnie R, Wallace R, eds: *Elder Abuse: Abuse, Neglect, and Exploitation in an Aging America*. Washington DC: National Academy Press, 2002.

Brannon GE, Bij S, Gentili A: Sleep disorders, Geriatrics. 2009. Retrieved June 9, 2010, from http://emedicine.medscape.com.

Breitbart W, Alici Y: Agitation and delirium at the end of life. *JAMA* 2008; 300: 2898–2910.

Breitbart W, Strout D: Delirium in the terminally ill. *Clinics in Geriatric Medicine* 2000; 16: 357–72.

Brekke M, Hunskaar S, Straand J: Self-reported drug utilization, health, and lifestyle factors among 70–74 year old community dwelling individuals in Western Norway: The Hordaland Health Study (HUSK). *BMC Public Health* 2006.

Bremner JD: Does stress damage the brain? Understanding trauma-related disorders from a mind-body perspective. *Directions in Psychiatry* 2004; 24: 167–76.

Brennan M, Horowitz A, Reinhardt JP: The September 11th attacks and depressive symptomatology among older adults with vision loss in New York City. *Journal of Gerontological Social Work* 2004; 40: 55–71.

Brennan PL: Functioning and health service use among elderly nursing home residents with alcohol use disorders: Findings from the national nursing home survey. *American Journal of Geriatric Psychiatry* 2005; 13: 475–83.

Brenner PR: The experience of Jacob Perlow Hospice: Hospice care of patients. In Volicer, L, Hurley A (eds.), *Hospice Care for Patients with Advanced Progressive Dementia*. New York: Springer, 1998, pp. 257–74.

Brenner PR: Palliative care and hospice: One approach. *American Journal of Hospice and Palliative Medicine* 2000; 17: 241–44.

Brew BJ: Evidence for a change in AIDS dementia complex in the era of highly active antiretroviral therapy and the possibility of new forms of AIDS dementia complex. *AIDS* 2004; 18: S75–78.

Broadway J, Mintzer J: The many faces of psychosis in the elderly. *Current Opinion in Psychiatry* 2007; 20: 551–58.

Brown AS, Derkits EJ: Prenatal infection and schizophrenia: A review of epidemiologic and translational studies. *American Journal of Psychiatry* 2010; 167: 261–80.

Brown L, Cohen D, Kohlmaier L: Older adults and terrorism. In B Bonger, L Brown, L Beutler, J Breckenridge, P Zimbardo (eds.), *Psychology of Terrorism*. New York: Oxford University Press, 2006, pp. 288–310.

Brown LM, Shiang J, Bongar B: Crisis intervention: Theory and practice. In G Stricker, TA Widiger (eds.), *Comprehensive Handbook of Psychology*. Volume 8: Clinical Psychology. New York: John Wiley & Sons, 2003, pp. 431–51.

Brown M, Barraclough B: Epidemiology of suicide pacts in England and Wales, 1988–92. *EMJ* 1997; 315: 286–87.

Brown P, Brandel J-P, Preese M, Sato T: Iatrogenic Creutzfeldt-Jakob disease: The waning of an era. *Neurology* 2006; 67: 389–93.

Bruce ML, Have TRT, Reynolds CF, Katz II, Schulberg HC, Mulsant BH, Alexopoulos GS: Reducing suicidal ideation and depressive symptoms in depressed older primary care patients: A randomized controlled trial. *JAMA* 2004; 291: 1081–91.

Bruce ML, Van Citters AD, Bartels SJ: Evidence-based mental health services for home and community. *Psychiatric Clinics of North America* 2005; 28: 1039–60.

Brunnhuber K, Nash S, Meir DE, Weissman DE: Putting evidence into practice: Palliative care. *British Medical Journal* 2008; 1–88.

Bruscoli M, Lovestone S: Is MCI really just early dementia? A systematic review of conversion studies. *International Psychogeriatrics* 2004; 16: 129–40.

Buchanan A: Mental capacity, legal competence and consent to treatment. *Journal of the Royal Society of Medicine* 2004; 97: 415–20.

Buchanan D, Tourigny-Rivard M-F, Cappeliez P, Frank C, Janikowski P, Spanjevic L, Herrmann N: National guidelines for seniors' mental health: The assessment and treatment of depression. *Canadian Journal of Geriatrics* 2006; 9: S52–58.

Buckley PF: Prevalence and consequences of the dual diagnosis of substance abuse and severe mental illness. *Journal of Clinical Psychiatry* 2006; 67: 5–9.

Budson AE, Price BH: Memory dysfunction. *New England Journal of Medicine* 2005a; 352: 692–99.

Budson AE, Price BH: Memory: Clinical disorders. In *Encyclopedia of Life Sciences* 2005b, pp. 1–9.

Budson AE, Sullivan AL, Solomon PR, Simons JS, Beier JS, Scinto LF: Memory and emotions for the September 11, 2001, terrorist attacks in patients with Alzheimer's disease, patients with mild cognitive impairment, and healthy older adults. *Neuropsychology* 2004; 8: 315–27.

Buhr GT, White HK: Difficult behaviors in long-term care patients with dementia. *Journal of the American Medical Directors Association* 2006; 7: 180–92.

Bulik CM, Sullivan PF, Wade TD, Kendler KS: Twin studies of eating disorders: A review. *International Journal of Eating Disorders* 1999; 27: 1–20.

Burchard EG, Ziv E, Coyle N, Gomez SL, Tang H, Karter AJ, Mountain JL, Pérez-Stable EJ, Sheppard D, Risch N: The importance of race and ethnic background in biomedical research and clinical practice. *Massachusetts Medical Society* 2003; 348: 1170–75.

Burdo JR, Chen Q, Calcutt NA, Schubert D: The pathological interaction between diabetes and pre-symptomatic Alzheimer's disease. *Neurobiology of Aging* 2009; 30: 1910–17.

Burgess, AW, Phillips SL: Sexual abuse, trauma, and dementia in the elderly: A retrospective study of 284 cases. *Victims and Offenders* 2006; 1:193–204.

Burgio L, Lichstein KL, Nichols L, Czaja S, Gallagher-Thompson D, Bourgeois M, Stevens A, Ory M, Schulz R: Judging outcomes in psychosocial interventions for dementia caregivers: The problem of treatment implementation. *The Gerontologist* 2001; 41: 481–89.

Burgio L, Stevens A, Guy D, Roth DL, Haley WE: Impact of two psychosocial interventions on White and African American family caregivers of individuals with dementia. *The Gerontologist* 2003; 43: 568–79.

Burkiewicz JS, Vesta KS, Hume AL: Improving effectiveness in communicating risk to patients. *Consultant Pharmacist* 2008; 23: 37–43.

Burn DJ: Parkinson's disease dementia: What's in a Lewy body? *Journal of Neural Transmission* 2006; 70: 361–65.

Burns A, Folstein S, Brandt J, Folstein M: Clinical assessment of irritability, aggression and apathy in Huntington and Alzheimer disease. *Journal of Nervous and Mental Disease* 1990; 178: 20–25.

Burns B, Larson D, Goldstrom I, Johnson W, Taube C, Miller N, Mathis E: Mental disorders among nursing home patients: Preliminary findings from the national nursing home survey pretest. *International Journal of Geriatric Psychiatry* 2004; 3: 22–35.

Burress JW, Kunik ME, Molinari V, Orengo CA, Rezabek P: Guardianship application for elderly patients: Why do they fail? *Psychiatric Services* 2000; 522–24.

Burston GR: Granny-battering. *British Medical Journal* 1975; 3: 592.

Buschke H, Kuslansky G, Katz M, Stewart WF, Sliwinski MJ, Eckholdt HM, Lipton RB: Screening for dementia with the Memory Impairment Screen. *Neurology* 1999; 52: 231.

Bush AI: The metal biology of Alzheimer's disease. *Trends in Neuroscience* 2003; 26: 207–14.

Busko M: Transcranial Magnetic Stimulation Effective for Depression in Large Trial. Retrieved from Medscape website 2007; http://www.medscape.com/viewarticle/567659.

Butler AC, Chapman JE, Forman EM, Beck AT: The empirical status of cognitive-behavioral therapy: A review of meta-analyses. *Clinical Psychology Review* 2006; 26: 17–31.

Butterwick SJ, Hommel PA, Keilitz I: *Evaluating Mediation as a Means of Resolving Adult Guardianship Cases*. Ann Arbor, MI: Center for Social Gerontology, 2001.

Buysse DJ, Germain A, Moul D, Nofzinger EA: Insomnia. *Focus* 2005; 3: 568–84.

Byard RW, Tsokos M: Forensic issues in cases of Diogenes syndrome. *American Journal of Forensic Medicine and Pathology* 2007; 28: 177–81.

Byrne S, McLean N: Eating disorders in athletes: A review of the literature. *Journal of Science and Medicine in Sport* 2001; 4: 145–59.

Cairney J, McCabe L, Veldhuizen S, Corna LM, Streiner D, Herrmann N: Epidemiology of social phobia in later life. *American Journal of Geriatric Psychiatry* 2007; 15: 224–33.

Cairney J, Corna LM, Veldhuizen S, Herrmann N, Streiner DL: Comorbid depression and anxiety in later life: Patterns of association, subjective well-being, and impairment. *American Journal of Geriatric Psychiatry* 2008; 16: 201–8.

Calhoun LG, Tedeschi RG (eds.): *Meaning Reconstruction and the Experience of Loss.* Washington, DC: American Psychological Association, 2001; 8: 359.

Calvert JF, Hollander-Rodriguez J, Kaye J, Leahy M: Dementia-free survival among centenarians: An evidence-based review. *Journal of Gerontology Biological Sciences Medical Sciences* 2006; 61: 951–56.

Camicioli R, Moore M, Kinney A, Corbridge E, Glassberg K, Kaye JA: Parkinson's disease is associated with hippocampal atrophy. *Movement Disorders* 2003; 18: 784–90.

Canadian Coalition for Seniors' Mental Health. National Guidelines for Seniors' Mental Health: The assessment and treatment of delirium. Toronto: author, 2006.

Cannon W: *The Wisdom of the Body.* New York: Norton, 1932.

Caplan G: *An Approach to Community Mental Health.* New York: Grune and Stratton, 1961.

Carey J: *Longevity: The Biology and Demography of Life Span.* Princeton, NJ: Princeton University Press, 2003.

Carney R, Freedland K, Miller G, Jaffe A: Depression as a risk factor for cardiac mortality and morbidity: A review of potential mechanisms. *Journal of Psychosomatic Research* 2002; 53: 897–902.

Carpenter WT, Gold JM, Lahti AC, Queern CA, Conley RR, Bartko JJ, Kocnick J, Appelbaum PS: Decisional capacity for informed consent in schizophrenia research. *Archives of General Psychiatry* 2000; 57: 533–38.

Cassel CK, Foley KM: *Principles for Care of Patients at the End of Life: An Emerging Consensus among the Specialties of Medicine.* New York: Milbank Memorial Fund, 1999.

Cassidy KL, Rector NA: The silent geriatric giant: Anxiety disorders in late life. *Geriatrics and Aging* 2008; 11: 150–56.

Cassity SA: Commentary: Study Note: To die or not to die: The history and future of assisted suicide laws in the US. *Journal of Law and Family Studies* 2009; 11: 467–75.

Castle NG: Citations and compliance with the nursing home reform act of 1987. *Journal of Health and Social Policy* 2001; 13: 73–95.

Catalano S, Dodson EC, Henze DA, Joyce JG, Kraft GA, Kinney GG: The role of amyloid-beta derived diffusible ligands (ADDLs) in Alzheimer's disease. *Current Topics in Medical Chemistry* 2006; 6: 597–608.

Cattell RB: *Intelligence: Its Structure, Growth and*

Action. Advances in Psychology, 35. Oxford, England: North-Holland, 1987.

Cavanagh JTO, Carson AJ, Sharpe M, Lawrie SM: Psychological autopsy studies of suicide: A systematic review. *Psychological Medicine* 2003; 33: 395–405.

Cegala D, Post D: On addressing racial and ethnic health disparities. *American Behavioral Scientist* 2006; 49: 853–67.

Centers for Disease Control: *Suicide Prevention Now: Linking Research to Practice.* Atlanta: Centers for Disease Control, National Center for Injury and Prevention and Control, 2001.

Centers for Disease Control and Prevention and Kimberly-Clark Corporation: *Assuring Healthy Caregivers, A Public Health Approach to Translating Research into Practice: The RE-AIM Framework.* Neenah, WI: Kimberly-Clark Corporation, 2008.

Cervo FA, Bryan L, Farber S: To PEG or not to PEG: A review of evidence for placing feeding tubes in advanced dementia and the decision-making process. *Geriatrics* 2006; 61: 30–35.

Chao MA: Semantic memory and the brain: Structure and processes. *Current Opinion in Neurobiology* 2001; 11: 194–201.

Charness N: Aging and human performance. *Human Factors* 2008; 50: 548–55.

Charney DS, Reynolds CF, Lewis L, Lebowitz BD, Sunderland T, Alexopoulos GS, Young RC: Depression and bipolar support alliance consensus statement on the unmet needs in diagnosis and treatment of mood disorders in late life. *Archives of General Psychiatry* 2003; 60: 664–72.

Chatterjee J: End-of-life care for patients with dementia. *Nursing for Older People* 2008; 20: 29–34.

Chen D, Cui QC, Yang H, Barrea RA, Sarkar FH, Sheng S, Yan B, Reddy GPV, Dou QP: Cliquinol, a therapeutic agent for Alzheimer's disease, has proteasome-inhibitory, androgen receptor-suppressing, apoptosis-inducing, and antitumor activities in human prostate cancer cells and xenografts. *Cancer Research* 2007; 67.

Chen H: Possible role of platelet gluR1 receptors in comorbid depression and cardiovascular disease. *Cardiovascular Psychiatry and Neurology* 2009; 1–3.

Chen H, Chung H, Chen T, Fang L, Chen JP: The emotional distress in a community after the terrorist attack on the World Trade Center. *Community Mental Health Journal* 2003; 39: 157–65.

Chen LY, Hardy CL: Alcohol consumption and health status in older adults. *Journal of Aging and Health* 2009; 12: 824–47.

Chernoff R: Tube feeding patients with dementia. *Nutrition in Clinical Practice* 2006; 21: 142–46.

Chertkow H, Massoud F, Nasreddine Z, Belleville S, Joanette Y, Bocti C, Bergman H: Diagnosis and treatment of dementia: Mild cognitive impairment and cognitive impairment without dementia. *Focus* 2009; 7: 64–78.

Chew-Graham CA, Baldwin R, Burns A: *Integrated Management of Depression in the Elderly*. Cambridge: Cambridge University Press, 2008.

Chochinov HM: Dying, dignity, and new horizons in palliative end-of-life care. *CA Cancer Journal for Clinicians* 2006; 56: 84–103.

Chochinov HM, Cann BJ: Interventions to enhance the spiritual aspects of dying. *Journal of Palliative Medicine* 2005; 8: S103–15.

Choi NG, Mayer J: Elder abuse, neglect, and exploitation: Risk factors and prevention strategies. *Journal of Gerontological Social Work* 2000; 33: 5–25.

Chrisakis NA: Social networks and collateral health effects have been ignored in medical care and clinical trials, but need to be studied. *British Medical Journal* 2004; 329: 184–85.

Christensen K, Vaupel JW: Determinants of longevity: Genetic, environmental and medical factors. *Journal of Internal Medicine* 1996; 240: 333–41.

Christianson S, Marren J: The impact of event scale—Revised (IES-R). *Annals of Long Term Care* 2009; 17: 25–26.

Chui HC, Mack W, Jackson JE, Mungas D, Reed BR, Tinklenberg J, Jagust WJ: Clinical criteria for the diagnosis of vascular dementia: A multicenter study of comparability and interrater reliability. *Archives of Neurology* 2000; 57: 191–96.

Chung I: The impact of the 9/11 attacks on the elderly in NYC Chinatown: Implications for culturally relevant services. *Journal of Gerontological Social Work* 2004; 40: 37–53.

Church M, Watts S: Assessment of mental capacity: A flow chart guide. *The Psychiatrist* 2007; 31: 304–7.

Cipriani A, Pretty H, Hawton K, Geddes JR: Lithium in the prevention of suicidal behavior and all-cause mortality in patients with mood disorders: A systematic review of randomized trials. *American Journal of Psychiatry* 2005; 162: 1805–19.

Citron M: β-Secretase inhibition for treatment of Alzheimer's disease: Promise and challenge. *Trends in Pharmacological Science* 2004; 25: 92–97.

Claessens P, Menten J, Schotsmans P, Broeckaert B: Palliative sedation: A review of the research literature. *Journal of Pain and Symptom Management* 2008; 36: 310–33.

Clancy CP, Graybeal A, Tompson WP, Badgett KS, Fekdman ME, Calhoun PS, Erkanil A, Hertzberg MA, Beckham JC: Lifetime trauma exposure in veterans with military-related posttraumatic stress disorder: Association with current symptomatology. *Journal of Clinical Psychiatry* 2006; 67: 1346–53.

Clardy SL, Connor JR: Restless leg syndrome. *Encyclopedia of Neuroscience* 2004; 131–35.

Clarke CE, Deane KH: Ropinirole for levodopa-induced complications in Parkinson's disease. *Cochrane Database Systematic Reviews* 2001; 1.

Clayton PJ: *Bereavement,* 2nd edition. Encyclopedia of Stress 2007; 317: 323.

Clever SL, Jin L, Levinson W, Meltzer DO: Does doctor-patient communication affect patient satisfaction with hospital care. *Health Research and Educational Trust* 2008; 43: 1505–19.

Cloninger R: Antisocial personality disorder: A review. In M Maj, H Akiskal, J Mezzich, A Okasha (eds.), *Personality Disorders*. West Sussex, England: John Wiley, 2005, pp. 125–69.

Cohen BA: Chronic meningitis. *Current Neurology and Neuroscience Reports* 2005; 5: 429–39.

Cohen CI (ed.): *Schizophrenia in Later Life: Treatment, Research, and Policy.* Washington, DC: American Psychiatric Publishing, 2003.

Cohen CI, Vahia I, Reyes P, Diwan S, Bankole AO, Palekar N, Ramirez P: Focus on geriatric psychiatry: Schizophrenia in later life: Clinical symptoms and social well-being. *Psychiatric Services* 2008; 59: 232–34.

Cohen D: Homicide-suicide in the aged: A growing public health problem. *Journal of Mental Health and Aging* 1995; 1: 83–84.

Cohen D: Homicide-suicide in older people. *Psychiatric Times* 2000; 17: 1–7.

Cohen D: Violent deaths and dementia. *Journal of Mental Health and Aging* 2004; 10: 83–86.

Cohen D, Eisdorfer C: *The Loss of Self: A Family Resource for Alzheimer's Disease and Related Dementias.* New York: Norton, 1986.

Cohen D, Eisdorfer C: *Caring for Your Aging Parents: A Planning and Action Guide.* New York: Penguin Group, 1995.

Cohen D, Eisdorfer C, Leverenz J: Alzheimer's disease and maternal age. *Journal of the American Geriatrics Society* 1982; 30: 656–59.

Cohen D, Eisdorfer C, Kennedy G: Phases of change in the patient with Alzheimer's dementia: A conceptual dimension for defining health care management. *Journal of the American Geriatrics Society* 1984; 32: 11–15.

Cohen D, Eisdorfer C, Gorelick P, Luchins D, Freels S, Semla T: Sex differences in the psychiatric manifestations of Alzheimer's disease. *Journal of the American Geriatrics Society* 1993; 41: 229–32.

Cohen D, Eisdorfer C, Paveza G, Ashford J, Luchins D, Gorelick P: Psychopathology associated with Alzheimer's disease and related disorders. *Journal of Gerontology* 1993; 48: M255–60.

Cohen D, Kallimanis BL: A geriatric mobile crisis response team: A resilience-promoting program to meet the mental health needs of community-residing older people. In Resnick B, Roberto K, Gwyther

L (eds.), *Resilience in Aging: Concepts, Research, and Outcomes.* New York: Springer, 2010.

Cohen D, Llorente M, Eisdorfer C: Homicide-suicide in older persons. *American Journal of Psychiatry* 1998; 155: 390–39.

Cohen D, Luchins D, Eisdorfer C, Paveza GJ: Caring for relatives with Alzheimer's disease: The mental health risks to spouses, adult children, and other family caregivers. *Behavior, Health, and Aging* 1990; 1: 171–82.

Cohen ST, Block S: Issues in psychotherapy with terminally ill patients. *Palliative and Supportive Care* 2004; 2: 181–89.

Cohen-Mansfield J: Nonpharmacological management of behavioral problems in persons with dementia: The TREA model. *Alzheimer's Care Today* 2000; 1: 22–34.

Cohen-Mansfield J: Nonpharmacologic interventions for inappropriate behaviors in dementia: A review, summary, and critique. *Focus* 2004; 2: 288–308.

Cohen-Mansfield J, Mintzer J: Time for change: The role of nonpharmacological interventions in treating behavior problems in nursing home residents with dementia. *Alzheimer Disease and Associated Disorders* 2005; 19: 37–40.

Cole MG: Delirium in elderly patients. *Focus* 2005; 3: 320–32.

Cole MG, Dendukuri N: Risk factors for depression among elderly community subjects: A systematic review and meta-analysis. *American Journal of Psychiatry* 2003; 160: 1147–56.

Cole MG, McCusker J: Improving the outcomes of delirium in older hospital inpatients. *International Psychogeriatrics* 2009; 21: 613–15.

Cole MG, McCusker J, Dendukuri N, Han L: Symptoms of delirium among elderly medical inpatients with or without dementia. *Journal of Neuropsychiatry and Clinical Neurosciences* 2002; 14: 167–75.

Colenda CC, Wagenaar DB, Mickus M, Marcus SC, Tanielian T, Pincus HA: Comparing clinical practice with guideline recommendations for the treatment of depression in geriatric patients: Findings from the APA practice research network. *American Journal of Geriatric Psychiatry* 2003; 11: 448–57.

Colombres M, Sagal JP, Inestrosa NC: An overview of the current and novel drugs for Alzheimer's disease with particular reference to anti-cholinesterase compounds. *Current Pharmaceutical Design* 2004; 10: 3121–30.

Combs CK, Johnson DE, Karlo JC, Cannady SB, Landreth GE: Inflammatory mechanisms in Alzheimer's disease: Inhibition of β-amyloid-stimulated proinflammatory responses and neurotoxicity by PPARγ agonists. *Journal of Neuroscience* 2000; 20: 558–67.

Comella CL: Sleep disorders in Parkinson's disease. *Sleep Medicine Clinics* 2008; 3: 325–35.

Comijs HC, Pot AM, Smit JH, Bouter LM, Jonker C: Elder abuse in the community: Prevalence and consequences. *Journal of the American Geriatric Society* 1998; 46: 885–88.

Compton WM, Thomas YF, Stinson FS, Grant BF: Prevalence, correlates, disability, and comorbidity of DSM-IV drug abuse and dependence in the United States: Results from the National Epidemiologic Survey on Alcohol and Related Conditions. *Archives of General Psychiatry* 2007; 64: 566–76.

Congdon N, O'Colmain B, Klaver CC, Klein R, Muñoz B, Friedman DS, Kempen J, Taylor HR, Mithcell P: Causes and prevalence of visual impairment among adults in the United States. *Archives of Opthalmology* 2004; 122: 477–85.

Conwell Y: Suicide in later life: A review and recommendations for prevention. *Suicide and Life-Threatening Behavior* 2001; 31: 32–47.

Conwell Y: Suicide prevention in later life: A glass half full, or half empty. *American Journal of Psychiatry* 2009; 166: 845–48.

Conwell Y, Pearson JL: Theme issue: Suicidal behaviors in older adults. *American Journal of Geriatric Psychiatry* 2002; 10: 359–61.

Conwell Y, Thompson C: Suicidal behavior in elders. *Psychiatric Clinics of North America* 2008; 31: 333–56.

Conwell Y, Lyness J, Duberstein P, Cox C, Seidlitz L, DiGiorgia A, Caine ED: Completed suicide among older patients in primary care practices: A controlled study. Journal of the American Geriatrics Society 2000; 48: 23–29.

Conwell Y, Duberstein PR, Caine ED: Risk factors for suicide in later life. *Biological Psychiatry* 2002; 52: 193–204.

Cook JM, Arean PA, Schnurr PP, Sheikh J: Symptom differences of older depressed primary care patients with and without history of trauma. *International Journal of Psychiatry in Medicine* 2001; 31: 415–28.

Cook JM, Marshall R, Masci C, Coyne JC: Physicians' perspectives on prescribing benzodiazepines for older adults: A qualitative study. *Journal of General Internal Medicine* 2007; 22: 303–7.

Cooke JR, Ancoli-Israel S: Sleep and its disorders in older adults. *Psychiatric Clinics of North America* 2006; 29: 1077–93.

Coon DW: *Lesbian, Gay, Bisexual and Transgender (LGBT) Issues and Family Caregiving.* San Francisco: Family Caregiver Alliance, 2003.

Coon DW: Exploring interventions for LGBT caregivers: Issues and examples. *Journal of Gay and Lesbian Social Services* 2007; 18: 109–28.

Coon KD, Myers AJ, Craig DW, Webster JA, Pearson

JV, Lince DH, Zismann VL, Beach TG, Leung D, Bryden L, Halperin RF, Marlowe L, Kaleem M, Walker DG, Ravid R, Heward CB, Rogers J, Papassotiropoulos A, Reiman EM, Hardy J, Stephan DA: A high density whole-genome association study reveals that APOE is the major susceptibility gene for sporadic late-onset Alzheimer's disease. *Journal of Clinical Psychiatry* 2007; 68: 613–18.

Cooper C, Selwood A, Livingston G: The prevalence of elder abuse and neglect: A systematic review. *Age and Ageing* 2008; 37: 151–60.

Costa DL: Changing chronic disease rates and long-term declines in functional limitation among older men. *Demography* 2002; 39: 119–37.

Costa P, Samuels J, Bagby M, Daffin L, Norton H: Obsessive-compulsive personality disorder: A review. In M Maj, H Akiskal, J Mezzich, A Okasha (eds.), *Personality Disorders*, volume 8. West Sussex, England: John Wiley, 2005, pp. 405–39.

Cotman CW, Poon WW, Rissman RA, Blurton-Jones M: The role of Caspase cleavage of tau in Alzheimer disease neuropathology. *Journal of Neuropathology and Experimental Neurology* 2005; 64: 2.

Covinsky KE, Newcomer R, Fox P, Wood J, Sands L, Dane K, Yaffe K: Patient and caregiver characteristics associated with depression in caregivers of patients with dementia. *Journal of General Internal Medicine* 2003; 18: 1006–14.

Cowan JD, Walsh D: Terminal sedation in palliative medicine: Definition and review of the literature. *Supportive Care in Cancer* 2001; 403–7.

Cowell DD: White House Conference on Aging: Abstracts of the Technical Committee Reports, Mini White House Conference Reports, and State White House Conference Reports. 1981.

Craddock N, Sklar P: Genetics of bipolar disorder: Successful start to a long journey. *Trends in Genetics* 2009; 25: 99–105.

Craig-Schapiro R, Fagan AM, Holtzman DM: Biomarkers of Alzheimer's disease. *Neurobiology of Disease* 2008; 35: 128–40.

Craik FIM, Salthouse TA: *The Handbook of Aging and Cognition*. Mahwah, NJ: Lawrence Erlbaum Associates, 2000.

Crawley LM: Racial, cultural, and ethnic factors influencing end-of-life care. *Journal of Palliative Medicine* 2005; 8: S58–69.

Creamer M, Parslow R: Trauma exposure and posttraumatic stress disorder in the elderly: A community prevalence study. *American Journal of Geriatric Psychiatry* 2008; 16: 853–56.

Crino R, Slade T, Andrews G: The changing prevalence and severity of obsessive-compulsive disorder criteria from DSM-III to DSM-IV. *American Journal of Psychiatry* 2005; 162: 876–82.

Crome I, Bloor R: Older substance misusers still deserve better treatment interventions: An update (Part 3). *Reviews in Clinical Gerontology* 2006; 16: 45–57.

Crome I, Sidhu H, Cromet P: No longer only a young man's disease: Illicit drugs and older people. *Journal of Nutrition, Health and Aging* 2009; 13: 141–43.

Crook TH, Bartus RT, Ferris SH, Whitehouse PJ, Cohen GD, Gershon S: Age-associated memory impairment: Proposed diagnostic criteria and measures of clinical change—report of a National Institute of Mental Health workgroup. *Developmental Neuropsychology* 1986; 2: 261–76.

Crosby NJ, Deane KH, Clarke CE: Amantadine for dyskinesia in Parkinson's disease. *Cochrane Database Systematic Reviews* 2003.

Crow SJ, Peterson CB, Swanson SA, Raymond NC, Specker S, Eckert ED, Mitchell JE: Increased mortality in bulimia nervosa and other eating disorders. *American Journal of Psychiatry* 2009; 166: 1342–46.

Culberson JW, Ziska M: Prescription drug misuse/abuse in the elderly. *Geriatrics* 2008; 63: 22–31.

Culpepper L: Generalized anxiety disorder and medical illness. *Journal of Clinical Psychiatry* 2009; 70: 20–24.

Cummings JL: The neuropsychiatric inventory: Assessing psychopathology in dementia patients. *Neurology* 1997; 48: S10–16.

Cummings JL: Use of cholinesterase inhibitors in clinical practice. *American Journal of Geriatric Psychiatry* 2003; 11: 131–45.

Cummings JL: Fluctuations in cognitive function in dementia with Lewy bodies. *Lancet Neurology* 2004; 3: 266.

Cummings JL, Mega M, Gray K, Rosenberg-Thompson S, Carusi DA, Gornbein J: The Neuropsychiatric Inventory: Comprehensive assessment of psychopathology in dementia. *Neurology* 1998; 44: 2308–14.

Cutchin MP: The process of mediated aging-in-place: A theoretically and empirically based model. *Social Science and Medicine* 2003; 57: 1077–90.

Daly M, Katzel L: *Health Promotion and Disease Prevention in the Elderly*. Washington, DC: Public Health Service (DHHS Publication), 2001 www.sergp.org/Educ2/Gertutor/Prevent/prevention.html.

Danysz W, Parsons CG: The NMDA receptor antagonist memantine as a symptomatological and neuroprotective treatment for Alzheimer's disease: Preclinical evidence. *International Journal of Geriatric Psychiatry* 2003; 18: S23–32.

Danysz W, Parsons CG, Möbius J, Stöffler A, Quack G: Neuroprotective and symptomatological action of memantine relevant for Alzheimer's disease: A unified glutamatergic hypothesis on the mechanism of action. *Neurotoxicity Research* 2000; 2: 85–97.

Dar K: Alcohol use disorders in elderly people: F Gfroerer act or fiction? *Advances in Psychiatric Treatment* 2006; 12: 173–81.

Dauer W, Przedborski S: Parkinson's disease: Mechanisms and models. *Neuron* 2003; 39: 889–909.

Davidson JR: Recognition and treatment of posttraumatic stress disorder. *JAMA* 2001; 286: 584–88.

De Asis JM, Stern E, Alexopoulos GS, Pan H, Van Gorp W, Blumberg H, Silbersweig DA: Hippocampal and anterior cingulate activation deficits in patients with geriatric depression. *American Journal of Psychiatry* 2001; 158: 1321–23.

Dedert EA, Green KT, Calhoun PS, Yoash-Gantz R, Taber KH, Mumford MM, Tupler LA, Morey RA, Marx CE, Weiner RD, Beckham JC: Association of trauma exposure with psychiatric morbidity in military veterans who have served since September 11, 2001. *Journal of Psychiatric Research* 2009; 43: 830–36.

Deeg DJH, Huizink AC, Comijs HC, Smid T: Disaster and associated changes in physical and mental health in older residents. *European Journal of Public Health* 2005; 15: 170–74.

Deisenhammer EA, Huber M, Kemmler G, Weiss EM, Hinterhuber H: Suicide victims' contacts with physicians during the year before death. *European Archives of Psychiatry and Clinical Neuroscience* 2007; 257: 480–85.

DeKosky ST, Fitzpatrick A, Ives DG, Saxton J, Williamson J, Lopez OL, Burke G, Fried L, Kuller LH, Robbins J, Tracy R, Woolard N, Dunn L, Kronmal R, Nahin R, Furberg C, for the Ginko Evaluation of Memory (GEM) Study Investigators: The ginkgo evaluation of memory (GEM) study: Design and baseline of a randomized trial of Ginkgo biloba extract in prevention of dementia. *Contemporary Clinical Trials* 2006; 27: 238–53.

DeKosky ST, Williamson JD, Fitzpatrick AL, Kronmal RA, Ives DG, Saxton JA, Lopez OL, Burke G, Carlson MC, Fried LP, KUller LH, Robbins JA, Tracy RP, Woolard NF, Dunn L, Snitz BE, Nahin RL, Furberg CD, for the Ginkgo Evaluation of Memory (GEM) Study Investigators: Ginkgo biloba for prevention of Dementia. *JAMA* 2008; 300: 2253–62.

Delacourte A, Buée, L: Tau pathology: A marker of neurodegenerative disorders. *Current Opinion in Neurology* 2000; 13: 371–76.

DeLamater J, Karraker A: Sexual functioning in older adults. *Current Psychiatry Reports* 2009; 11: 6–11.

Dennerstein L, Dudley E, Burger H: Are changes in sexual functioning during midlife due to aging or menopause? *Fertility and Sterility* 2001; 76: 456–60.

Dennis NA, Cabeza R: Neuroimaging of healthy cognitive aging. In Craik FIM, Salthouse, TA (eds.), *The Handbook of Aging and Cognition,* 3rd edition. East Sussex, UK: Psychology Press, 2007, pp. 1–54.

De Oliveira e Silva ER, Foster D, Harper MM, Seidman CE, Smith JD, Breslow JL, Brinton EA: Alcohol consumption raises HDL cholesterol levels by increasing the transport rate of apolipoproteins A-I and A-II. *Circulation* 2000; 102: 2347–52.

Depp CA, Jeste DV: Bipolar disorder in older adults: A critical review. *Bipolar Disorder* 2004; 6: 343–67.

Depp CA, Jeste DV: Definitions and predictors of successful aging: A comprehensive review of larger quantitative studies. *Focus* 2009; 7: 137–50.

Depp C, Vahia IV, Jeste D: Successful aging: Focus on cognitive and emotional health. *Annual Review of Clinical Psychology* 2010; 6.

Desikan RS, Cabral HJ, Hess CP, Dillon WP, Glastonbury CM, Weiner MW, Fischl B: Automated MRI measures identify individuals with mild cognitive impairment and Alzheimer's disease. *Brain* 2009; 132: 2048–57.

Devanand DP: Comorbid psychiatric disorders in late life depression. *Biological Psychiatry* 2002; 52: 236–42.

De Waal MWM, Arnold IA, Eekhof JAH: Somatoform disorders in general practice: Prevalence, functional impairment, and comorbidity with anxiety and depressive disorders. *British Journal of Psychiatry* 2004; 184: 470–76.

Di Castelnuovo A, Costanzo S, Bagnardi V, Donati MB, Iacoviello L, de Gaetano G: Alcohol dosing and total mortality in men and women: An updated meta-analysis of 34 prospective studies. *Archives of Internal Medicine* 2006; 166: 2437–45.

Dilworth-Anderson P, Gibson BE: The cultural influence of values, norms, meanings, and perceptions in understanding dementia in ethnic minorities. *Alzheimer Disease and Associated Disorders* 2002; 16: 56–63.

Dombrovski AY, Mulsant BH: ECT: The preferred treatment for severe depression in late life. *International Psychogeriatrics* 2007; 19: 10–14.

Doody RS: Cholinesterase inhibitors and memantine: Best practices. *CNS Spectrums* 2008; 10S16: 34–35.

Doody RS, Stevens JC, Beck RM, Dubinsky JA, Kaye JA, Gwyther L, Mohs RC, Thal LJ, Whitehouse PJ, DeKosky ST, Cummings JL: Practice parameter: Management of dementia (an evidence-based review). Report of the Quality Standards Subcommittee of the American Academy of Neurology. *American Academy of Neurology* 2001; 56: 1154–66.

Draper B, MacCuspie-Moore C, Brodaty H: Suicidal ideation and the "wish to die" in dementia patients: The role of depression. *Age and Ageing* 1998; 27: 503–7.

Druss B, Bradford D, Rosenheck R, Radford M, Krumholz H: Quality of care and excess mortality in older patients. *Archives of General Psychiatry* 2001; 58: 565–72.

Duara R, Barker W, Luis CA: Frontotemporal dementia and Alzheimer's disease: Differential diagnosis. *Dementia and Geriatric Cognitive Disorders* 1999; 10: 37–42.

Dube SR, Asman K, Malarcher A, Carabollo R: Cigarette smoking among adults and trends in smoking cessation, United States, 2008. *Morbidity and Mortality Weekly Report* 2009; 58: 1227–32.

Duberstein PR, Heisel MJ, Conwell Y: Suicide. In Agronin ME, Maletta GJ (eds.), *Principles and Practice of Geriatric Psychiatry*. Philadelphia: Lippincott Williams & Wilkins, 2005, pp. 393–405.

Dubler N, Nimmons D: *Ethics on Call: A Medical Ethicist Shows How to Take Charge of Life-and-Death Choices*. New York: Harmony Books, 1982.

Dubnov G, Berry EM: Stress in the pathogenesis of eating disorders and obesity. In Yehuda S, Mostofsky DI (eds.), *Nutrients, Stress, and Medical Disorders*. Totowa, NJ, Humana Press, 2006, pp. 253–63.

Dubois B, Pillon B: Cognitive deficits in Parkinson's disease. *Journal of Neurology* 1997; 244: 2–8.

Dubois B, Feldman HH, Jacova C, DeKosky ST, Barberger-Gateau P, Cummings J, Delacourte A, Galasko D, Gauthier S, Jicha G, Meguro K, O'Brien J, Pasquier F, Robert P, Rossor M, Salloway S, Stern Y, Visser PJ, Scheltens P: Research criteria for the diagnosis of Alzheimer's disease: Revising the NINCDC-ADRDA criteria. *The Lancet* 2007; 6: 734–36.

Dufour M, Fuller RK: Alcohol in the elderly. *Annual Review of Medicine* 2003; 46: 123–32.

Dunlop BW, Nemeroff CB: The role of dopamine in the pathophysiology of depression. *Archives of General Psychiatry* 2007; 64: 327–37.

Dunn LB, Jeste DV: Enhancing informed consent for research and treatment. *Neuropsychopharmacology* 2001; 24: 595–607.

Dunn LB, Nowrangi MA, Palmer BW, Jeste DV, Saks ER: Assessing decisional capacity for clinical research or treatment: A review of instruments. *American Journal of Psychiatry* 2006; 163: 1323–34.

Dworkin RH, O'Connor AB, Backonja M, Farrar JT, Finnerup NB, Jensen TS, Kalso EA, Loeser JD, Miaskowski C, Nurmikko TJ, Portenoy RK, Rice ASC, Stacey BR, Treede R, Turk DC, Wallace MS: Pharmacologic management of neuropathic pain: Evidence-based recommendations. *Pain* 2007; 132: 237–51.

Dy SM, Lorenz KA, Naeim A, Sanati H, Walling A, Asch SM: Evidence-based recommendations for cancer fatigue, anorexia, depression, and dyspnea. *Journal of Clinical Oncology* 2008; 26: 3886–95.

Dyer CB, Goodwin JS, Pickens-Pace S, Burnett J, Kelly PA: Self-neglect among the elderly: A model based on more than 500 patients seen by a geriatric medicine team. *American Journal of Public Health* 2007; 97: 1671–76.

Dyer CB, Regev M, Burnett J, Festa N, Cloyd B: SWIFT: A rapid triage tool for vulnerable older adults in disaster situations. *Disaster Medicine and Public Health Preparedness* 2008; 2: S45–50.

Dyer CB, Toronjo C, Cunningham M, Festa NA, Pavlik VN, Hyman DJ, Poythress EL, Searle NS: The key elements of elder neglect: A survey of adult protective service workers. *Journal of Elder Abuse and Neglect* 2005; 17: 1–10.

Eardley I, Cartledge J: Tadalafil (Cialis) for men with erectile dysfunction. *International Journal of Clinical Practice* 2002; 56: 300–304.

Edge MD, Ramel W, Drabant EM, Kuo JR, Parker KJ, Gross JJ: For better or worse? Stress inoculation effects for implicit but not explicit anxiety. *Depression and Anxiety* 2009; 26: 831–37.

Eggermont L, Swaab D, Luiten P, Scerder E: Exercise, cognition, and Alzheimer's disease: More is not necessarily better. *Neuroscience and Biobehavioral Reviews* 2006; 30: 562–75.

Eisdorfer C, Czaja SJ, Loewenstein DA, Rubert MP, Arguelles S, Mitrani VB, Szapocznik, J: The effect of a family therapy and technology-based intervention on caregiver depression. *The Gerontologist* 2003; 43: 521–31.

Eisenberg L: Psychiatry and society: A sociobiologic synthesis. *New England Journal of Medicine* 1977; 296: 903–10.

Eliason S: Murder-suicide: A review of the recent literature. *Journal of the American Academy of Psychiatry Law* 2009; 37: 371–76.

Elliott GR, Eisdorfer C: *Stress and Human Health*. New York: Springer, 1982.

Ellison JM: Pharmacotherapy for mild cognitive impairment: Are we there yet? *Psychiatric Times* 2008; 25.

Ellison J, Kyomen H, Verma S (eds.): *Depression in Later Life: A Multidisciplinary Psychiatric Approach*. New York: Informa Healthcare, 2008.

Ellman L, Yolken R, Buka S, Torrey F, Cannon T: Cognitive functioning prior to the onset of psychosis: The role of fetal exposure to serologically determined influenza. *Biological Psychiatry* 2009; 65: 1040–47.

Elmer L: Cognitive issues in Parkinson's disease. *Neurologic Clinics* 2004; 22: S91–106.

Elzinga BM, Roelofs K, Tollenaar MS, Bakvis P, van Pelt J, Spinhoven P: Diminished cortisol responses to psychosocial stress associated with lifetime adverse events: A study among healthy young subjects. *Psychoneuroendocrinology* 2008; 33: 227–37.

Emanuel EJ, Emanuel LL: The promise of a good death. *Lancet* 1998; 351: 21–29.

Emanuel E, Librach L: *Palliative Care: Core Skills and Clinical Competencies.* Philadelphia: Saunders, 2007.

Emanuel LL, von Gunten CF, Ferris FD: Advance care planning. *Archives of Family Medicine* 2000; 9: 1181–87.

Emre M: Dementia associated with Parkinson's disease. *Neurology* 2003; 2: 229–37.

Enck RE: Hospice palliative medicine: A look back and into the future. *American Journal of Hospice and Palliative Care* 2009; 26: 429.

Engberg H, Christensen K, Andersen-Ranberg K, Jeune B: Cohort changes in cognitive function among Danish centenarians. *Dementia and Geriatric Cognitive Disorders* 2008; 26: 153–60.

Erikson E: Problems of ego identity. *Journal of the American Psychoanalytical Society* 1956; 4: 56–121.

Erikson E, Arve S, Lauri S: Informational and emotional support received by relatives before and after the cancer patient's death. *European Journal of Oncological Nursing* 2006; 10: 48–58.

Erkinjuntti T, Roman G, Gauthier S: Treatment of vascular dementia: Evidence from clinical trials with cholinesterase inhibitors. *Journal of the Neurological Sciences* 2004; 226: 63–66.

Erlingsson CL, Saveman BI, Berg AC: Perceptions of elder abuse in Sweden: Voices of older persons. *Brief Treatment and Crisis Intervention* 2005; 5: 213–27.

Espeland MA, Rapp SR, Shumaker SA, Brunner R, Manson JE, Sherwin BB, Hsia J, Margolis KL, Hogan PE, Wallace R, Dailey M, Freeman R, Hayes J, the Women's Health Initiative Memory Study: Conjugated Equine estrogens and global cognitive function in postmenopausal women. *JAMA* 2004; 291: 2959–98.

Esposito D, Rouillon F, Limosin F: Diogenes syndrome in a pair of siblings. *Canadian Journal of Psychiatry* 2003; 48: 571–72.

Etchells E, Darzins P, Silberfeld M, Singer PA, McKenny J, Naglie G, Katz M, Hyatt GH, Strang D: Assessment of patient capacity to consent to treatment. *Journal of General Internal Medicine* 1999; 14: 27–34.

Etminan M, Gill S, Sami A: Effect of non-steroidal anti-inflammatory drugs on risk of Alzheimer's disease: Systematic review and meta-analysis of observational studies. *British Medical Journal* 2003; 327: 128–32.

Evans BC, Crogan NL, Shultz JA: The meaning of mealtimes: Connection to the social world of the nursing home. *Journal of Gerontological Nursing* 2006; 21: 11–17.

Evans DL, Charney DS, Lewis L, Golden RN, Gorman JM, Krishnan KRR, Valvo WJ: Mood disorders in the medically ill: Scientific review and recommendations. *Biological Psychiatry* 2005; 58: 175–89.

Everly Jr. GS, Hamilton SE, Tyiskac CG, Ellersd K: Mental health response to disaster: Consensus recommendations: Early Psychological Intervention Subcommittee (EPI), National Volunteer Organizations Active in Disaster (NVOAD). *Aggression and Violent Behavior* 2008; 13: 407–12.

Ewing JA: Detecting alcoholism: The CAGE questionnaire. *JAMA* 1984; 252: 1905–7.

Faggiani FT, Schroeter G, Pacheco SL, Araujo de Souza AC, Werlang MC, Attilio de Carli G, Beuno Morrone F: Profile of drug utilization in the elderly living in Porto Alegre, Brazil. *Pharmacy Practice* 2007; 5: 179–84.

Fahn S, Oakes D, Shoulson I, Kieburtz K, Rudolph A, Lang A, Marek K: Levodopa and the progression of Parkinson's disease. *New England Journal of Medicine* 2004; 351: 2498–508.

Farrer LA, Bowirratm A, Friedland RP, Waraska K, Korczyn AD, Baldwin, CT: Identification of multiple loci for Alzheimer disease in a consanguineous Israeli-Arab community. *Human Molecular Genetics* 2003; 12: 415–22.

Fava M: Diagnosis and definition of treatment-resistant depression. *Biological Psychiatry* 2003; 53: 649–59.

Fazio L, Brock G: Erectile dysfunction: Management update. *Canadian Medical Association Journal* 2004; 170: 1429–37.

Federal Interagency Forum on Aging Related Statistics: *Older Americans, 2008: Key Indicators of Well-Being.* Washington, DC: FIFARS, 2008.

Feinberg LF, Wolkwitz K, Goldstein C: *Ahead of the Curve: Emerging Trends and Practices in Family Caregiver Support.* Washington, DC: AARP, 2006.

Ferman TJ, Smith GE, Boeve BF: DLB fluctuations: Specific features that reliably differentiate from AD and normal aging. *Neurology* 2004; 62: 181–87.

Fernandez LS, Byard D, Lin CC, Benson S, Barbera JA: Frail elderly as disaster victims: Emergency management strategies. *Prehospital and Disaster Medicine* 2002; 17: 67–74.

Ferraro RF: Psychological resilience in older adults following the 1997 flood. *Clinical Gerontologist* 2003; 26: 139–43.

Ferrell BR: Overview of the domains of variables relevant to end-of-life care. *Journal of Palliative Medicine* 2005; 8: S22–29.

Ferrer I, Santepere G, van Leeuwen FW: Argyrophilic grain disease. *Brain* 2008; 131: 1416–32.

Ferri CP, Prince M, Brayne C, Brodaty H, Fratiglioni L, Ganguli M, Hall K, Hasegawa K, Hendrie H, Huang Y, Jorm A, Mathers C, Menezes PR, Rimmer E, Scazufca: Global prevalence of dementia:

A Delphi consensus study. *The Lancet* 2006; 366: 2112–17.

Ferris FD: Competency in end-of-life care: Last hours of life. *Journal of Palliative Medicine* 2004; 6: 605–13.

Fetter JC: Psychosocial response to mass casualty terrorism: Guidelines for physicians. *Journal of Clinical Psychiatry* 2005; 7: 49–52.

Fick D, Cooper J, Wade W, Waller J, Maclean R, Beers M: Updating the Beers criteria for potentially inappropriate medication use in older adults: Results of a US consensus panel of experts. *Archives of Internal Medicine* 2003; 163: 2716–24.

Fick DM, Maclean JR, Rodriguez NA, Short L, Heuvel RV, Waller JL, Rogers RL: A randomized study to decrease the use of potentially inappropriate medications among community-dwelling older adults in a southeastern managed care organization. *American Journal of Managed Care* 2004; 10: 761–68.

Field D: Palliative medicine and the medicalization of death. *European Journal of Cancer Care* 2010; 3: 58–62.

Field MJ, Behram RE (eds): *When Children Die: Improving Palliative and End-of-Life Care for Children and Their Families.* Washington, DC: National Academies Press, 2003.

Field MJ, Cassel CK (eds): *Approaching Death: Improving Care at the End of Life.* Washington DC: National Academy Press.

Fillenbaum GG: *Multidimensional Functional Assessment of Older Adults: The Duke Older Americans Resources and Services Procedures.* Mahwah, NJ: Lawrence Erlbaum Associates, 1988; 12: 179.

Fillit HM, Butler RN, O'Connell AW, Albert MS, Birren JE, Cotman CW, Greenough WT, Gold PE, Kramer AF, Kuller LH, Perls TT, Sahagan BG, Tully T: Achieving and maintaining cognitive vitality with aging. *Mayo Clinic Proceedings* 2002; 77: 681–96.

Fillit HM, Doody RS, Binaso K, Crooks GM, Ferris SH, Farlow MR, Leifer B, Mills C, Minkoff N, Orland B, Reichman WE, Salloway S: Recommendations for best practices in the treatment of Alzheimer's disease in managed care. *American Journal of Geriatric Pharmacotherapy* 2006; 4: S9–24.

Finkel S, Burns A: Behavioral and psychological symptoms of dementia (BPSD): A clinical and research update. *International Psychogeriatrics* 2000; 12: 9–12.

Firoz S, Carlson G: Characteristics and treatment outcome of older methadone-maintenance patients. *American Journal of Geriatric Psychiatry* 2004; 12: 539–41.

First M, Pincus H: The DSM-IV text revision: Rationale and potential impact on clinical practice. *Psychiatric Services* 2002; 53: 288–92.

First MB, Spitzer RL, Gibbon M, Williams JBW: *Structured Clinical Interview for DSM-IV Axis I Disorders: Patient Education.* New York: New York State Psychiatry Institute, 1997.

Fischer P, Jungwirth S, Zehetmayer S, Weissgram S, Hoenigschnabl S, Gelpi E, Tragl, KH: Conversion from subtypes of mild cognitive impairment to Alzheimer dementia. *Neurology* 2007; 68: 288–91.

Fisher A, Pittel Z, Haring R, Bar-Ber N, Kliger-Spatz M, Natan N, Egozi I, Sonego H, Marcovitch I, Brandeis, R: M1 muscarinic agonists can modulate some of the hallmarks in Alzheimer's disease. *Journal of Molecular Neuroscience* 2003; 20: 1559–66.

Fisk A, Rogers W, Charness S, Czaja S, Sharit J (eds.): *Design for Older Adults: Principles and Creative Human Factors.* Boca Raton, FL: CRC Press, 2009.

Fleisher AS, Raman R, Siemers ER, Becerra L, Clark CM, Dean RA, Farlow MR, Galvin JE, Peskind ER, Quinn JF, Sherzai A, Sowell BB, Aisen PS, Thal LJ: Phase 2 safety trial targeting amyloid β production with a γ-secretase inhibitor in Alzheimer disease. *Archives of Neurology* 2008; 65: 1031–38.

Fleminger S, Oliver DL, Lovestone S, Rabe-Hesketh S, Giora A: Head injury as a risk factor for Alzheimer's disease: The evidence 10 years on; a partial replication. *Journal of Neurology, Neurosurgery, and Psychiatry* 2003; 74: 857–62.

Fletcher PC, Henson RNA: Frontal lobes and human memory: Insights from functional neuroimaging. *Brain* 2001; 124: 849–81.

Flint AJ: Anxiety disorders in later life: From epidemiology to treatment. *American Journal of Geriatric Psychiatry* 2007; 15: 635–38.

Flory J, Emanuel E: Interventions to improve research participants' understanding in informed consent for research. *JAMA* 2004; 292: 1593–1601.

Fochtmann J, Gelenberg AJ: *Guideline Watch: Practice Guideline for the Treatment of Patients with Major Depressive Disorder,* 2nd edition. Washington, DC: American Psychiatric Association, 2005.

Folsom D, McCahill M, Bartels S, Ganiats T, Jeste DV: Medical comorbidity and receipt of medical care by older homeless people with schizophrenia or depression. *Psychiatric Services* 2002; 53: 1456–60.

Folsom DP, Lebowitz BD, Lindamer LA, Palmer BW, Patterson TL, Jeste DV: Schizophrenia in late life: Emerging issues. *Dialogues in Clinical Neuroscience* 2006; 8: 45–52.

Folstein MF, Folstein SE, McHugh PR: "Mini-mental state": A practical method for grading the cognitive state of patients for the clinician. *Journal of Psychiatric Research* 1975; 12: 189–98.

Ford BC, Bullard KM, Taylor RJ, Toler AK, Neighbors H, Jackson JS: Lifetime and 12-month prevalence of DSM-IV disorders among older African

Americans: Findings from the National Survey of American Life. *American Journal of Geriatric Psychiatry* 2007; 15: 652–59.

Frank D, DeBenedetti AF, Volk RJ, Williams EC, Kivlahan DR, Bradley KA: Effectiveness of the AUDIT-C as a screening test for alcohol misuse in three race/ethnic groups. *Journal of General Internal Medicine* 2008; 23: 781–87.

Frank G, Blackhall LJ, Michel V, Murphy ST, Azen SP, Park K: A discourse of relationship in bioethics: Patient autonomy and end-of-life decision making among elderly Korean Americans. *Medical Anthropology Quarterly* 2008; 12: 403–23.

Fratiglioni L, Winblad B, von Strauss E: Prevention of Alzheimer's disease and dementia: Major findings from the Kungsholmen project. *Physiology and Behavior* 2007; 92: 98–104.

Freeman MP, Freeman SA: Lithium: Clinical considerations in internal medicine. *American Journal of Medicine* 2006; 119: 478–81.

Friedlander AH, Norman DC: Geriatric alcoholism: Pathophysiology and dental implications. *Journal of the American Dental Association* 2006; 137: 330–38.

Fries JF: Aging, natural death, and the compression of morbidity. *New England Journal of Medicine* 1980; 303: 130–35.

Fuchs FD, Chambless LE, Folsom AR, Eigenbrodt ML, Duncan BB, Gilbert A, Szkło M: Association between alcoholic beverage consumption and incidence of coronary heart disease in whites and blacks: The atherosclerosis risk in communities study. *American Journal of Epidemiology* 2004; 160: 466–74.

Fuh JL, Teng EL, Lin KN, Larson EB, Wang SJ, Liu CY, Liu HC: The Informant Questionnaire on Cognitive Decline in the Elderly (IQCODE) as a screening tool for dementia for a predominantly illiterate Chinese population. *Neurology* 1995; 45: 92–96.

Fullerton CS, Ursano RJ, Norwood AE, Holloway HH: Trauma, terrorism, and disaster. In RJ Ursano, CS Fullerton, AE Norwood (eds.), *Terrorism and Disaster: Individual and Community Mental Health Interventions*. Cambridge: Cambridge University Press, 2003, pp. 1–20.

Fulmer T, Guadagno L, Dyer CB, Connolly MT: Progress in elder abuse screening and assessment instruments. *Journal of the American Geriatrics Society* 2004; 52: 297–304.

Fulmer T, Paveza G, VandeWeerd C, Fairchild S, Guadagno L, Bolton-Blatt M, Norman R: Dyadic vulnerability and risk profiling for elder neglect. *The Gerontologist* 2005; 45: 525–34.

Gadalla TM: Eating disorders and associated psychiatric comorbidity in elderly Canadian women.

Archive of Women's Mental Health 2008; 5–6: 357–62.

Gajdusek DC: Unconventional Viruses and the Origin and Disappearance of Kuru. Nobel Lecture presented at the National Institutes of Health, Bethesda, MD, 1976.

Galasko D: Dementia with Lewy bodies. *Continuum of Lifelong Learning in Neurology* 2007; 13: 69–86.

Gallagher-Thompson D, Coon DW: Evidence-based psychological treatments for distress in family caregivers of older adults. *Psychology and Aging* 2007; 22: 37–51.

Gallo J, Fulmer T, Paveza G, Reichel W (eds.): *Handbook of Geriatric Assessment,* 3rd edition. Gaithersburg: Aspen Publication, 2000.

Gallo JJ, Zubritsky C, Maxwell J, Nazar M, Bogner HR, Quijano LM, Levkoff SE: Primary care clinicians evaluate integrated and referral models of behavioral health care for older adults: Results from a multisite effectiveness trial (PRISM-E). *Annals of Family Medicine* 2004; 2: 305–9.

Gallo JJ, Bogner HR, Morales KH, Post EP, Lin JY, Bruce ML: The effect of a primary care practice-based depression intervention on mortality in older adults: A randomized trial. *Annals of Internal Medicine* 2007; 146: 689–98.

Galvez-Andres A, Blanco-Fontecilla H, Gonzalez-Parra S, de Dios Molina J, Padin JM, Rodriguez RH: Secondary bipolar disorder and Diogenes syndrome in frontotemporal dementia: Behavioral improvement with Quetiapine and Sodium Valproate. *Journal of Clinical Psychopharmacology* 2007; 27: 722–23.

Gamblin TC, Chen F, Zambrano A, Abraha A, Lagalwar S, Guillozet AL, Lu M, Fu Y, Garcia-Sierra F, LaPointe N, Miller R, Berry RW, Binder LI, Cryns VL: Caspase cleavage of tau: Linking amyloid and neurofibrillary tangles in Alzheimer's disease. *Proceedings of the National Academy of Sciences of the United States of America* 2003; 100: 10032–37.

Ganguli M, Dodge HH, Shen C, DeKosky ST: Mild cognitive impairment, amnestic type: An epidemiologic study. *Neurology* 2004; 63: 115–21.

Gans KM, Ross E, Barner CW, Wylie-Rosett J, McMurray J, Eaton C: REAP and WAVE: New tools to rapidly assess/discuss nutrition with patients. *Journal of Nutrition* 2003; 133: 556–62S.

Ganz M: The Medicare Prescription Drug, Improvement, and Modernization Act of 2003: Are we playing the lottery with health care reform? *Duke Law and Technology Review* 2004; 11: 1–19.

Garrett M: Medicare chronic care improvement program puts the spotlight on case management. *Case Manager* 2005; 16: 56–58.

Gatz, M: Commentary on evidence-based psychological treatments for older adults. *Psychology and Aging* 2007; 22: 52–55.

Gauthier S, Reisberg B, Zaudig M, Petersen RC, Ritchie K, Broich K, Winblad, B: Mild cognitive impairment. *The Lancet* 2006; 367: 1262–70.

Gavier-Widen D, Stack MJ, Baron T, Balachandran A, Simmons M: Diagnosis of transmissible spongiform encephalopathies in animals: A review. *Journal of Veterinary Diagnostic Investigation* 2005; 17: 509–27.

Gavrilov L, Gavrilov N: Evolutionary theory of aging and longevity. *Scientific World Journal* 2002; 2: 339–56.

Geldmacher DS, Provenzano G, McRae T, Mastey V, Ieni JR: Donepezil is associated with delayed nursing home replacement in patients with Alzheimer's disease. *Journal of the American Geriatrics Society* 2003; 51: 937–44.

Geller J, Brown KE, Zaitsoff SL, Goodrich S, Hastings F: Collaborative versus directive interventions in the treatment of eating disorders: Implications for care providers. *Professional Psychology: Research and Practice* 2003; 34: 406–13.

Gellis ZD, Bruce ML: Problem-solving therapy for subthreshold depression in home healthcare patients with cardiovascular disease. *American Journal of Geriatric Psychiatry* 2010; 18: 464–74.

Gellis ZD, Kenaley B: Problem-solving therapy for depression in adults: A systematic review. *Research on Social Work Practice* 2008; 18: 117–31.

Genazzani AR, Gambacciani M, Simoncini T: Menopause and aging, quality of life and sexuality. *Climacteric* 2007; 10: 88–96.

George LK, Fillenbaum GG: OARS methodology: A decade of experience in geriatric assessment. *Journal of the American Geriatrics Society* 1985; 33: 607–15.

Georgi S: Nicotinic Acetylcholine receptors and Alzheimer's disease therapeutics: A review of current literature. *Journal of Young Investigators* 2005; 12.

Gerretsen P, Pollock BG: Pharmacogenetics and the serotonin transporter in late-life depression. *Expert Opinion on Drug Metabolism and Toxicology* 2008; 4: 1465–78.

Gershon AA, Dannon PN, Grunhaus L: Transcranial magnetic stimulation in the treatment of depression. *American Journal of Psychiatry* 2003; 160: 835–45.

Gertz HJ, Kiefer M: Review about ginkgo biloba extract Egb 761 (Ginkgo). *Current Pharmaceutical Design* 2004; 10: 261–64.

Gfroerer J, Penne M, Pemberton M, Folsom R: Substance abuse treatment need among older adults in 2020: The impact of the aging baby-boom cohort. *Drug and Alcohol Dependence* 2003; 69: 127–35.

Ghezzi EM, Ship JA: Dementia and oral health. *Oral Surgery, Oral Medicine, Oral Pathology, Oral Radiology, and Endodontology* 2000; 89: 2–5.

Gibbons S, Lauder W, Ludwick R: Self-neglect: A proposed new NANDA diagnosis. *International Journal of Nursing Terminologies and Classifications* 2006; 17: 110–18.

Gildengers AG, Whyte EM, Drayer RA, Soreca I, Fagiolini A, Kilbourne AM, Mulsant BH: Medical burden in late-life bipolar and major depressive disorders. *American Journal of Geriatric Psychiatry* 2008; 16: 194–200.

Gillespie CF, Nemeroff CB: Hypercortisolemia and depression. *Psychosomatic Medicine* 2005; 67: S26–28.

Gilley D, Wilson R, Beckett L, Evans D: Psychotic symptoms and physically aggressive behavior in Alzheimer's disease. *Journal of the American Geriatrics Society* 1997; 45: 1074–79.

Gillick MR, Volandes AE: The standard of caring: Why do we still use feeding tubes in patients with advanced dementia? *Journal of the American Medical Directors Association* 2008; 9: 364–67.

Gillies J, Neimeyer RA: Loss, grief, and the search for significance: Toward a model of meaning reconstruction in bereavement. *Journal of Constructivist Psychology* 2006; 19: 31–65.

Ginsberg SD, Che S, Wuu J, Counts SE, Mufson EJ: Down regulation of trk but no p75^{NTR} gene expression in single cholinergic basal forebrain neurons mark the progression of Alzheimer's disease. *Journal of Neurochemistry* 2006; 97: 475–87.

Gitlin LN, Belle SH, Burgio LD, Czaja SJ, Mahoney D, Gallagher-Thompson D, Burns R, Hauck WW, Zhang S, Schulz R, Ory MG: Effect of multicomponent interventions on caregiver burden and depression: The REACH multisite initiative at 6-month follow-up. *Psychology and Aging* 2003; 18: 361–74.

Glanz K, Rimer B, Viswanath K (eds.): *Health Behavior and Health Education: Theory, Research, and Practice.* New York: John Wiley & Sons, 2001.

Glock C: Resident-on-resident violence in long term care. *STAT: Chubbs Health Care Newsletter* 2005.

Goblirsch MJ, Zwolak PP, Clohisy DR: Biology of bone cancer pain. *Clinical Cancer Research* 2006; 12: 6231–35s.

Godart NT, Flament MF, Curt F, Perdereau F, Lang F, Venisse JL, Fermanian J: Anxiety disorders in subjects seeking treatment for eating disorders: A DSM-IV controlled study. *Psychiatry Research* 2003; 117: 245–58.

Golbe LI: Progressive supranuclear palsy. *Current Treatment Options in Neurology* 2001; 3: 473–77.

Goldfarb LG: Kuru: The old epidemic in a new mirror. *Microbes and Infection* 2002; 4: 875–82.

Gong Y, Chang L, Viola K, Lacor PN, Lamert MP, Finch CE, Krafft GA, Klein, WL: Alzheimer's disease-affected brain: Presence of oligomeric alpha-beta ligands (ADDLs) suggests a molecular basis for reversible memory loss. *Proceedings of the National Academy of Sciences* 2003; 100: 10417–22.

Good P: Re: Efficacy, safety, and ethical validity of palliative sedation therapy. *Journal of Pain and Symptom Management* 2006; 31: 196–97.

Gordon RM, Brill D: The abuse and neglect of the elderly. *International Journal of Law and Psychiatry* 2001; 24: 183–97.

Gore TA, Lucas JZ: (2009 December). Posttraumatic stress disorder. Retrieved from Emedicine from WebMd website 2009, February 22: http:// emedicine.medscape.com/article/288154-overview.

Gorelick PB: Risk factors for vascular dementia and Alzheimer disease. *Stroke* 2004; 35: 2620–26.

Gorman JM, Kent JM, Sullivan GM, Coplan JD: Neuroanatomical hypothesis of panic disorder, revised. *Focus* 2004; 2: 426–39.

Gozes I, Steingart RA, Spier AD: NAP mechanisms of neuroprotection. *Journal of Neuroscience* 2004; 24: 67–72.

Gracon S, Knapp MJ, Berghoff WG, Pierce M, De-Jong R, Lobbestael SJ, Symons J, Dombey SL, Luscombe FA, Kraemer D: Safety of Tacrine: Clinical trials, treatment IND, and postmarketing experience. *Alzheimer's Disease and Associated Disorders* 1998; 12.

Graff-Radford NR, Woodruff BK: Frontotemporal dementia. *Seminars in Neurology* 2007; 27: 48–57.

Graham NL, Emery T, Hodges JR: Distinctive cognitive profiles in Alzheimer's disease and subcortical vascular dementia. *Journal of Neurology, Neurosurgery, and Psychiatry* 2004; 75: 61–71.

Granholm E, McQuaid JR, McClure FS: A randomized, controlled trial of cognitive behavioral social skills training for middle-aged and older outpatients with chronic schizophrenia. *American Journal of Psychiatry* 2005; 162: 520–29.

Green BL, Goodman LA, Krupnick JL, Corcoran CB, Petty RM, Stockton P: Outcomes of single versus multiple trauma exposure in a screening sample. *Journal of Traumatic Stress* 2000; 13: 271–86.

Grinage, BD: Diagnosis and management of posttraumatic stress disorder. *American Family Physician* 2003; 68: 2401–8.

Grisso T: *Evaluating Competencies: Forensic Assessments and Investments.* New York: Plenum Press, 2003.

Grisso T, Appelbaum PS: *Assessing Competence to Consent to Treatment: A Guide for Physicians and Other Health Professionals.* New York: Oxford University Press, 1998.

Grisso T, Appelbaum P, Hill-Fotouhi C: The Mac-CAT-T: A clinical tool to assess patients' capacities to make treatment decisions. *Psychiatric Services* 1997; 48: 1415–19.

Grossman M, Ash S: Primary progressive aphasia: A review. *Neurocase* 2004; 10: 3–18.

Grover S, Mattoo SK, Gupta N: Theories on mechanism of action of electroconvulsive therapy. *German Journal of Psychiatry* 2005; 8: 70–84.

Grundman M, Petersen RC, Ferris SH, Thomas RG, Aisen PS, Bennett DA, Thal LJ: Mild cognitive impairment can be distinguished from Alzheimer disease and normal aging for clinical trials. *Archives of Neurology* 2004; 61: 59–66.

Guay DRP: Inappropriate sexual behaviors in cognitively impaired older individuals. *American Journal of Geriatric Pharmacotherapy* 2008; 6: 269–88.

Gum AM, Arean PA, Hunkeler E, Tang L, Katon W, Hitchcock P, Unutzer J: Depression treatment preferences in older primary care patients. *The Gerontologist* 2006; 46: 14–22.

Gupta M: Mandatory reporting laws and the emergency physician. *Annals of Emergency Medicine* 2007; 49: 369–76.

Gupta N, de Jonghe J, Schieveld J, Leonard M, Meagher D: Delirium phenomenology: What can we learn from the symptoms of delirium? *Journal of Psychosomatic Research* 2008; 65: 215–22.

Guskiewicz KM, Marshall SW, Bailes J, McCrea M, Cantu RC, Randolph C, Jordan BD: Association between recurrent concussion and late-life impairment in retired professional football players. *Neurosurgery* 2005; 57: 719–26.

Gutheil TG: Common pitfalls in the evaluation of testamentary capacity. *Journal of the American Academy of Psychiatry* 2007; 35: 514–17.

Hachinski VC, Iliff LD, Zilhka E, Du Boulay GH, McAllister VL, Marshall J, Symon L: Cerebral blood flow in dementia. *Archives of Neurology* 1975; 32: 632–37.

Hafner H: Gender differences in schizophrenia. *Psychoneuroendocrinology* 2003; 28, 17–54.

Hagberg B, Alfredson B, Poon L, Homma A: Cognitive functioning in centenarians: A coordinated analysis of results from three countries. *Journal of Gerontology: Psychological Sciences* 2001; 56B: P141–51.

Hajjar ER, Hanlon JT, Sloane R, Linblad CI, Peiper CF, Ruby CM, Branch LC, Schmader KE: Unnecessary drug use in frail older people at hospital discharge. *Journal of the American Geriatrics Society* 2005; 53: 1518–23.

Hakim S, Adams RD: The special clinical problem of symptomatic hydrocephalus with normal cerebrospinal fluid pressure: Observations on cerebrospinal fluid hydrodynamics. *Journal of Neurological Sciences* 1965; 2: 307.

Haley WE, Lamonde LA, Han B, Narramoer S, Schonwetter R: Effects on psychological and health functioning among spousal caregivers of hospice patients with lung cancer or dementia. *Hospice Journal* 2001; 15: 1–18.

Haley WE, Kasl-Goldley J, Larson DG, Neimeyer RA, Kwislosz DM: Roles for psychologists in end-of-life care: Emerging models of practice. *Professional Psychology: Research and Practice* 2003; 24: 626–33.

Halter JB, Ouslander JG, Tinetti ME, Studenski S, High KP, Asthana S: Hazzard's *Geriatric Medicine and Gerontology,* 6th edition. New York: McGraw-Hill, 2009.

Hamilton SP, Fyer AJ, Durner M, Heiman GA, de Leon AB, Hodge SE, Knowles JA, Weissman MM: Further genetic evidence for a panic disorder syndrome mapping to chromosome 13q. *National Academy of Sciences* 2002; 100: 2550–55.

Hamilton SP, Slage SL, de Leon AB, Heiman GA, Klein DF, Hodge SE, Weissman MM, Knowles JA: Evidence for genetic linkage between polymorphism in the adenosine 2A receptor and panic disorder. *Neuropsychopharmacology* 2004; 29: 558–65.

Han B, Gfroerer J, Colliver J: An examination of trends in illicit drug use among adults aged 50 to 59 in the United States. *OAS Data Review* 2009; 1–10.

Hancock K, Chang E, Johnson A, Harrison K, Daly J, Easterbrook SB, Noel M, Luhr-Taylor M, Davidson P: Palliative care for people with advanced dementia: The need for a collaborative, evidence-based approach. *Alzheimer's Care Quarterly* 2006; 7: 49–57.

Hanlon JT, Shimp LA, Semla TP: Recent advances in geriatrics: Drug-related problems in the elderly. *Annals of Pharmacotherapy* 2000; 34: 360–65.

Hanlon JT, Schmader KE, Ruby CM, Weinberger M: Suboptimal prescribing in older inpatients and outpatients. *Journal of the American Geriatrics Society* 2001; 49: 200–209.

Hanlon JT, Pieper CF, Hajjar ER, Sloane RJ, Lindblad CI, Schumader KE: Incidence and predictors of all and preventable adverse drug reactions in frail elderly persons after hospital stay. *Journals of Gerontology, Series A, Biological Sciences and Medical sciences* 2006; 61: 511–15.

Hanrahan P, Luchins DJ: Access to hospice programs in end-stage dementia: A national survey of hospice programs. *Journal of the American Geriatrics Society* 1995; 43: 1174–76.

Harris D: Forget me not: Palliative care for people with dementia. *Postgraduate Medical Journal* 2007; 83: 362–66.

Hanzlick R, Koponen M: Murder-suicide in Fulton County, Georgia, 1988–1991: Comparison with a recent report and proposed typology. *American Journal of Forensic Medicine and Pathology* 1994; 15: 168–73.

Harciarek M, Kertesz A: The prevalence of misidentification syndromes in neurodegenerative diseases. *Alzheimer Disease and Associated Disorders* 2008; 22: 163–69.

Harding AJ, Kril JJ, Halliday GM: Practical measures to simplify the Braak tangle staging method for routine pathological screening. *Acta Neurologica Scandinavica* 2000; 99: 199–208.

Hardy J: The amyloid hypothesis for Alzheimer's disease: A critical reappraisal. *Journal of Neurochemistry* 2009; 110: 1129–34.

Hardy J, Selkoe D: The amyloid hypothesis of Alzheimer's disease: Progress and problems on the road to therapeutics. *Science* 2002; 297: 353–56.

Harman SM, Metter EJ, Tobin JD, Pearson J, Blackman MR: Longitudinal effects of aging on serum total and free testosterone levels in healthy men. *Journal of Clinical Endocrinology and Metabolism* 2001; 86: 724–31.

Harold D, Abraham R, Hollingworth P, Sims R, Gerish A, Hamshere ML, Pahwa JS, Moskvina V, Dowzell K, Williams A, Jones N, Thomas C, Stretton A, Morgan AR, Lovestone S, Powell J, Proitsi P, Lupton MK, Brayne C, Rubinsztein DC, Gill M, Lawlor B, Lynch A, Morgan K, et al. Genome-wide association study identifies variants at CLU and PICALM associated with Alzheimer's disease. *Nature Genetics* 2009; 41: 1088–93.

Harr SD, Uint L, Hollister R, Hyman BT, Mendez AJ: Brain expression of apolipoproteins E, J, and A-I in Alzheimer's disease. *Journal of Neurochemistry* 2002; 66: 2429–35.

Hassing L, Johansson B, Nilsson SE, Berg S, Pedersen NL, Gatz M, McClearn G: Diabetes mellitus is a risk factor for vascular dementia, but not for Alzheimer's disease: A population-based study of the oldest old. *International Psychogeriatrics* 2002; 14: 239–48.

Hauser RA, Pahwa R: Parkinson Disease. Retrieved from eMedicine from WebMD, 2009. http://emedicine.medscape.com/article/1151267-overview.

Havighurst RJ: Successful aging. *The Gerontologist* 1961; 1: 8–13.

Haw C, Harwood D, Hawton K: Dementia and suicidal behavior: A review of the literature. *International Psychogeriatrics* 2009; 21: 440–53.

Haxby JV, Petit L, Ungerleider LG, Courtney SM: Distinguishing the functional roles of multiple regions in distributed neural systems for visual working memory. *Neuroimage* 2000; 11: 380–91.

Hayes R, Dennerstein L: The impact of aging on sexual function and sexual dysfunction in women: A review of population-based studies. *Journal of Sexual Medicine* 2005; 2: 317–30.

Hebert LE, Scherr PA, Bienias JL, Bennett DA,

Evans DA: Alzheimer disease in the US population. *Archives of Neurology* 2003; 60: 1119–22.

Hedden T, Gabrieli JDE: Insights into the ageing mind: A view from cognitive neuroscience. *Nature Reviews: Neuroscience* 2004; 5: 87–97.

Heisel MJ, Duberstein PR: Suicide prevention in older adults. *Clinical Psychology: Science and Practice* 2006; 12: 242–59.

Heisler CJ: Elder abuse and the criminal justice system: New awareness, new responses. *Generations* 2000; 24: 52–58.

Heisler CJ, Stiegel LA: Enhancing the justice system's response to elder abuse: Discussions and recommendations of the "Improving Prosecution" working group of the National Policy Summit on Elder Abuse. *Journal of Elder Abuse and Neglect* 2004; 14: 31–54.

Hendrie HC, Albert MS, Butters MA, Gao S, Knopman DS, Launer LJ, Wagster MV: The NIH Cognitive and Emotional Health Project: Report of the Critical Evaluation Study Committee. *Alzheimer's and Dementia* 2006; 2: 12–32.

Hendrie HC, Ogunniyi A, Hall KS, Baiyewu O, Unverzagt FW, Gureje O, Gao S, Evans RM, Ogunseyinde AO, Adeyinka AO, Musick B, Hui, S: Incidence of dementia and Alzheimer disease in two communities. *JAMA* 2001; 285: 739–47.

Hendriks GJ, Oude Voshaar RC, Keijsers GP, Hoogduin CA, van Balkom AJ: Cognitive-behavioral therapy for late-life anxiety disorders: A systematic review and meta-analysis. *Acta Psychiatrica Scandinavica* 2008; 117: 403–11.

Heppler J: The 1981 White House Conference on Aging: Impetus for decision-making for and by seniors. *Journal of Gerontological Nursing* 1981; 7: 9.

Herman JP, Mueller NK, Figueiredo H, Cullinan WE: Chapter 4.1 Neurocircuit regulation of the hypothalamo-pituitary-adrenocortical stress response: An overview. *Techniques in the Behavioral and Neural Sciences* 2005; 15: 405–18.

Hesley JD, Vanin SK: Geriatric anxiety and anxiety disorders. In Vanin JR, Hesley JD DM (eds.), *Anxiety Disorders: A pocket guide for primary care.* Totowa, NJ: Humana Press, 2008, pp. 221–42.

Hetényi C, Körtvélyesi T, Penke B: Mapping of possible binding sequences of two beta-sheet breaker peptides on beta amyloid peptide of Alzheimer disease. *Bioorganic and Medicinal Chemistry* 2002; 10: 15874–93.

Hettema JM, Neale MC, Kendler KS: A review and meta-analysis of the genetic epidemiology of anxiety disorders. *American Journal of Psychiatry* 2001; 158: 1568–78.

Hickson GB, Federspiel CF, Pichert JW, Miller CS, Gauld-Jaeger J, Bost P: Patient complaints and malpractice risk. *JAMA* 2002; 287: 2951–57.

Hinrichsen GA: Interpersonal psychotherapy for late life depression: Current status and new applications. *Journal of Rational-Emotive and Cognitive-Behavioral Therapy* 2008; 26: 263–75.

Hinrichsen GA, Clougherty KF: *Interpersonal Psychotherapy for Depressed Older Adults.* Washington, DC: American Psychological Association, 2006.

Hirai K, Morita T, Kashiwagi T: Professionally perceived effectiveness of psychosocial interventions for existential suffering of terminally ill cancer patients. *Palliative Medicine* 2003; 17: 688–94.

Hirschfeld RMA, Bowden CL, Gitlin MJ, Keck PE, Perlis RH, Suppes T, Wagner KD: Practice guideline for the treatment of patients with bipolar disorder. *Focus* 2003; 1: 64–110.

Hoch DB: Creutzfeldt-Jakob disease. Retrieved from MedlinePlus website 2009: www.nlm.nih.gov/medlineplus/ency/article/000788.htm.

Hodges J, Davies R, Xuereb J, Casey B, Broe M, Bak T, Kril J, Halliday G: Clinicopathological correlates in frontotemporal dementia. *Annals of Neurology* 2004; 56: 399–406.

Hoek HW: Incidence, prevalence, and mortality of anorexia nervosa and other eating disorders. *Current Opinion in Psychiatry* 2006; 19: 389–94.

Hofer S, Alwin D (eds.): *Handbook of Cognitive Aging: Interdisciplinary Perspectives.* Thousand Oaks, CA: Sage, 2008.

Hofmann SG, Smits JAJ: Cognitive-behavioral therapy for adult anxiety disorders: A meta-analysis of randomized placebo-controlled trials. *Journal of Clinical Psychiatry* 2008; 69: 621–32.

Holderness CC, Brooks-Gunn J, Warren MP: Co-morbidity of eating disorders and substance abuse. A review of the literature. *International Journal of Eating Disorders* 2006; 16: 1–34.

Hollon SD, Jarrett RB, Nierenberg AA, Thase ME, Trivedi M, Rush AJ: Psychotherapy and medication in the treatment of adult and geriatric depression: Which monotherapy or combined treatment? *Journal of Clinical Psychiatry* 2005; 66: 455–68.

Holmes S: Treatment of male sexual dysfunction. *British Medical Bulletin* 2000; 56: 798–808.

Holtzer R, Tang M, Devanand DP, Albert SM, Wegesin DJ, Marder K, Bell K, Albert M, Brandt J, Stern Y: Psychopathological features in Alzheimer's disease: Course and relationship with cognitive status. *Journal of the American Geriatrics Society* 2003; 51: 953–60.

Horn JL, Cattell RB: Age differences in fluid and crystallized intelligence. *Acta Psychologica* 1967; 26: 107–29.

Horowitz GR: What is a complete work-up for dementia? *Clinical Geriatric Medicine* 1988; 4: 163–80.

Horowitz MJ, Siegel B, Holen A, Bonanno GA, Milbrath C, Stinson CH: Diagnostic criteria for complicated grief disorder. *Focus* 2003; 1: 290–98.

Howard R: Late-onset schizophrenia and very late-onset schizophrenia-like psychosis. *Reviews in Clinical Gerontology* 2001; 11: 337–52.

Howard R, Rapins PV, Seeman MV, Jeste DV, International Late-onset Schizophrenia Group: Late-onset schizophrenia and very-late-onset schizophrenia-like psychosis: An international consensus. *American Journal of Psychiatry* 2000; 157: 172–78.

Howes OD, McDonald C, Cannon M, Arseneault L, Boydell J, Murray RM: Pathways to schizophrenia: The impact of environmental factors. *International Journal of Neuropsychopharmacology* 2004; 7: S7–13.

Huang N, Marie SK, Livramento JA, Chammas R, Nitrini R: 14-3-3 protein in the CSF of patients with rapidly progressive dementia. *Neurology* 2003; 61: 354–57.

Huang X, Moir RD, Tanzi RE, Bush AI, Rogers JT: Redox-Active metals, oxidative stress, and Alzheimer's disease pathology. *Annals of the New York Academy of Sciences* 2006; 1012: 153–63.

Hudson JI, Hiripi E, Pope HG, Kessler RC: The prevalence and correlates of eating disorders in the National Comorbidity Survey replication. *Biological Psychiatry* 2007; 61: 348–58.

Hughes K, Reynolds R: Evolutionary and mechanistic theories of aging. *Annual Review of Entomology* 2005; 50: 421–25.

Hunkler EM, Katon W, Tang L, Williams JW, Kroenke K, Lin EHB, Unutzer J: Long term outcomes from the IMPACT randomised trial for depressed elderly patients in primary care. *British Medical Journal* 2006; 332: 259–63.

Hunt IM, While D, Windfuhr K, Swinson N, Shaw J, Appelby L, Kapur N: Suicide pacts in the mentally ill: A national clinical survey. *Psychiatry Research* 2009; 167: 131–38.

Hurley AC, Volicer L: Alzheimer disease: It's OK, mama, if you want to go, it's okay. *JAMA* 2002; 288: 2324–31.

Hurley AC, Volicer L, Rempusheski VF, Fry ST: Reaching consensus: The process of recommending treatment decisions for Alzheimer's patients. *Advances in Nursing Science* 1995; 18: 33–43.

Hurme SB, Wood E: Guardian accountability then and now: Tracing tenets for an active court role. *Stetson Law Review* 2002; 31: 867.

Huskamp HA, Stevenson DG, Chernew ME, Newhouse JP: A new Medicare end-of-life benefit for nursing home residents. *Health Affairs* 2009; 29: 130–35.

Hwalek MA, Sengstock MC: Assessing the probability of abuse in the elderly: Toward development of a clinical screening instrument. *Journal of Applied Gerontology* 1986; 5: 153–73.

Hybels CF, Pieper CF, Blazer DG, Steffens DC: The course of depressive symptoms in older adults with comorbid major depression and dysthymia. *American Journal of Geriatric Psychiatry* 2008; 16: 300–309.

Hyer L, Sacks A: PTSD (Post-traumatic stress disorder) in later life. In Gallagher-Thompson D, Steffen AM, Thompson LW (eds.), *Handbook of Behavioral and Cognitive Therapies with Older Adults.* New York: Springer, 2008, pp. 278–94.

Illa L, Brickman A, Saint-Jean G, Echenique M, Metsch L, Eisdorfer C, Sanchez-Martinez M: Sexual risk behaviors in late middle age and older HIV seropositive adults. *AIDS Behavior* 2008; 12: 935–42.

Ineichen B: The epidemiology of dementia in Africa: A review. *Social Science and Medicine* 2000; 50: 1673–77.

Inouye SK: *The Confusion Assessment Method (CAM): Training Manual and Coding Guide.* New Haven, CT: Yale University School of Medicine, 2003.

Inouye S, Studensk S, Tinetti M, Kuchel G: Geriatric syndromes: Clinical, research, and policy implications of a core geriatric concept. *Journal of the American Geriatrics Society* 2007; 55: 780–91.

Institute of Medicine: *Nursing Staff in Hospitals and Nursing Homes: Is It Adequate?* Washington, DC: National Academy Press, 1996.

Institute of Medicine: *Crossing the Quality Chasm: A New Health System for the Twenty-first Century.* Washington, DC: National Academy Press, 2001a.

Institute of Medicine: *Improving the Quality of Long-term Care.* Washington, DC: National Academy Press, 2001b.

Institute of Medicine: *Reducing Suicide: A National Imperative.* Washington, DC: National Academies Press, 2002.

Institute of Medicine: *Preparing for the Psychological Consequences of Terrorism: A Public Health Strategy.* Washington DC: National Academies Press, 2003a.

Institute of Medicine: *Unequal Treatment: Confronting Racial and Ethnic Disparities in Healthcare.* Washington, DC: National Academy Press, 2003b.

Institute of Medicine: *Public Health Risks of Disasters: Communication, Infrastructure, and Preparedness.* Washington DC: National Academies Press, 2005.

Institute of Medicine: *Retooling for an Aging America: Building the Health Care Workforce.* Washington, DC: National Academies Press, 2008.

Iqbal K, del C Alonso A, Chohan MO, El-Akkad E, Gong C-X, Khatoon S, Grundke-Iqbal I: Tau pathology in Alzheimer disease and other tauopathies. *Biochimica et Biophysica Acta* 2005; 1739: 198–210.

Ishihara Y, Goto G, Miyamoto M: Central selective acetylcholinesterase inhibitor with neurotrophic activity structure-activity relationships of TAK-147 and related compounds. *Current Medicinal Chemistry* 2000; 7: 341–54.

Ismail-Beigi F, Catalano PM, Hanson RW: Metabolic programming: Fetal origins of obesity and metabolic syndrome in the adult. *American Journal of Physiology—Endocrinology and Metabolism* 2006; 291: E439–40.

Jackson KC, Lipman AG: Drug therapy for anxiety in adult palliative care patients. *Cochrane Database of Systematic Reviews* 2004.

Jackson JS, Torres M, Caldwell CH, Neighbors HW, Nesse RM, Taylor RJ, Trierweiler SJ, Williams DR: The National Survey of American Life: A study of racial, ethnic, and cultural influences on mental disorders and mental health. *International Journals of Methods in Psychiatric Research* 2004; 13: 196–207.

Jacobi C, Hayward C, de Zwaan M, Kraemer HC, Agras WS: Coming to terms with risk factors for eating disorders: Application of risk terminology and suggestions for a general taxonomy. *Psychological Bulletin* 2004; 130: 19–65.

Jacobsen G, Anderson G: Medicare Part D: Ongoing challenges for doctors and patients. *Annual Review of Medicine* 2010; 61: 469–76.

Jacobs S, Prigerson H: Psychotherapy of traumatic grief: A review of evidence for psychotherapeutic treatments. *Death Studies* 2000; 24: 479–95.

Janca A: Rethinking somatoform disorders. *Current Opinion in Psychiatry* 2005; 18: 65–71.

Jennings B, Ryndes T, D'Onofrio C, Baily MA: Access to hospice care: Expanding boundaries, overcoming barriers. *Hastings Center Report* 2003; 33: S3–7.

Jeste DV, Finkel SI: Psychosis of Alzheimer's disease and related dementias: Diagnostic criteria for a distinct syndrome. *American Journal of Geriatric Psychiatry* 2000; 8: 29–34.

Jeste DV, Nasrallah HA: Schizophrenia and aging: No more dearth of data? *American Journal of Geriatric Psychiatry* 2003; 11: 584–88.

Jeste DV, Alexopoulos GS, Bartels SJ, Cummings JL, Gallo JJ, Gottlieb GL, Halpain MC, Palmer BW, Patterson TL, Reynolds CF, Lebowitz BD: Consensus statement on the upcoming crisis in geriatric mental health: Research agenda for the next two decades. *Archives of General Psychiatry* 1999; 56: 848–53.

Jeste DV, Barak Y, Madhusoodanan S, Grossman F, Gharabawi G: An international multisite double-blind trial of the atypical antipsychotic risperidone and olanzapine in 175 elderly patients with chronic schizophrenia. *American Journal of Geriatric Psychiatry* 2003a; 11: 638–47.

Jeste DV, Dunn LB, Palmer BW, Saks E, Halpain M, Cook A, Appelbaum P, Scneiderman, L: A collaborative model for research on decisional capacity and informed consent in older patients with schizophrenia: Bioethics unit of a geriatric psychiatry intervention research center. *Psychopharmacology* 2003b; 171: 68–74.

Jeste DV, Blazer DG, First M: Aging-related diagnostic variations: Need for diagnostic criteria appropriate for elderly psychiatric patients. *Biological Psychiatry* 2005; 58: 265–71.

Jeste DV, Meeks TW, Kim DS, Zubenko GS: Research Agenda for DSM-V: Diagnostic categories and criteria for Neuropsychiatric syndromes in dementia. *Journal of Geriatric Psychiatry and Neurology* 2006; 19: 160–71.

Jhee SS, Fabbri L, Piccinno A, Monici P, Moran S, Zarotsky V, Tan EY, Shiovitz, T: First clinical evaluation of Gangstigmine in patients with probable Alzheimer's disease. *Clinical Neuropharmacology* 2003; 26: 164–69.

Jhoo JH, Huh Y, Lee SB, Park JH, Lee JJ, Choi EA, Han C, Choo IH, Youn JC, Lee DY, Woo JI: Prevalence of dementia and its subtypes in an elderly urban Korean population: Results from the Korean longitudinal study on health and aging. *Dementia and Geriatric Cognitive Disorders* 2008; 26: 270–76.

Jiang W, Krishnan C, Conner C: Depression and heart disease: Evidence of a link and therapeutic implications. *CNS Drugs* 2002; 16: 111–12.

Jogerst G, Daly J, Hartz A: Ombudsman program characteristics related to nursing home abuse reporting. *Journal of Gerontological Social Work* 2005; 46: 85–98.

Johnson A, Roush Jr. RE, Howe JL, Sanders M, McBride MR, Sherman A, Palmisano B, Tumosa N, Perweiler EA, Weiss J: Bioterrorism and emergency preparedness in aging (BTEPA), HRSA-funded GEC collaboration for curricula and training. *Gerontology and Geriatrics Education* 2006; 26: 63–86.

Johnson PB, Sung H-E: Substance abuse among aging baby boomers: Health and treatment implications. *Journal of Addictions Nursing* 2009; 20: 124–26.

Joshi S, Flaherty JH: Elder abuse and neglect in long-term care. *Clinics in Geriatric Medicine* 2005; 21: 333–54.

Joynt KE, Whellan DJ, O'Connor CM: Why is depression bad for the failing heart? A review of the mechanistic relationship between depression and heart failure. *Journal of Cardiac Failure* 2004; 10: 258–71.

Kafetz K: What happens when elderly people die? *Journal of the Royal Society of Medicine* 2002; 95: 536–38.

Kahana B, Dan A, Kahana E, Kercher K: The personal and social context of planning for end-of-life care. *Journal of the American Geriatrics Society* 2004; 52: 1163–67.

Kaiser Family Foundation: *Prescription Drug Trends.* 2007. www.kff.org/rxdrugs/upload/3057-08.pdf.

Kalaria R: Similarities between Alzheimer's disease and vascular dementia. *Journal of the Neurological Sciences* 2002; 203–4: 29–34.

Kalaria RN, Viitanen M, Kalimo M, Dichgans M, Tabira T: The pathogenesis of CADASIL: An update. *Journal of the Neurological Sciences* 2004; 226: 35–39.

Kales H, Blow F, Bingham C, Roberts J, Copeland L, Mellow A: Race, psychiatric diagnosis, and mental health care utilization in older patients. *American Journal of Geriatric Psychiatry* 2000; 8: 301–8.

Kallimanis-King B, Schonfeld L, Molinari VA, Algase D, Brown LM, Kearns WD, Davis DM, Werner DH, Beattie ER, Nelson AL: Longitudinal investigation of wandering behaviors in Department of Veterans Affairs nursing home care units. *International Journal of Geriatric Psychiatry* 2009; 25:166–74.

Kaltman S, Bonanno GA: Trauma and bereavement: Examining the impact of sudden and violent deaths. *Journal of Anxiety Disorders* 2003; 17: 131–47.

Kamel HK, Hajjar RR: Sexuality in the nursing home, part 2: Managing abnormal behavior: Legal and ethical issues. *Journal of the American Medical Directors Association* 2004; 4: 203–6.

Kane R: The future history of geriatrics: Geriatrics at the crossroads. *Journal of Gerontology: Medical Sciences* 2002; 57A: M803–5.

Kane R, Kane R: *Assessing Older Persons: Meaning and Practical Applications.* New York: Oxford University Press, 2000.

Kaniasty K, Norris FH: A test of the support deterioration model in the context of natural disaster. *Journal of Personality and Social Psychology* 1993; 64: 395–408.

Karlamangla AS, Sarkisian CA, Kado DM, Dedes H, Liao DH, Kim S, Moore AA: Light to moderate alcohol consumption and disability: Variable benefits by health status. *American Journal of Epidemiology* 2009; 169: 96–104.

Karlawish J: Measuring decision-making capacity in cognitively impaired individuals. *Neurosignals* 2008; 16: 91–98.

Karlawish JA: Neuroethics in daily practice and in clinical trials focused on special populations. *Journal of the Neurological Sciences* 2009; 285: S16–17.

Karlawish JHT, Quill T, Meier DE: A consensus-based approach to providing palliative care to patients who lack decision-making capacity. *Annals of Internal Medicine* 1999; 130: 835–40.

Karlawish JH, Bonnie RJ, Appelbaum PS, Lyketsos C, James B, Knopman D, Patusky C, Kane RA, Karlan PS: Addressing the ethical, legal, and social issues raised by voting by persons with dementia. *JAMA* 2004; 292: 1345–50.

Karlin BE, Duffy M: Geriatric mental health policy: Impact on service delivery and directions for effecting change. *Professional Psychology: Research and Practice* 2004; 35: 509–19.

Karp N, Wood E: *Incapacitated and Alone: Healthcare Decision Making for Unbefriended Older People.* Washington, DC: American Bar Association, 2003.

Kaspar S, Heiden A: Do SSRIs differ in their anti-depressant efficacy? *Human Psychopharmacology: Clinical and Experimental* 2004; 10: S163–S172.

Katon WJ, Lin E, Russo J, Unutzer J: Increased medical costs of a population-based sample of depressed elderly patients. *Archives of General Psychiatry* 2003; 60: 897–903.

Katona C, Livingston G, Cooper C, Ames D, Brodaty H, Chiu E: International Psychogeriatric Association consensus statement on defining and measuring treatment benefits in dementia. *International Psychogeriatrics* 2007; 19: 345–54.

Katz S, Ford AB, Moskowitz RW, Jackson BA, Jaffee MW: Studies of the illness in the aged. The index of ADL: A standardized measure of biological and psychosocial function. *JAMA* 1963; 185: 914–19.

Katzenschlager R, Sampaio C, Costa J, Lees A: Anticholinergics for symptomatic management of Parkinson's disease. *ACP Journal Club* 2004; 140: 15.

Katzman R: The prevalence and malignancy of Alzheimer's disease: A major killer. *Alzheimer's and Dementia* 1976; 33: 217–18.

Katzman R: Education and prevalence of dementia and Alzheimer's disease. *Neurology* 1993; 43: 13–20.

Katzman R, Bick K: The rediscovery of Alzheimer's disease in the 1960s and 1910s. In Whitehouse P, Maurer K, Ballenger J (eds.): *Concepts of Alzheimer's Disease: Biological, Clinical, and Cultural Perspectives.* Baltimore: Johns Hopkins University Press, 2000.

Kaufman AS, McLean JE, Kaufman-Packer JL, Reynolds CR: Is the pattern of intellectual growth and decline across the adult life span different for men and women? *Journal of Clinical Psychology* 2006; 47: 801–12.

Kaufman S: *The Ageless Self: Sources of Meaning in Late Life.* Madison: University of Wisconsin Press, 1994.

Kaufman S: And a time to die: How American hospitals shape the end of life. *Oncology Times* 2005; 27: 16–20.

Keane TM, Marshall AD, Taft CT: Posttraumatic stress disorder: Etiology, epidemiology, and treatment outcome. *Annual Review of Clinical Psychology* 2006; 2: 161–97.

Keel PK, Dorer DJ, Eddy KT, Franko D, Charatan DL, Herzog DB: Predictors of mortality in eating disorders. *Archives of General Psychiatry* 2003; 60: 179–83.

Kelly KG, Zisselman M: Update on electroconvulsive therapy (ECT) in older adults. *Journal of the American Geriatrics Society* 2000; 48: 560–66.

Kendal WS: Suicide and cancer: A gender-comparative study. *Annals of Oncology* 2007; 18: 381–87.

Kennedy G: *Geriatric Mental Health Care: A Treatment Guide for Health Professionals.* New York: Guilford Press, 2001.

Kennedy MS: The 2005 White House conference on aging: Real policymaking—or rubber stamping? *American Journal of Nursing* 2006; 106: 33–34.

Kent JM, Rauch SL: Neurocircuitry of Anxiety Disorders. *American Psychiatric Association* 2004; 2: 402–9.

Kerani RP, Handsfield HH, Stenger MS, Shafii T, Zick E, Brewer D, Golden MR: Rising rates of syphilis in the era of syphilis elimination. *Sexually Transmitted Diseases* 2007; 34: 154–61.

Kertesz A, Kalvach P: Arnold Pick and German neuropsychiatry in Prague. *Archives of Neurology* 1996; 53: 935–38.

Kertesz A, McMonagle P, Blair M, Davidson W, Munoz DG: The evolution and pathology of frontotemporal dementia. *Brain* 2005; 128: 1996–2005.

Kessler RC: The epidemiology of dual diagnosis. *Biological Psychiatry* 2004; 56: 730–37.

Kessler RC, Berglund P, Demler O, Jin R, Koretz D, Merikangas KR, Wang PS: The epidemiology of major depressive disorder: Results from the National Comorbidity Survey Replication (NCS-R). *JAMA* 2003; 289: 3095–3105.

Kessler RC, Demler O, Frank RG, Olfson M, Pincas HA, Walters EE, Wang P, Wells KB, Zaslavsky AM: Prevalence and treatment of mental disorders, 1990 to 2003. *New England Journal of Medicine* 2005; 352: 2515–23.

Kim D, Nguyen MD, Dobbin MM, Fischer A, Sananbenesi F, Rodgers JT, Delalle I, Baur JA, Sui G, Armour SM, Puigserver P, Sinclair DA, Tsai, L: SIRT1 deacetylase protects against neurodegeneration in models of Alzheimer's disease and amyotrophic schlerosis. *EMBO Journal* 2007; 26: 3169–79.

Kim KY, Yeaman PA, Keene RL: Practical geriatrics: End-of-life care for persons with Alzheimer's disease. *Psychiatric Services* 2005; 56: 139–41.

Kim SYH, Caine ED: Utility and limits of the Mini-Mental State Examination in evaluating consent capacity in Alzheimer's disease. *Psychiatric Services* 2002; 53: 1322–24.

Kim SYH, Caine ED, Currier GW, Leibovici A, Ryan JM: Assessing the competence of persons with Alzheimer's disease in providing informed consent for participation in research. *American Journal of Psychiatry* 2001; 158: 712–17.

Kinsella K, Wan H: *An Aging World, 2008.* U.S. Census Bureau, International Population Reports, P95/09-1. Washington, DC: U.S. Government Printing Office, 2009.

Kirkwood T: *Time of Our Lives: The Science of Human Aging.* Oxford: Oxford University Press, 1999.

Kirkwood T: Evolution of aging. *Mechanisms of Aging and Human Development* 2002; 123: 737–40.

Kivipelto M, Helkala E, Laakso M, Hänninen T, Hallikainen M, Alhainen K, Soininen H, Tuomilehto J, Soininen, H: Apolopoprotein E ε4 allele, elevated midlife total cholesterol level, and high midlife systolic blood pressure are independent risk factors for late-life Alzheimer disease. *Annals of Internal Medicine* 2002; 137: 149–55.

Klauber M, Wright B: *The 1987 Nursing Home Reform Act.* Washington, DC: AARP Public Policy Institute, 2001.

Klegeris A, McGeer PL: Non-steroidal anti-inflammatory drugs (NSAIDs) and other anti-inflammatory agents in the treatment of neurodegenerative disease. *Current Alzheimer Research* 2005; 2: 355–65.

Klein WC, Jess C: One last pleasure? Alcohol use among elderly people in nursing homes. *Health and Social Work* 2002; 27: 193–203.

Kleinman A: Anthropology and psychiatry: The role of culture in cross-cultural research on illness. *British Journal of Psychiatry* 1987; 151: 447–54.

Kleinman A: *The Illness Narratives: Suffering, Healing, and the Human Condition.* New York: Basic Books, 1988.

Kleinman A: *What Really Matters: Living a Moral Life amidst Uncertainty and Danger.* New York: Oxford University Press, 2007.

Kleinman A, Eisenberg L, Good B: Culture, illness, and care: Clinical lessons from anthropologic and cross-cultural research. *Focus* 2006; 4: 140–49.

Kleinman LS, Lowin A, Flood E, Gandhi G, Edgell E, Revicki DA: Costs of bipolar disorder. *Pharmaco-Economics* 2003; 21: 601–22.

Klerman G, Weissman M (eds.): *New Applications of Interpersonal Psychotherapy.* Washington, DC: American Psychiatric Association, 1993.

Klerman G, Weissman M, Rounsaville B: *Interpersonal Psychotherapy of Depression.* New York: Basic Books, 1984.

Klunk WE, Lopresti BJ, Ikonomovic MD, Lefterov IM, Koldamova RP, Abrahamson EE: Binding of the positron emission tomography tracer Pittsburgh compound-B reflects the amount for amyloid-β in Alzheimer's disease brain but not in transgenic mouse brain. *Journal of Neuroscience* 2005; 25: 10598–606.

Knapp M, Thorgrimsen L, Patel A, Spector A, Hallam A, Woods B, Orrell M: Cognitive stimulation therapy for people with dementia: Cost-effectiveness analysis. *British Journal of Psychiatry* 2006; 188: 574–80.

Knaus WA, Draper EA, Wagner DP, Zimmerman JE: APACHE II: A severity of disease classification system. *Critical Care Medicine* 1985; 13: 818–29.

Knaus WA, Wagner DP, Draper EA, Zimmerman JE, Bergner M, Bastos PG, Sirio CA, Murphy DJ, Otring T, Damiano A: The APACHE III prognostic system: Risk prediction of hospitality mortality for critically ill hospitalized adults. *Chest* 1991; 100: 1619–36.

Knight B, Karel M, Hinrichsen G, Qualls S, Duffy M: Pikes Peak model for training in professional geropsychology. *American Psychologist* 2009; 64: 204–14.

Knight BG, Gatz M, Heller K, Bengston VL: Age and emotional response to the Northridge Earthquake: A longitudinal analysis. *Psychology and Aging* 2000; 15: 627–34.

Knight MM, Houseman EA: A collaborative model for the treatment of depression in homebound elders. *Issues in Mental Health Nursing* 2008; 29: 974–91.

Knoll JL: The psychological autopsy, Part 1: Applications and methods. *Journal of Psychiatric Practice* 2008; 14: 393–97.

Kohn L, Corrigan J, Donaldson M (eds.): *To Err Is Human: Building a Safer Health Care System.* Washington, DC: National Academy Press, 2000.

Kohn NA: Preserving voting rights in long-term care institutions: Facilitating resident voting while maintaining election integrity. *McGeorge Law Review* 2007; 38: 1065–1111.

Kokemen E, Smith GE, Petersen RC, Tangalos E, Ivnik RC: The short test of mental status: Correlations with standardized psychometric testing. *Archives of Neurology* 1991; 48: 725–28.

Kominski G, Andersen R, Bastani R, Gould R, Hackman C, Huang D, Jarvik L, Maxwell A, Moye J, Olsen E, Rohrbaugh R, Rosansky J, Taylor S, Van Stone W: UPBEAT: The impact of a psychogeriatric intervention in VA medical centers. *Medical Care* 2001; 39: 500–512.

Korenchevsky V: Natural relative hypoplasia of organs and the process of ageing. *Journal of Pathology and Bacteriology* 1942; 54: 13–24.

Korenchevsky V: *Physiological and Pathological Ageing.* New York: Hafner Publishing, 1961.

Koster S, Hensens AG, van der Palen J: The long-term cognitive and functional outcomes of postoperative delirium after cardiac surgery. *Annals of Thoracic Surgery* 2009; 87: 1469–74.

Kovach CR, Weissman DE, Griffie J, Matson S, Muchka S: Assessment and treatment of discomfort for people with late-stage dementia. *Journal of Pain and Symptom Management* 1999; 18: 412–19.

Kovach CR, Noonan PE, Griffie J, Muchka S, Weissman DE: The assessment of discomfort in dementia protocol. *Pain Management Nursing* 2002; 3: 16–27.

Kövari E, Gold G, Herrmann FR, Canuto A, Hof PR, Bouras C, Giannakopoulos P: Lewy body densities in the entorhinal and anterior cingulate cortex predict cognitive deficits in Parkinson's disease. *Acta Neurologica Scandinavica* 2003; 106: 83–88.

Kowalski A, Jamrozik Z, Kwieciński H: Progressive supranuclear palsy: parkinsonian disorder with tau pathology. *Folia Neuropathologica* 2004; 42: 119–23.

Kraepelin E: Psychiatrie: *Ein Lehrbuch fur Studierende ud Artz.* Leipzig, Verlag V.: Johann mbrosius Barth, 1910.

Krakauer EL, Crenner C, Fox K: Barriers to optimum end-of-life care for minority patients. *Journal of the American Geriatrics Society* 2002; 50: 182–90.

Kral VA: Senescent forgetfulness: Benign and malignant. *Canadian Medical Association Journal* 1962; 86: 257–60.

Kresevic DM: Assessment of function. In Capezuti E, Zwicker D, Mezey M, Fulmer T (eds.), *Evidence-based Geriatric Nursing Protocols for Best Practice,* 3rd edition. New York: Springer, 2008, pp. 23–40.

Kroenke K: Efficacy of treatment for somatoform disorders: A review of randomized controlled trials. *Psychosomatic Medicine* 2007; 69: 881–88.

Kroenke K, Spitzer RL, Williams JBW, Monahan PO, Löwe B: Anxiety disorders in primary care: Prevalence, impairment, comorbidity, and detection. *Annals of Internal Medicine* 2007; 146: 317–25.

Krug E, Dahlberg L, Mercy J, Zwi A, Lozano R (eds.): *World Report on Violence and Health.* Geneva: World Health Organization, 2002.

Kudielka BM, Kirschbaum C: Biological bases of the stress response. *Stress and Addiction* 2007; 3–19.

Kupelian V, Shabsigh R, Travison TG, Page ST, Araujo AB, McKinlay JB: Is there a relationship between sex hormones and erectile dysfunction? Results from the Massachusetts Male Aging Study. *Journal of Urology* 2006; 176: 2584–88.

Kyomen HK, Whitfield TH: Psychosis in the elderly. *American Journal of Psychiatry* 2009; 166: 146–50.

Lachs M, Bachman R, Williams CS, O'Leary J: Resident-to-resident elder mistreatment and police contact in nursing homes: Findings from a population-based cohort. *Journal of the American Geriatrics Society* 2007; 55: 840–45.

Lachs MS, Pillemer K: Abuse and neglect of elderly persons. *New England Journal of Medicine* 1995; 332: 437–43.

Lachs MS, Pillemer K: Elder abuse. *Lancet* 2004; 364: 1263–72.

Lachs MS, Williams CS, O'Brien S, Pillemer KA, Charlson ME: The mortality of elder mistreatment. *JAMA* 1998; 280: 428–32.

Lachs MS, Williams CS, O'Brien S, Pillemer KA: Adult protective service use and nursing home placement. *The Gerontologist* 2000; 42: 734–39.

Lack SA: *First American Hospice.* New Haven, CT: Hospice, 1978.

Lacor PN, Buniel MC, Chang L, Fernandez SJ, Gong Y, Viola KL, Lambert MP, Velasco PT, Bigio EH, Finch CE, Krafft GA, Klein WL: Synaptic targeting by Alzheimer-related amyloid β oligomers. *Journal of Neuroscience* 2004; 24: 10191–200.

Ladin K, Daniels N, Kawachi I: Exploring the relationships between absolute and relative position and late-life depression: Evidence from 10 European Countries. *The Gerontologist* 2009; 50: 48–59.

Laditka JN, Beard RL, Bryant LL, Fetterman D, Hunter R, Ivey S, Logsdon RG, Sharkey JR, Wu B: Promoting cognitive health: A formative research collaboration of the healthy aging research network. *The Gerontologist* 2009; 49: S12–17.

Ladogana A, Puopolo M, Croes EA, Budka H, Jarius C, Collins S, Zerr I: Mortality from Creutzfeldt–Jakob disease and related disorders in Europe, Australia, and Canada. *Neurology* 2005; 64: 1586–91.

Lai JM, Karlawish J: Assessing the capacity to make everyday decisions: A guide for clinicians and an agenda for future research. *American Journal of Geriatric Psychiatry* 2007; 15: 101–11.

Lair L, Naidech AM: Modern neuropsychiatric presentation of neurosyphilis. *Neurology* 2004; 63: 1331–33.

Lander M, Wilson K, Chochinov HM: Depression and the dying older patient. *Clinics in Geriatric Medicine* 2000; 16: 335–56.

Langbaum JBS, Rebok GW, Bandeen-Roche K, Carlson MC: Predicting memory training response patterns: Results from ACTIVE. *Journals of Gerontology* 2009; 64B: 14–23.

Lapid MI, Prom MC, Burton MC, McAlpine DE, Sutor B, Rummans TA. Eating disorders in the elderly. *International Psychogeriatrics* 2010; doi:10.1017/S1041610210000104.

Larsen R, Thorpe C: Elder mediation: Optimizing major family transitions. *Marquette Elder's Advisor* 2006; 7: 293–312.

Larson DG, Tobin DR: End-of-life conversations: Evolving practice and theory. *JAMA* 2000; 284: 1573–78.

Lasmezas CI: The transmissible spongiform encephalopathies. *Revue Scientifique et Technique* 2003; 22: 23–89.

Laumann EO, Das A, Waite LJ: Sexual dysfunction among older adults: Prevalence and risk factors from a nationally representative U.S. probability sample of men and women 57–85 years of age. *Journal of Sexual Medicine* 2008; 5: 2300–311.

Lavretsky H, Siddarth P, Kumar A, Reynolds CF: The effects of the dopamine and serotonin transporter polymorphisms on clinical features and treatment response in geriatric depression: A pilot study. *International Journal of Geriatric Psychiatry* 2008; 23: 55–59.

Lawton MP, Brody EM: Assessment of older people: Self-maintaining and instrumental activities of daily living. *The Gerontologist* 1969; 9: 179–86.

Lazarou J, Pomeranz B, Corey P: Incidence of adverse drug reactions in hospitalized patients: A meta-analysis of prospective studies. *JAMA* 1998; 279: 1200–205.

Leach MJ: Rapport: A key to treatment success. *Contemporary Therapies in Clinical Practice* 2005; 11: 262–65.

Lee R: Rethinking the evolutionary theory of aging: Transfers not births. *Proceedings of the National Academy of Sciences* 2003; 100: 9637–42.

le Grange D, Lock J: The dearth of psychological treatment studies for anorexia nervosa. *International Journal of Eating Disorders* 2005; 37: 79–91.

Leichsenring F, Leibing E: Psychodynamic psychotherapy: A systematic review of techniques, indications and empirical evidence. *Psychology and Psychotherapy: Theory, Research and Practice* 2007; 80: 217–28.

Leigh PN, Abrahams S, Al-Chalabi A, Ampong M-A, Goldstein LH, Johnson J, Willey E: The management of motor neurone disease. *Journal of Neurology, Neurosurgery, and Psychiatry* 2003; 74: iv32–iv47.

Leiknes KA, Finset A, Moum T, Sandanger I: Overlap, comorbidity, and stability of somatoform disorders and the use of current versus lifetime criteria. *Psychosomatics* 2008; 49: 152–62.

Lemke MR, Brecht HM, Koester J, Reichman H: Effects of the dopamine agonist pramipexole on depression, anhedonia and motor functioning in Parkinson's disease. *Journal of the Neurological Science* 2006; 248: 266–70.

Lenzenweger MF, Lane MC, Loranger AW, Kessler RC: DSM-IV personality disorders in the National Comorbidity Survey replication. *Biological Psychiatry* 2007; 62: 553–64.

Leonard BE: Changes in biogenic amine neurotransmitters in panic disorder. *Stress Medicine* 2006; 6: 267–74.

Leroi I, Voulgari A, Breitner J, Lyketsos CG: The epidemiology of psychosis in dementia. *American Journal of Geriatric Psychiatry* 2003; 11: 83–91.

Levin A: When does hoarding cross the line into obsessive-compulsive disorder? *Psychiatric News* 2008; 43: 35.

Levin S, Kruger J: *Substance Abuse among Older Adults: Physicians Guide.* DHHS Publication No. (SMA) 04-3937. Treatment Improvement Protocol series. Rockville, MD: Substance Abuse and Mental Health Services Administration, 2000.

Levine C, Zuckerman C: The trouble with families: Toward an ethic of accommodation. *Annals of Internal Medicine* 1999; 130: 148–52.

Leyhe T, Wiendl H, Buchkremer G, Wormstall H: CADASIL: Underdiagnosed in psychiatric patients? Acta Neurologica *Scandinavica* 2005; 111: 392–97.

Lia KZH, Lindenberger U: Relations between aging sensory/sensorimotor and cognitive functions. *Neuroscience and Biobehavioral Reviews* 2002; 26: 777–83.

Lief S, Kirwin P, Colenda C: Proposed geriatric psychiatry core competencies for subspecialty training. *American Journal of Geriatric Psychiatry* 2005; 13: 815–21.

Lichtman JH, Bigger JT, Blumenthal JA, Frasure-Smith N, Kaufmann PG, Lesperance F, Froelicher ES: Depression and coronary heart disease: Recommendations for screening, referral, and treatment. A science advisory from the American Heart Association Prevention Committee of the Council on Cardiovascular Nursing, Council on Clinical Cardiology, Council on Epidemiology and Prevention, and Interdisciplinary Council on Quality of Care and Outcomes Research endorsed by the American Psychiatric Association. *Circulation* 2008; 118: 1768–75.

Lieberman JA, Stroup TS, McEvoy JP: Effectiveness of antipsychotic drugs in patients with chronic schizophrenia. *New England Journal of Medicine* 2005; 353: 1209–23.

Liebowitz B: Diagnosis and treatment of depression in late life: An overview of the NIH consensus statement. *American Journal of Geriatric Psychiatry* 1996; 4: S3–6.

Liem M, Postulart M, Nieuwbeerta P: Homicide-Suicide in the Netherlands. *Homicide Studies* 2009; 13: 99–123.

Light SA, Holroyd S: The use of medroxyprogesterone acetate for the treatment of sexually inappropriate behavior in patients with dementia. *Journal of Psychiatry and Neuroscience* 2006, 31: 132–34.

Lindau ST, Schumm P, Laumann EO, Levinson W, O'Muircheartaigh CA, Waite LJ: A study of sexual-

ity and health among older adults in the United States. *New England Journal of Medicine* 2007; 357: 762–74.

Lindblad CI, Hanlon JT, Gross CR, Sloane RJ, Pieper CF, Hajjar ER: Multidisciplinary Consensus Panel. Clinically important drug-disease interactions and their prevalence in older adults. *Clinical Therapeutics* 2006; 28: 1133–43.

Lingler JH, Sherwood PR, Crighton MH, Song MK, Happ MB: Conceptual challenges in the study of caregiver-care recipient relationships. *Nursing Research* 2008; 57: 367–72.

Linsk NL: HIV among older adults: Age-specific issues in prevention and treatment. *AIDS Read* 2000; 10.

Livingston G, Johnston K, Katona C, Paton J, Lyketsos CG, Old Age Task Force of the World Federation of Biological Psychiatry: Systematic Review of Psychological Approaches to the management of neuropsychiatric symptoms of dementia. *American Journal of Psychiatry* 2005; 162: 1996–2021.

LoboPrabhu S, Molinari V, Pate J, Lomax J: The after-death call to family members: Academic perspectives. *Academic Psychiatry* 2008; 32: 132–35.

Lockwood P, Ewy W, Hermann DM, Holford N: Application of clinical trial simulation to compare proof-of-concept study designs for drugs with a slow onset of effect: An example in Alzheimer's disease. *Pharmaceutical Research* 2006; 23: 2050–59.

Loebel JP: Practical geriatrics: Completed suicide in late life. *Psychiatric Services* 2005; 56: 260–62.

Loewenstein DA, Acevedo A, Czaja SJ, Duara R: Cognitive rehabilitation of mildly impaired Alzheimer disease patients on cholinesterase inhibitors. *American Journal of Geriatric Psychiatry* 2004; 12: 395–402.

Loewy EH: Euthanasia, physician assisted suicide, and other methods of helping along death. *Health Care Analysis* 2004; 12: 181–93.

Logsdon RG: Dementia: Psychosocial interventions for family caregivers. *The Lancet* 2008; 372: 182–83.

Logsdon RG, McCurry SM, Teri L: Evidence-based psychological treatments for disruptive behaviors in individuals with dementia. *Psychology and Aging* 2007; 22: 28–36.

Logsdon RG, Teri L, McCurry SM: Non-pharmacological treatment of severe dementia: The Seattle protocols. In Burns A, Winblad B (eds.), *Severe Dementia.* West Sussex, England: John Wiley, 2006.

Londos E, Boschian K, Linden A, Persson C, Minthon L, Lexell J: Effects of a goal-oriented rehabilitation program in mild cognitive impairment: A pilot study. *American Journal of Alzheimer's Disease and Other Dementias* 2008; 23: 177–83.

Lonergan E, Luxenberg J, Colford J: Haloperidol for

agitation in dementia. *Cochrane Database Systematic Reviews* 2002; 2.

Loo CK, Mitchell PB: A review of the efficacy of transcranial magnetic stimulation (TMS) treatment for depression, and current and future strategies to optimize efficacy. *Journal of Affective Disorders* 2005; 88: 255–67.

Lopes MA, Furtado EF, Ferrioli E, Litvoc J, de Campos Bottino CM: Prevalence of alcohol-related problems in an elderly population and their association with cognitive impairment and dementia. *Alcoholism: Clinical and Experimental Research* 2010.

Lopez J, Crespo M, Zarit SH: Assessment of the efficacy of a stress management program for informal caregivers of dependent older adults. *The Gerontologist* 2007; 47: 205–14.

Lopez OL, Jagust WJ, DeKosky ST, Becker JT, Fitzpatrick A, Dulberg C, Kuller LH: Prevalence and classification of mild cognitive impairment in the cardiovascular health study cognition study. *Archives of Neurology* 2003; 60: 1385–89.

Lopez OL, Kuller LH, Becker JT, Jagust WJ, DeKosky ST, Fitzpatrick A, Carlson M: Classification of vascular dementia in the Cardiovascular Health Study Cognition Study. *Neurology* 2005; 64: 1539–47.

Lorenz KA, Lynn J, Dy SM, Shugarman SR, Wilkinson A, Mularski RA, Morton SC, Hughes RG, Hilton LK, Maglione M, Rhodes SL, Rolon C, Sun VC, Shekelle PG: Evidence for improving palliative care at the end of life: A systematic review. *Annals of Internal Medicine* 2008; 148: 147–59.

Loveman E, Green C, Kirby J, Takeda A, Picot J, Payne E, Clegg A: The clinical and cost-effectiveness of donepezil, rivastigmine, galantamine and memantine for Alzheimer's disease. *Health Technology Assessment* 2006; 10.

Lowenstein A, Eisikovitz Z, Band-Winterstein T, Enosh G: Is elder abuse and neglect a social phenomenon? Data from the First National Prevalence Survey in Israel. *Journal of Elder Abuse and Neglect* 2009; 21: 253–77.

Lowy M: Disorders of male sexual function. *Obstetrics and Gynaecology* 2006; 8: 30–31.

Loy C, Schneider L: Galantamine for Alzheimer's disease and mild cognitive impairment. *Cochrane Database Systematic Reviews* 2006; 25.

Luchsinger JA, Tang M, Shea S, Mayeux R: Hyperinsulinemia and risk of Alzheimer disease. *Neurology* 2004; 63: 1187–92.

Lue TF: Erectile dysfunction. *New England Journal of Medicine* 2000; 342: 1802–13.

Luecke LJ, Kraft A, Appelhans BM, Enders C: Emotional and cardiovascular sensitization to daily stress following childhood parental loss. *Developmental Psychology* 2009; 45: 296–302.

Luger A, Schmidt B, Kaulich M: Significance of laboratory findings for the diagnosis of neurosyphilis. *International Journal of STD and AIDS* 2000; 11: 224–34.

Lund and Manchester Groups: Clinical and neuroathological criteria for frontotemporal dementia. *Journal of Neurology, Neurosurgery, and Psychiatry* 1994; 57: 416–18.

Luoma JB, Martin CE, Pearson JL: Contact with mental health and primary care providers before suicide: A review of the evidence. *American Journal of Psychiatry* 2002; 159: 909–16.

Lyketsos CG: Neuropsychiatric symptoms (behavioral and psychological symptoms of dementia) and the development of dementia treatments. *International Psychogeriatrics* 2007; 19: 409–20.

Lyketsos CG, Lee HB: Diagnosis and treatment of depression in Alzheimer's disease: A practical update for the clinician. *Dementia and Geriatric Cognitive Disorders* 2004; 17: 55–64.

Lyketsos CG, Lopez O, Jones B, Fitzpatrick A, Breitner J, DeKosky S: Prevalence of neuropsychiatric symptoms in dementia and mild cognitive impairment. *JAMA* 2002; 288: 1475–83.

Lyketsos C, Colenda C, Beck C, Blank K, Doraiswamy M, Kalunian D, Yaffe K: Position statement of the American Association for Geriatric Psychiatry regarding principles of care for patients with dementia resulting from Alzheimer's disease. *American Journal of Geriatric Psychiatry* 2006; 14: 561–73.

Lyness JM: End-of-life care: Issues relevant to the geriatric psychiatrist. *Journal of the American Psychiatric Association* 2007; 5: 459–71.

Lyness JM, Niculescu A, Tu X, Reynolds CF, Caine ED: The relationship of medical comorbidity and depression in older, primary care patients. *Psychosomatics* 2006; 47: 435–39.

Lyons WL: Delirium in postacute and long-term care. *Journal of the American Medical Directors Association* 2006; 7: 254–61.

Lyoo IK, Kim MJ, Stoll AL, Demopulos CM, Parow AM, Dager SR, Renshaw PF: Frontal lobe gray matter density decreases in bipolar I disorder. *Biological Psychiatry* 2004; 55: 648–51.

Maciejewski PK, Zhang B, Block SD, Prigerson HG: An empirical examination of the stage theory of grief. *JAMA* 2007; 297: 716–23.

Mackin RS, Arean PA: Evidence-based psychotherapeutic interventions for geriatric depression. *Psychiatric Clinics of North America* 2005; 28: 805–20.

Madaan V: Assessment of panic disorder across the life span. *Focus* 2008; 6: 438–44.

Mahapatra RK, Edwards MJ, Schott JM, Bhatia KP: Corticobasal degeneration. *Lancet Neurology* 2004; 3: 736–43.

Mahoney F, Barthel DW: Functional evaluation: The

Barthel index. *Maryland State Medical Journal* 1965; 14: 61–65.

Mai E, Buysse DJ: Insomnia: Prevalence, impact, pathogenesis, differential diagnosis, and evaluation. *Focus* 2009; 7: 491–98.

Maia L, de Mendonca A: Does caffeine intake protect from Alzheimer's disease? *Journal of the European Federation of Neurological Societies* 2002; 9: 377–82.

Maier M, Seabrook TJ, Lazo ND, Jiang L, Das P, James C, Lemere CA: Short amyloid-β (Aβ) immunogens reduce cerebral Aβ load and learning deficits in an Alzheimer's disease mouse model in the absence of an Aβ-specific cellular immune response. *Journal of Neuroscience* 2006; 26: 4717–28.

Maj M, Akiskal H, Mezzich J, Okasha A: *Personality Disorders.* West Sussex, England: John Wiley, 2005.

Malphurs JE, Cohen D: A statewide case-control study of spousal homicide-suicide in older persons. *American Journal of Geriatric Psychiatry* 2005; 13: 211–17.

Mangweth-Matzek B, Rupp CI, Hausmann A, Assmayr K, Mariacher E, Kemmler G, Whitworth AB, Biebl W: Never too old for eating disorders or body dissatisfaction: A community study of elderly women. *International Journal of Eating Disorders* 2006; 39: 583–86.

Mann JJ, Apter A, Bertolote J, Beautrais S, Currier D, Haas A, Hegerl U, Lonnqvist J, Malone K, Marusic A, Mehlum L, Patton G, Phillips M, Rutz W, Rihmer Z, Schmidtke A, Shaffer D, Silverman M, Takahashi Y, Varnik A, Wasserman D, Yip P, Hendin H: Suicide prevention strategies: A systematic review. *JAMA* 2005; 294: 2064–74.

Manton KG, Gu X, Lamb VL: Change in chronic disability from 1982 to 2004/2005 as measured by long-term changes in function and health in the U.S. elderly population. *Proceedings of the National Academy of Sciences* 2006; 103: 18374–79.

Mariani SM: Spongiform encephalopathies: A tale of cannibals, cattle, and prions. *Medscape General Medicine* 2003; 5: 42.

Maris RW, Berman AL, Silverman MM: *Comprehensive Textbook of Suicidology.* New York: Guilford Press, 2000.

Marra CM: Update on neurosyphilis. *Current Infectious Disease Reports* 2009; 11: 127–34.

Marshall BL: The new virility: Viagra, male aging and sexual function. *Sexualities* 2006; 9: 345–62.

Martin BK, Frangakis CE, Rosenberg PB, Mintzer JE, Katz IR, Porsteinsson AP, Lyketsos CG: Design of depression in Alzheimer's disease study-2. *American Journal of Geriatric Psychiatry* 2006; 14: 920–30.

Martin M, Hofer SM: Intraindividual variability, change, and aging: Conceptual and analytical issues. Gerontology 2004; 50: 7–11.

Martinez-Martin P, Gil-Nagel P, Morlan Gracia J, Balseiro Gomez J, Martinez-Sarries J, Bermejo F: Unified Parkinson's disease rating scale characteristics and structure. *Movement Disorders* 2004; 9: 76–83.

Martinon-Torres G, Fioravanti, M, Grimley EJ: Trazodone for agitation in dementia. *Cochrane Database Systematic Reviews* 2004; 18.

Martire LM, Lustig AP, Schulz R, Miller GE, Helgeson VS: Is it beneficial to involve a family member? A meta-analysis of psychosocial interventions for chronic illness. *Health Psychology* 2004; 23: 599–611.

Marzuk P, Tardiff K, Hirsch C: The epidemiology of homicide-suicide. *JAMA* 1992; 267: 3179–83.

Mason BJ, Lehert P: Effects of nicotine and illicit substance use on alcoholism treatment outcomes and acamprosate efficacy. *Journal of Addiction Medicine* 2009; 3: 164–71.

Massey BA: Victims or survivors? A three-part approach to working with older adults in disaster. *Journal of Geriatric Psychiatry* 1997; 30: 193–202.

Mast KR, Salama M, Silverman GK, Arnold RM: End-of-life content in treatment guidelines for life-limiting diseases. *Journal of Palliative Medicine* 2004; 7: 754–73.

Matais-Cols D, Campos M, Leckman J: A multidimentional model of obsessive compulsive disorder. *American Journal of Psychiatry* 2005; 162: 228–38.

Mathes M, Reifsnyder J, Gibney M: Commitment, relationship, voice: Cornerstones for an ethics of long-term care. *Ethics, Law, and Aging Review* 2004; 10: 3–22.

Matthews DA: Dr. Marjory Warren and the origin of British geriatrics. *Journal of the American Geriatrics Society* 1984; 32: 253–58.

Maurizi CP: Why was the 1918 influenza pandemic so lethal? The possible role of a neurovirulent neuraminidase. *Medical Hypotheses* 1985; 16: 1–5.

Mayo AM, Walhagen MI: Methodological reviews: Consideration of informed consent and decision-making competence in older adults with cognitive impairment. *Research in Gerontological Nursing* 2009; 2.

McAlpine CH: Elder abuse and neglect. *Age and Ageing* 2008; 37: 132–33.

McArthur JC, Brew BJ, Nath A: Neurological complications of HIV infection. *The Lancet Neurology* 2005; 4: 543–55.

McCabe L, Cairney J, Veldhuizen S, Herrmann N, Streiner DL: Prevalence and correlates of agoraphobia in older adults. *American Journal of Geriatric Psychiatry* 2006; 14: 515–52.

McCarty CE, Volicer L: Hospice access for individuals with dementia. *American Journal of Alzheimer's Disease and Other Dementias* 2009; 24: 476–85.

McCurry SM, Gibbons LE, Logsdon RG, Teri L: Anxiety and nighttime behavioral disturbances: Awakenings in patients with Alzheimer's disease. *Journal of Gerontological Nursing* 2004; 30: 12–20.

McCurry SM, Gibbons LE, Logsdon RG, Vitiello MV, Teri L. Nighttime insomnia treatment and education for Alzheimer's disease: A randomized controlled trial. *Journal of the American Geriatrics Society* 2005; 53: 793–802.

McCurry SM, Vitiello MV, Gibbons LE, Logsdon RG, Teri L: Factors associated with caregiver reports of sleep disturbances in persons with dementia. *American Journal of Geriatric Psychiatry* 2006; 14: 112–20.

McDougall GJ, Becker H, Vaughan PW, Acee TW, Delville CL: The revised direct assessment of functional status for independent older adults. *The Gerontologist* 2010; 50: 363–70.

McGarity TO: Federal regulation of mad cow disease. *Administrative Law Review* 2005; 57: 289–410.

McIntosh JL, Santos JF, Hubbard RW, Overholser JC: *Elder Suicide: Research, Theory, and Treatment.* Washington, DC: American Psychological Association, 1994.

McKee A, Cantu R, Nowinski CJ, Hedley-Whyte ET, Gavett BE, Budson AE, Santini VE, Lee H, Kubilus C, Stern RA: Chronic traumatic encephalopathy in athletes: Progressive tauopathy after repetitive head injury. *Journal of Neuropathology and Experimental Neurology* 2009; 68: 709–35.

McKeith I: Consensus guidelines for the clinical and pathologic diagnosis of dementia with Lewy bodies (DLB): Report of the Consortium on DLB International Workshop. *Journal of Alzheimer's Disease* 2006; 9: 417–23.

McKeith IG, Burn D: Spectrum of Parkinson's disease, Parkinson's dementia, and Lewy body dementia. *Neurologic Clinics* 2000; 18: 865–83.

McKeith IG, Galasko D, Kosaka K: Consensus guidelines for the clinical and pathologic diagnosis of dementia with Lewy bodies (DLB). Report of the consortium on DLB international workshop. *Neurology* 1996; 47: 1113–24.

McKeith IG, Perry EK, Perry RH: Report of the second dementia with Lewy body international workshop. *Neurology* 1999; 35: 902–5.

McKeith I, Del Ser T, Spano P, Emre M, Wesnes K, Anand R, Cicin-Sain A, Ferrara R, Spiegel, R: Efficacy of rivastigmine in dementia with Lewy bodies: A randomized, double-blinded, placebo controlled international study. *The Lancet* 2000; 356: 2031–36.

McKeith IG, Mintzer J, Aarsland D, Burn D, Chiu H, Cohen-Mansfield J, Reid W: Dementia with Lewy bodies. *The Lancet Neurology* 2004; 3: 19–28.

McKeith IG, Dickson DW, Lowe J, Emre M, O'Brien JT, Feldman H, Yamada M: Diagnosis and management of dementia with Lewy bodies. *Neurology* 2005; 65: 1863–72.

McKhann G, Drachman D, Folstein M, Katzman R, Price D, Stadlan EM: Clinical diagnosis of Alzheimer's disease: Report of the NINCDS-ADRDA Work Group under the auspices of Department of Health and Human Services Task Force on Alzheimer's Disease. *Neurology* 1984; 34: 939.

McKhann GM, Albert MS, Grossman M, Miller B, Dickson D, Trojanowski JQ: Clinical and pathological diagnosis of frontotemporal dementia. Report of the Work Group on Frontotemporal Dementia and Pick's Disease. *Archives of Neurology* 2001; 58: 1803–9.

McNichol E, Horowicz-Mehler N, Fisk RA, Bennett K, Gialeli-Goudas M, Chew PW, Lau J, Carr D: Management of opioid side effects in cancer-related and chronic noncancer pain: A systematic review. *Journal of Pain* 2003; 4: 231–56.

McShane R, Areosa SA, Minakaran N: Memantine for dementia. *Cochrane Database Systematic Reviews* 2006; 19.

Mechanic D: *Mental Health and Social Policy: Beyond Managed Care,* 5th edition. Boston: Pearson Education, 2007.

Mechanic D, McAlpine DD: Use of nursing homes in the care of persons with severe mental illness: 1985 to 1995. *Psychiatric Services* 2000; 51: 354–58.

Medawar P: *An Unsolved Problem of Biology.* London: Lewis, 1952.

Mehler P, Andersen A: *Eating Disorders: A Guide to Medical Care and Complications.* Baltimore: Johns Hopkins University Press, 2000.

Mehta K, Yaffe K, Lange K, Sands L, Whooley M, Covinski K: Additive effects of cognitive functioning and depression symptoms on mortality in community-living elderly. *Journal of Gerontology: Biological Sciences and Medical Sciences* 2003; 58: M461–67.

Meisel A, Jennings B: Ethics, end-of-life care and the law: Overview. In Doka KJ, Jennings B (eds.), *Living with Grief: Ethical Dilemmas at the End of Life.* Washington, DC: Hospice Foundation of America, 2005.

Meisel A, Snyder L, Quill T: Seven legal barriers to end-of-life care: Myths, realities, and grains of truth. *JAMA* 2000; 284: 2495–2501.

Menefee LA, Monti DA: Nonpharmacologic and complementary approaches to cancer pain management. *Journal of the American Osteopathic Association* 2005; 105: 15–20.

Menninger JA: Assessment and treatment of alcoholism and substance-related disorders in the elderly. *Bulletin of the Menninger Clinic* 2002; 66: 166–83.

Messer SB: Evidence-based practice: Beyond empirically supported treatments. *Professional Psychology: Research and Practice* 2004; 35: 580–88.

Mesulam MM: Primary progressive aphasia: A language-based dementia. *New England Journal of Medicine* 2003; 349: 1535–42.

Mesulam MM: Primary progressive aphasia: A 25-year retrospective. *Alzheimer Disease and Associated Disorders* 2007; 21: S8–11.

Meyer JS, Huang J, Chowdhury M: MRI abnormalities associated with mild cognitive impairments of vascular (VMCI) versus neurodegenerative (NMCI) types prodromal for vascular and Alzheimer's dementias. *Current Alzheimer Research* 2005; 2: 579–85.

Michaud L, Burnand B, Stiefel F: Taking care of the terminally ill cancer patient: Delirium as a symptom of terminal disease. *Annals of Oncology* 2004; 15: iv199–203.

Miklowitz DJ, Otto MW: New psychosocial interventions for bipolar disorder: A review of literature and introduction of the systematic treatment enhancement program. *Journal of Cognitive Psychotherapy* 2006; 20: 215–30.

Millar HR, Wardell F, Vyvyan JP, Naji SA, Prescott GJ, Eagles JM: Anorexia nervosa mortality in Northeast Scotland, 1965–1999. *American Journal of Psychiatry* 2005; 162: 753–57.

Miller G: A late hit for pro football players. *Science* 2009; 325: 670–72.

Miller MD: *Clinician's Guide to Interpersonal Psychotherapy in Late Life: Helping Cognitively Impaired or Depressed Elders and Their Caregivers.* Oxford: Oxford University Press, 2009.

Miovic M, Block S: Psychiatric disorders in advanced cancer. *Cancer* 2007; 110: 1665–75.

Mirra SS, Heyman A, McKeel D: The Consortium to Establish a Registry for Alzheimer's Disease (CERAD) II. Standardisation of the neuropathological assessment of Alzheimer's disease. *Neurology* 1991; 41: 479–86.

Mitchell SL, Kiely DK, Miller SC, Connor SR, Spence S, Teno SM: Hospice care for patients with dementia. *Journal of Pain and Symptom Management* 2007; 34: 7–16.

Mitrani VB, Lewis JE, Feaster DJ, Czaja SJ, Eisdorfer C, Schulz R, Szapocznik J: The role of family functioning in the stress process of dementia caregivers: A structural family framework. *The Gerontologist* 2006; 46: 97–105.

Mittelman MS, Roth DL, Clay OJ, Haley WE: Preserving health of Alzheimer caregivers: Impact of a spouse caregiver intervention. *American Journal of Geriatric Psychiatry* 2007; 15: 780–89.

Mittelman MS, Roth DL, Coon DW, Haley WE: Sustained benefit of supportive intervention for depressive symptoms in caregivers of patients with Alzheimer's disease. *American Journal of Psychiatry* 2004; 161: 850–56.

Mockenhaupt M, Viboud C, Dunant A, Naldi L, Halevy S, Nico J, Flahault A: Stevens-Johnson syndrome and toxic epidermal necrolysis: Assessment of medication risks with emphasis on recently marketed drugs. The EuroSCAR-study. *Journal of Investigative Dermatology* 2008; 128: 35–44.

Mojtabai R: Unmet need for treatment of major depression in the United States. *Psychiatric Services* 2009; 60: 297–305.

Molinari V, Karel M, Jones Sr S, Zeiss A, Cooley SG, Wray L, Brown E, Gallagher-Thompson D: Recommendations about the knowledge and skills required of psychologists working with older adults. *Professional Psychology: Research and Practice* 2003; 34: 435–43.

Molinuevo JL, Lladó A, Rami L: Memantine: Targeting glutamate excitotoxicity in Alzheimer's disease and other dementias. *American Journal of Alzheimer's Disease and Other Dementias* 2005; 20: 77–85.

Monteleoni C, Clark E: Using rapid-cycle quality improvement methodology to reduce feeding tubes in patients with advanced dementia: Before and after study. *British Medical Journal* 2004; 329: 491–94.

Moore AA, Seeman T, Morgenstern H, Beck JC, Reuben DB: Are there differences between older persons who screen positive on the CAGE Questionnaire and the Short Michigan Alcoholism Screening Test-Geriatric Version? *Journal of the American Geriatrics Society* 2002; 50: 858–62.

Moos RH, Schutte KK, Brennan PL, Moos BS: Older adults' alcohol consumption and late-life drinking problems: A 20-year perspective. *Addiction* 2009; 104: 1293–1302.

Morales A: Erectile dysfunction: An overview. *Clinics in Geriatric Medicine* 2003; 19: 529–38.

Moran M, Lawlor B: Late-life schizophrenia. *Psychiatry* 2005; 4: 51–55.

Moreira T, Hughes JC, Kirkwood T, May C, McKeith I, Bond J: What explains variations in the clinical use of mild cognitive impairment (MCI) as a diagnostic category? *International Psychogeriatrics* 2008; 20: 697–709.

Morgan AC: Practical geriatrics: Psychodynamic psychotherapy with older adults. *Psychiatric Services* 2003; 54: 1592–94.

Morgan RC: The uniform guardianship and protective proceedings act of 1997: Ten years of developments. *Stetson Law Review* 2007; 37: 1–5.

Moriguchi S, Shioda N, Maejima H, Zhao X, Marszalec W, Yeh JZ, Fukunaga K, Narahashi T: Nefiracetam potentiates *N*-Methyl-D-aspartate (NMDA) receptor function via protein kinase C activation and reduces magnesium block of NMDA receptor. *Molecular Pharmacology* 2007; 71: 580–87.

Morita T, Hirai K, Sakaguchi Y, Tsuneto S, Shima Y: Family-perceived distress from delirium-related symptoms of terminally ill cancer patients. *Psychosomatics* 2004; 45: 107–13.

Morley JE: Is the hormonal fountain of youth drying up? *Journals of Gerontology Series A: Biological Sciences and Medical Sciences* 2004; 59: 458–60.

Morley JE, Thomas DR: *Geriatric Nutrition.* Boca Raton, FL: CRC Press, 2007.

Moroney JT, Bagiella E, Desmond DW, Hachinski VC, Molsa PK, Gustafron L, Tatemichi TK: Meta-analysis of the Hachinski Ischemic Score in pathologically verified dementias. *Neurology* 1997; 49: 1069–1105.

Morris JC: Clinical dementia rating: A reliable and valid diagnostic and staging measure for dementia of the Alzheimer type. *International Psychogeriatrics* 1997; 9: 173–76.

Morrison LJ, Morrison RS: Palliative care and pain management. *Medical Clinics of North America* 2006; 90: 983–1004.

Mossakowska M, Barcikowska M, Broczek K, Grodzicki T, Klich-Raczka A, Kupisz-Urbanska M, Podsiadly-Moczydlowska T, Sikora E, Szybinska A, Wieczortowska-Tobis K, Zyckowska J, Kuznicki J: Polish centenarians programme—multidisciplinary studies of successful aging: Aims, methods, and preliminary results. *Experimental Gerontology* 2008; 43: 238–44.

Motzer SA, Hertig V: Stress, stress response, and health. *Nursing Clinics of North America* 2004; 39: 1–17.

Moussavi S, Chatterji S, Verdes E, Tandon A, Patel V, Ustun B: Depression, chronic diseases, and decrements in health: Results from the world health surveys. *Lancet,* 2007; 370: 851–58.

Moutier C, Wetherell JL, Zisook S: Combined psychotherapy and pharmacotherapy for late-life depression. *Geriatric Times* 2003; IV.

Moye J, Marson DC: Assessment of decision-making capacity in older adults: An emerging area of practice and research. *Focus* 2009; 7: 88–97.

Muckart DJJ, Bhagwanjee S, Neijenhuis PA: Prediction of the risk of death by APACHE II scoring in critically ill trauma patients without head injury. *British Journal of Surgery* 2005; 83: 1123–27.

Mueller PS, Hook C, Fleming KC: Ethical issues in geriatrics: A guide for clinicians. *Mayo Foundation for Medical Education and Research* 2004; 79: 554–62.

Muller N, Schwarz MJ: The immune-mediated alteration of serotonin and glutamate: Towards an integrated view of depression. *Molecular Psychiatry* 2007; 12: 988–1000.

Mulsant BH, Whyte E, Lenze EJ, Lotrich F, Karp JF, Pollock BG, Reynolds III CF: Achieving long-term optimal outcomes in geriatric depression. *CNS Spectra* 2003; 8: 27–34.

Mulsant BH, Alexopoulos GS, Reynolds CF, Katz IR, Abrams R, Oslin D, Schulberg HC: Pharmacological treatment of depression in older primary care patients: The PROSPECT algorithm. *Focus* 2004; 2: 253–59.

Mykletun A, Bjerkeset O, Dewey M, Prince M, Overland S, Stewart R: Anxiety, depression, and cause-specific mortality: The HUNT study. *Psychosomatic Medicine* 2007; 69: 323–31.

Mynors-Wallis LM, Gath DH, Day A, Baker F: Randomised controlled trial of problem solving treatment, antidepressant medication, and combined treatment for major depression in primary care. *British Medical Journal* 2000; 320: 26–30.

Naegle M: Substance misuse and alcohol use disorders. In E Capezuti, D Zwicker, M Mezey, T Fulmer (eds.), *Evidence-based Geriatric Nursing Protocols for Best Practice,* 3rd edition. New York: Springer, 2008, pp. 649–76.

Nagata K, Saito H, Ueno T, Sato M, Nakase T, Maeda T, Satoh Y, Komatsu H, Suzuki M, Kondoh Y: Clinical diagnosis of vascular dementia. *Journal of Neurological Sciences* 2007; 15: 44–48.

Nasreddine ZS, Phillips NA, Bédirian V, Charbonneau S, Whitehead V, Collin I, Cummings JL, Chertkow H: The Montreal Cognitive Assessment, MoCA: A brief screening tool for mild cognitive impairment. *Journal of the American Geriatrics Society* 2005; 53: 695–69.

Natan Z, Gimelfarb Y, Barak Y, Baruch Y: Prevalence of dual diagnosis elderly inpatients: Is the phenomenon rare? *European Psychiatry* 2007; 22: S194.

Narumoto J, Nakamura K, Kitbayashi Y, Shibata K, Nakamae T, Fukui K. Relationships among burnout, coping style, and personality: Study of Japanese professional caregivers for elderly. *Psychiatry and Clinical Neurosciences* 2008; 62: 174–76.

National Alliance for Caregiving (NAC) and American Association of Retired Persons (AARP). *Caregiving in the US.* Washington, DC: NAC and AARP, 2004.

National Alliance for Caregiving and United Hospital Fund. *Young Caregivers in the U.S.: Report of Findings.* Washington, DC: NAC and UHF, 2005.

National Consensus Project (NCP): *Clinical Practice Guidelines for Quality Palliative Care,* 2nd edition. Pittsburgh, PA: National Consensus Project, 2009.

National Hospice and Palliative Care Organization (NHPCO): *Caring for Persons with Alzheimer's and Other Dementias: Guidelines for Hospice Providers.*

Alexandria, VA: National Hospice and Palliative Care Organization, 2007.

National Institute on Alcohol Abuse and Alcoholism: *Helping Patients That Drink Too Much: A Clinician's Guide.* Bethesda, MD: National Institute on Alcohol Abuse and Alcoholism, 2005.

National Institute of Mental Health and Substance Abuse and Mental Health Services Administration: *State Implementation of Evidence-Based Practices: Bridging Science and Service.* Bethesda, MD: National Institute of Mental Health, 2002.

Neal AV, Hwalek MA, Scott RO, Stahl C: Validation of the Hwalek-Sengstock elder abuse screening test. *Journal of Applied Gerontology* 1991; 10: 406–15.

Neary D, Snowden J, Mann D: Frontotemporal dementia. *The Lancet Neurology* 2005; 4: 771–80.

Neil W, Curran S, Wattis J: Antipsychotic prescribing in older people. *Age and Ageing* 2003; 32: 475–83.

Neimeyer RA: Searching for the meaning of meaning: Grief therapy and the process of reconstruction. *Death Studies* 2000; 24: 541–58.

Neimeyer RA, Herrero O, Botella LO: Chaos to coherence: Psychotherapeutic integration of traumatic loss. *Journal of Constructivist Psychology* 2006; 19: 127–45.

Nelson A, Algase D: *Evidence-based Practices for the Management of Wandering Behaviors.* New York: Springer, 2007.

Nelson A, Powell-Cope G, Gavin-Dreschnack D, Quigley P, Bulat T, Baptiste AS, Applegarth S, Friedman Y: Technology to promote safe mobility in the elderly. *Nursing Clinics of North America* 2004; 39: 649–71.

Nelson HD, Nygren P, McInerney Y, Klein J: Screening women and elderly adults for family and intimate partner violence: A review of the evidence for the U.S. Preventive Services Task Force. *Annals of Internal Medicine* 2004; 140: 387–96.

Nelson MM, Smith MA, Martinson BC, Kind A, Luepker RV: Declining patient functioning and caregiver burden/health: The Minnesota Stroke Survey—quality of life after stroke study. *The Gerontologist* 2008; 48: 573–83.

Nemeroff CB: Recent findings in the pathophysiology of depression. *Focus* 2008; 6: 3–14.

Nemeroff CB, Owens MJ: The role of serotonin in the pathophysiology of depression: As important as ever. *Clinical Chemistry* 2009; 55: 1578–79.

Ness-Abramof R, Apovian CM: Drug-induced weight gain. *Drugs Today* 2005; 41: 547.

Nestor PJ, Scheltens P, Hodges JR: Advances in the early detection of Alzheimer's disease. *Neurodegeneration* 2004; S34–41.

Neugarten B: The future and the young-old. *The Gerontologist* 1975; 15: 4–9.

Nezu AM, D'Zurilla TJ: Problem-solving therapy—General. In Freeman A, Felgoise SH, Nezu CM, Nezu AM, Reinecke MA (eds.), *Encyclopedia of Cognitive Behavior Therapy.* New York: Springer, 2006.

NIA: Consensus recommendations for the postmortem diagnosis of Alzheimer's disease. The National Institute on Aging, and Reagan Institute Working Group on Diagnostic Criteria for the Neuropathological Assessment of Alzheimer's disease. *Neurobiological Aging* 1997; 18: s1–2.

Nicoll JAR, Yamada M, Frackowiak J, Mazur-Kolecka B, Weller RO: Cerebral amyloid angiopathy plays a direct role in the pathogenesis of Alzheimer's disease: Pro-CAA position statement. *Neurobiology of Aging* 2004; 25: 589–97.

Nierenberg AA, Katz J, Fava M: A critical overview of the pharmacologic management of treatment-resistant depression. *Psychiatric Clinics of North America* 2007; 30: 13–29.

Nieves L: *La verdadere muerte de Juan Ponce de Leon.* Puerto Rico: Editorial Cordillera, 2007.

Norman D, Loredo JS: Obstructive sleep apnea in older adults. *Clinics in Geriatric Medicine* 2008; 24: 151–65.

Norris FH, Byrne CM, Diaz E, Kaniasty K: The range, magnitude, and duration of effects of natural and human-caused disasters: A review of the empirical literature. A National Center for PTSD Fact Sheet, 2001, www.ncptsd.org/facts/disasters/fs_range.html [accessed November 12, 2004].

Norris FH, Friedman MJ, Watson PJ: 60,000 disaster victims speak: part II. Summary and implications of the disaster mental health research. *Psychiatry* 2002a; 65: 240–60.

Norris FH, Friedman MJ, Watson PJ, Byrne CM, Diaz E, Kaniasty K: 60,000 disaster victims speak: part I. an empirical review of the empirical literature, 1981–2001. *Psychiatry* 2002b; 65: 207–39.

Noyes Jr N, Carney CP, Langbehn DR: Specific phobia of illness: Search for a new subtype. *Journal of Anxiety Disorders* 2003; 18: 531–45.

Nuland SB: *How We Die.* London: Chatto and Windus, 1994.

Nutt D, Argyropoulos S, Hood S, Potokar J: Generalized anxiety disorder: A comorbid disease. *European Neuropsychopharmacology* 2006; 16: S109–18.

O'Brien JT, Colloby SJ, Fenwick J: Dopamine transporter loss visualized with FP-CIT SPECT in dementia with Lewy bodies. *Archives of Neurology* 2004; 61: 919–25.

O'Brien N: *Emergency Preparedness for Older People.* Issue Brief January–February 2003. New York: International Longevity Center–USA, 2003.

O'Connell H, Chin A-V, Cunningham C, Lawlor B: Alcohol use disorders in elderly people: Redefining an age old problem in old age. *British Medical Journal* 2003; 327: 664–67.

Odeshoo JR: Note: No brainer? The USDA's regulatory response to the discovery of "mad cow" disease in the United States. *Stanford Law and Policy Review* 2005; 16: 277–315.

Oeppen J, Vaupel J: Broken limits to life expectancy. *Science* 2003; 296: 1029–31.

Office of Inspector General: *Medicare Hospice Care: A Comparison of Beneficiaries in Nursing Facilities and Beneficiaries in Other Settings.* OIG, Department of Health and Human Services, 2007.

Ohlén J, Andershed B, Berg C, Frid I, Palm CA, Ternestedt BM, Segesten K: Relatives in end-of-life care—part 2: A theory for enabling safety. *Journal of Clinical Nursing* 2007; 16: 382–90.

Okura Y, Miyakoshi A, Kohyama K: Nonviral αβ DNA vaccine therapy against Alzheimer's disease: Long-term effects and safety. *Proceedings of the National Academy of Sciences* 2006; 103: 9619–24.

Olfson M, Pincus H: Outpatient mental health care in nonhospital settings: Distribution of patients across provider groups. *American Journal of Psychiatry* 1996; 153: 1353–56.

Olin JT, Katz IR, Meyers BS, Schneider LS, Lebowitz BD: Provisional diagnostic criteria for depression of Alzheimer disease: Rationale and background. *American Journal of Geriatric Psychiatry* 2002; 10: 129–41.

Olshansky J, Carnes B: *The Quest for Immortality: Science at the Frontiers of Aging.* New York: Norton, 2002.

Olshansky SJ, Goldman DP, Zheng Y, Rowe JW: Aging in America in the twenty-first century: Demographic forecasts from the MacArthur Foundation Research Network on an aging society. *Milbank Quarterly* 2009; 87: 842–62.

Ory MG, Hoffman RR, Yee JL, Tennstedt S, Schulz R: Prevalence and impact of caregiving: A detailed comparison between dementia and nondementia caregivers. *The Gerontologist* 1999; 39: 177–86.

Oslin DW, Mavandadi S: Alcohol and drug problems. In Blazer DG, Steffans DC (eds.), *The American Psychiatric Publishing Textbook of Geriatric Psychiatry,* 4th edition. Washington, DC: American Psychiatric Publishing, 2009.

Oslin DW, Thompson R, Kallan MJ, TenHave T, Blow FC, Bastani R, Gould RL, Maxwell AE, Rosansky J, Van Stone W, Jarvik L: Treatment effects from UPBEAT: A randomized trial of care management for behavioral health problems in hospitalized elderly patients. *Journal of Geriatric Psychiatry and Neurology* 2004; 17: 99–106.

Osterweil D, Brummel-Smith K, Beck J, Osterweil D: *Comprehensive Geriatric Assessment.* New York: McGraw Hill Professional, 2000.

Ostling S, Skoog I: Psychotic symptoms and paranoid ideation in a nondemented population-based sample of the very old. *Archives of General Psychiatry* 2002; 59; 53–59.

Otero JL: Dementia and Parkinson's disease: Clinical diagnosis, neuropsychological aspects and treatment. *Dementia and Neuropsychologia* 2008; 2: 261–66.

Ouimet S, Kavanagh BP, Gottfried SB, Skrobik Y: Incidence, risk factors and consequences of ICU delirium. *Intensive Care Medicine* 2007; 33: 66–73.

Overall J, Gorham D: The brief psychiatric rating scale. *Psychological Reports* 1962; 10: 799–812.

Pachana NA, Byrne GJ, Siddle H, Koloski N, Harley E, Arnold E: Development and validation of the geriatric anxiety inventory. *International Psychogeriatrics* 2007; 19: 103–14.

Paech D, Weston A: Problematic substance use in older adults: A rapid literature scan. *HSAC Report* 2009; 2.

Paganini-Hill A, Kawas CH, Corrada MM: Type of alcohol consumed, changes in intake over time and mortality: The Leisure World Cohort Study. *Age and Ageing* 2007; 36: 203–9.

Palmer BW, Jeste DV: Relationship of individual cognitive abilities to specific components of decisional capacity among middle-aged and older patients with schizophrenia. *Schizophrenia Bulletin* 2006; 32: 98–106.

Palmer BW, Bondi MW, Twamley EW, Thal L, Golshan S, Jeste DV: Are late-onset schizophrenia-spectrum disorders a neurodegenerative condition? Annual rates of change on two dementia measures. *Journal of Neuropsychiatry Clinical Neuroscience* 2003; 15: 45–52.

Pandi-Perumal SR, Monti JM, Monjan AA: *Principles and Practice of Geriatric Sleep Medicine.* New York: Cambridge University Press, 2010.

Pandya M, Kubu CS, Giroux ML: Parkinson disease: Not just a movement disorder. *Cleveland Clinic Journal of Medicine* 2008; 75: 856–64.

Panza F, D'Introno A, Colacicco AM, Capurso C, Pichichero G, Capuro SA, Capuro SA, Solfrizzi V: Lipid metabolism in cognitive decline and dementia. *Brain Research Reviews* 2006; 51: 275–92.

Papadopoulos FC, Ekbom A, Brandt L, Ekselius L: Excess mortality, causes of death, and prognostic factors in anorexia nervosa. *British Journal of Psychiatry* 2009; 194: 10–17.

Pardini DA, Plante TG, Sherman A, Stump JE: Religious faith and spirituality in substance abuse recovery: Determining the mental health benefits. *Journal of Substance Abuse Treatment* 2000; 19: 347–54.

Park D, Schwartz N (eds.): *Cognitive Aging: A Primer.* Philadelphia: Psychology Press, 2000.

Parker SM, Clayton JM, Hancock K, Walder S, Butow PN, Carrick S, Currow D, Ghersi D, Glare P, Hagerty R, Tattersail MHN: A systematic review of prognostic/end-of-life communication with adults in the advances stages of a life-limiting illness: Patient/caregiver preferences for the content, style, and timing of information. *Journal of Pain and Symptom Management* 2007; 34: 81–93.

Parnas J, Licht D, Bovet P: Cluster A disorders: A review. In Maj M, Akiskal H, Mezzich J, Okasha A (eds.), *Personality Disorders.* West Sussex, England: John Wiley, 2005, pp. 1–74.

Patterson GT: An examination of evidenced-based practice interventions for public emergencies. *Journal of Evidence-Based Social Work* 2009; 6: 274–87.

Patterson TL, McKibbin CL, Taylor MJ: Functional Adaptation Skills Training (FAST): A pilot psychosocial intervention study in middle-aged and older patients with chronic psychotic disorders. *American Journal of Geriatric Psychiatry* 2003; 11, 17–23.

Paul T, Schroeder K, Dahmer B, Nutzinger D: Self-injurious behaviors in women with eating disorders. *American Journal of Psychiatry* 2002; 159: 408–11.

Paulsen JS, Salmon DP, Thal LJ, Romero R, Weisstein-Jenkins C, Galasko D, Hofstetter CR, Grant I, Jeste DV: Incidence of and risk factors for hallucinations and delusions in patients with probable AD. *Neurology* 2000; 54: 1965–71.

Paveza GJ, Cohen D, Eisdorfer C, Freels S, Semla T, Ashford JW, Gorelick P, Hirschman R, Luchins D, Levy P: Severe family violence and Alzheimer's disease: Prevalence and risk factors. *The Gerontologist* 1992; 32: 493–97.

Payne BK, Fletcher LB: Elder abuse in nursing homes: prevention and resolution strategies and barriers. *Journal of Criminal Justice* 2005; 33: 119–125.

Peabody F: The care of the patient. *JAMA* 1927; 88: 877–82.

Pearson JL: Progress in identifying risk and protective factors in older suicidal adults. *American Journal of Geriatric Psychiatry* 2006; 14: 721–23.

Peat CM, Peyerl NL, Muehlenkamp JJ: Body image and eating disorders in older adults: A review. *Journal of General Psychology* 2008; 135: 343–58.

Penner NR: Collaborating with relief agencies: A guide for hospice. In Lattanzi-Licht M, Doka KJ (eds.), *Living with Grief: Coping with Public Tragedy.* New York: Brunner-Routledge, 2003, pp. 277–88.

Pergolizzi J, Böger RH, Budd K, Dahan A, Erdine S, Hans G, Kress HG, Langford R, Likar R, Raffa RB, Sacerdote P: Opioids and the management of chronic severe pain in the elderly: Consensus statement of an International Expert Panel with focus on the six clinically most often used World Health Organization Step III opioids (buprenorphine, fentanyl, hydromorphone, methadone, morphine, oxycodone). *Pain Practice* 2008; 8: 287–313.

Perlis RH, Ostacher MJ, Patel JK, Marangell LB, Zhang H, Wisniewski SR, Thase ME: Predictors of recurrence in bipolar disorder: Primary outcomes from the systematic treatment enhancement program for bipolar disorder (STEP-BD). *Focus* 2006; 4: 553–61.

Peters N, Opherk C, Bergmann T, Castro M, Herzog J, Dichgans M: Spectrum of mutations in biopsy-proven CADASIL: Implications for diagnostic strategies. *Archives of Neurology* 2005; 62: 1091–94.

Petersen RC: *Mild Cognitive Impairment: Aging to Alzheimer's Disease.* New York: Oxford University Press, 2003.

Petersen RC, Morris JC: Mild cognitive impairment as a clinical entity and treatment target. *Archives of Neurology* 2005; 62: 1160–63.

Petersen RC, Stevens JC, Ganguli M, Tangalos EG, Cummings JL, DeKosky ST: Practice parameter: Early detection of dementia: mild cognitive impairment (an evidence-based review). Report of the Quality Standards Subcommittee of the American Academy of Neurology. *Neurology* 2001; 56: 1133–42.

Petrozzi L, Ricci G, Giglioli NJ, Sicilliano G, Mancuso M: Mitochondria and neurodegeneration. *Bioscience Reports* 2007; 27: 87–104.

Pillemer K, Finkelhor D: The prevalence of elder abuse: A random sample survey. *The Gerontologist* 1988; 28: 51–57.

Pillemer KA, Wolf RS: *Elder Abuse: Conflict in the Family.* Westport, CT: Auburn House Publishing Company, 1986.

Pinholt EM, Kroenke K, Hanley JF, Kussman MJ, Twyman PL, Carpenter JL: Functional assessment of the elderly: A comparison of standard instruments with clinical judgment. *Archives of Internal Medicine* 1987; 147: 484–88.

Pinquart M, Duberstein PR: Treatment of anxiety disorders in older adults: A meta-analytic comparison of behavioral and pharmacological interventions. *American Journal of Geriatric Psychiatry* 2007; 15: 639–51.

Pinquart M, Sorensen S: Ethnic differences in stressors, resources, and psychological outcomes of family caregiving: A meta-analysis. *The Gerontologist* 2005; 45: 90–106.

Pinquart M, Duberstein PR, Lyness JM: Treatments for later-life depressive conditions: A meta-analytic comparison of pharmacotherapy and psychotherapy. *American Journal of Psychiatry* 2006; 163: 1493–1501.

Pirkis J, Pfaff J, Williamson M, Tyson O, Stocks N, Goldney R, Almeida OP: The community prevalence of depression in older Australians. *Journal of Affective Disorders* 2009; 115: 54–61.

Plassman BL, Havlik RJ, Steffens DC, Helms MJ, Newman TN, Drosdick D, Phillips C, Gau BA, Welsh-Bohmer KA, Burke JR, Guralnik JM, Breitner JCS: Documented head injury in early adulthood and risk of Alzheimer's disease and other dementia. *Neurology* 2000; 55: 1158–66.

Plosker GL, Keating GM: Management of mild to moderate Alzheimer disease: Defining the role of Rivastigmine. *AIDS International* 2004; 12: 55–72.

Podnieks E, Pillemer K, Nicholson JP, Shillington T, Frizzel A: *National Survey on Abuse of the Elderly in Canada: The Ryerson study.* Toronto: Ryerson Polytechnical Institute, 1990.

Podsiadlo D, Richardson S: The timed "Up and Go": A test of basic functional mobility for frail elderly persons. *Journal of the American Geriatrics Society* 1991; 39: 142–48.

Pohjasvaara T, Mäntylä R, Ylikoski R, Kaste M, Erkinjuntti T: Comparison of different clinical criteria (DSM-III, ADDTC, ICD-10, NINDS-AIREN, DSM-IV) for the diagnosis of vascular dementia. *Stroke* 2000; 31: 2952–57.

Polinski JM, Wang PS, Fischer MA: Medicaid's prior authorization program and access to atypical antipsychotic medications. *Health Affairs* 2007; 26: 750–60.

Pollack J, Kutzin MS, Warjone R, Armstrong D, Aldridge RL, Johns AF, Hommel P: Guardianships over the elderly: Security provided or freedoms denied? Committee on Aging, 2003, pp. 108–11.

Pollack SJ, Lewis H: Secretase inhibitors for Alzheimer's disease: Challenges of a promiscuous protease. *Current Opinion in Investigational Drugs* 2005; 6: 35–47.

Poon L, Perls D (eds.): *Biopsychosocial Approaches to Longevity.* Annual Review of Gerontology and Geriatrics. New York: Springer, 2007.

Poon LW, Martin P, Margrett J: Cognition and Emotion in Centenarians. In Depp CA, Jeste DV (eds.), *Successful Cognitive and Emotional Aging.* Arlington, VA: American Psychiatric Publishing, 2010, pp. 115–33.

Port CL, Engdahl B, Frazier P: A longitudinal and retrospective study of PTSD among older prisoners of war. *American Journal of Psychiatry* 2001; 158: 1474–79.

Port CL, Engdahl B, Frazier P, Eberly R: Factors related to the long-term course of PTSD in older ex-prisoners of war. *Journal of Clinical Geropsychology* 2002; 8: 203–14.

Portet F, Ousset PJ, Visser PJ, Frisoni GB, Nobili F, Scheltens P, Touchon J: Mild cognitive impairment (MCI) in medical practice: A critical review of the concept and new diagnostic procedure. Report of the MCI Working Group of the European consortium on Alzheimer's disease. *Journal of Neurology, Neurosurgery, and Psychiatry* 2006; 77: 714–18.

The Presidential Commission for the Study of Bioethical Issues: *Beyond Therapy: Biotechnology and the Pursuit of Happiness.* Washington, DC: Presidential Commission for the Study of Bioethical Issues, 2003.

President's New Freedom Commission on Mental Health: *Achieving the Promise: Transforming Mental Health Care in America.* Washington, DC: Substance Abuse and Mental Health Services Administration, 2003.

Preti A, Girolamo G, Vilagut G, Alonso J, Graaf R, Bruffaerts R, Demyttenaere K, Pinto-Meza A, Haro JM, Morosini P: The epidemiology of eating disorders in six European countries: Results of the ESEMeD-WMH project. *Journal of Psychiatric Research* 2009; 43:1125–32.

Price JC, Klunk WE, Lopresti BJ, Lu X, Hoge JA, Ziolko SK, Holt DP, Meltzer CC, DeKosky ST, Mathis CA: Kinetic modeling of amyloid binding in humans using PET imaging and Pittsburgh Compound-B. *Journal of Cerebral Blood Flow and Metabolism* 2005; 25: 1528–47.

Prince JA, Zetterberg H, Andreasen N, Marcusson J, Blennow K: APOE ε4 allele is associated with reduced cerebrospinal fluid levels of Aβ42. *Neurology* 2004; 62: 2116–18.

Pritchard J: *The Needs of Older Women: Services for Victims of Elder Abuse and Other Abuse.* Bristol: Policy Press, 2000.

Pritts SD, Susman J: Diagnosis of eating disorders in primary care. *American Family Physician* 2003; 67: 297–304.

Purandare N, Voshaar RCO, Rodway C, Burns A, Kapur N: Suicide in dementia: 9-year national clinical survey in England and Wales. *British Journal of Psychiatry* 2009; 194: 175–80.

Quereshi A, Johri A: Issues involving informed consent for research participants with Alzheimer's disease. *Journal of Academic Ethics* 2008; 6: 197–203.

Qureshi KA, Merrill JA, Gershon RM, Calero-Breckheimer A: Emergency preparedness training for public health nurses: A pilot study. *Journal of Urban Health: Bulletin of the New York Academy of Medicine* 2002; 79: 413–16.

Quill TE, Lo B, Brock DW: Palliative options of last resort: A comparison of voluntarily stopping eating and drinking, terminal sedation, physician-assisted suicide, and voluntary active euthanasia. In Birnbacher D, Dahl E (eds.), *International Library of Ethics, Law, and the New Medicine.* Netherlands: Springer, 2008, 38: 49–64.

Rabbitt P, Lunn M, Wong D: Understanding terminal decline in cognition and risk of death: Methodological and theoretical implications of practice and dropout effects. *European Psychologist* 2006; 11: 164–71.

Rabinowitz T, Hirdes JP, Desjardins I: Somatoform disorders. In Agronin ME, Maletta GJ (eds.), *Principles and Practice of Geriatric Psychiatry*. Philadelphia: Lippincott Williams & Wilkins, 2006, pp. 489–504.

Rabins PV, Blacker D, Rovner BW, Rummans T, Schneider LS, Tariot PN, Blass DM: Practice Guideline for the Treatment of Patients with Alzheimer's Disease and Other Dementias. APA (Psychiatric Practice Section) 2007; 7–64.

Rademakers R, Cruts M, van Broeckhoven C: The role of tau (MAPT) in frontotemporal dementia and related tauopathies. *Human Mutation* 2004; 24: 277–95.

Radloff LS: The CES-D scale. *Applied Psychological Measurement* 1977; 1: 385–401.

Raginwala NA, Hynan LS, Weiner MF, White III CL: Clinical criteria for the diagnosis of Alzheimer disease: Still good after all these years. *American Journal of Geriatric Psychiatry* 2008; 16: 384–88.

Rahilly CR, Farwell WR: Prevalence of smoking in the United States: A focus on age, sex, ethnicity, and geographic patterns. *Current Cardiovascular Risk Reports* 2007; 1: 379–83.

Raina P, Santaguida P, Ismaila A, Patterson C, Cowan D, Levine M, Oremus M: Effectiveness of cholinesterase inhibitors and Memantine for treating dementia: Evidence review for a clinical practice guideline. *Annals of Internal Medicine* 2008; 148: 379–97.

Raine A: Sexual behaviour of nursing home residents: Staff perceptions and responses. *Journal of Advanced Nursing* 2006; 48: 371–79.

Rao GS, Blake LM: Decision-making capacity in the elderly. *Primary Care Updates for OB/GYNS* 2002; 9: 71–75.

Rao TS, Reid RT, Correa LD, Santori EM, Gardner MF, Sacaan AI, Lorrain D, Vernier JM: In vivo pharacological characterization of (±)-4-[2-(1-methyl-2-pyrrolidinyl)ethyl]thio phenol hydrochloride (SIB-1553A), a novel cholinergic ligand: microdialysis studies. *Brain Research* 2003; 986: 71–81.

Rao V, Lyketsos CG: The benefits and risks of ECT for patients with primary dementia who also suffer from depression. *International Journal of Geriatric Psychiatry* 2000; 15: 729–35.

Rapaport MH, Judd LL, Schettler PJ, Yonkers KA, Thase ME, Kupfer DJ, Rush AJ: A descriptive analysis of minor depression. *Focus* 2005; 3: 98–105.

Rapp S, Espeland MA, Shumaker SA, Henderson VW, Brunner RL, Manson JE, Gass MLS, Stefanick ML, Lane DS, Hays J, Johnson KC, Coker LH, Dailey M, Bowen D: Effect of estrogen plus progestin on global cognitive function in post-menopausal women. *JAMA* 2003; 289: 2663–72.

Raschetti R, Albanese E, Vanacore N, Maggini M: Cholinesterase inhibitors in mild cognitive impairment: A systematic review of randomised trials. *PLoS Medicine* 2007; 4: 1818–28.

Rascol O, Brooks DJ, Melamed E, Oertel W, Poewe W, Stocchi F, Tolosa E: Rasagiline as an adjunct to levodopa in patients with Parkinson's disease and motor fluctuations (LARGO, Lasting effect in Adjunct therapy with Rasagiline Given Once daily, study): A randomised, double-blind, parallel-group trial. *Lancet* 2005; 365: 947–54.

Rau R, Soroko E, Jasilionis D, Vaupel JW: Continued reductions in mortality at advanced ages. *Population and Development Review* 2008; 34: 747–68.

Rayner L, Price A, Evans A, Valsrag K, Higgonson I, Hotopf M: *Antidepressants for Depression in Physically Ill People.* New York: John Wiley & Sons, 2010.

Raz N: Decline and compensation in aging brain and cognition: Promises and constraints. *Neuropsychology Review* 2009; 19: 411–14.

Raz N, Lindenberger U, Rodrigue KM, Kennedy KM, Head D, Williamson A, Dahle C, Gerstorf D, Acker JD: Regional brain changes in aging healthy adults: General trends, individual differences and modifiers. *Cerebral Cortex* 2005; 15: 1676–89.

Rea MM, Tompson MC, Miklowitz DJ, Goldstein MJ, Hwang S, Mintz J: Family-focused treatment versus individual treatment for bipolar disorder: Results of a randomized clinical trial. *Journal of Consulting and Clinical Psychology* 2003; 71: 482–92.

Reisberg B, Auer SR, Monteiro IM: Behavioral pathology in Alzheimer's disease (BEHAVE-AD) rating scale. *International Psychogeriatrics* 1997; 8: 301–8.

Reisberg B, Borenstein J, Salob SP, Ferris SH, Franssen E, Georgotas A: Behavioral symptoms in Alzheimer's disease: Phenomenology and treatment. *Journal of Clinical Psychiatry* 1987; 48: S9–15.

Reisberg B, Doody R, Stöffler A, Schmitt F, Ferris S, Möbius HJ: Memantine in moderate-to-severe Alzheimer's disease. *New England Journal of Medicine* 2003; 348: 1333–41.

Repetto L, Audisio RA: Elderly patients have become the leading drug consumers: It's high time to properly evaluate new drugs within the real targeted population. *Journal of Clinical Oncology* 2006; 24: e62–63.

Report of the 2005 White House Conference on Aging: *The Booming Dynamics of Aging: From Awareness to Action.* 2005.

Reuter-Lorenz PA, Lustig C: Brain aging: Reorganizing discoveries about the aging mind. *Current Opinion in Neurobiology* 2005; 15: 245–51.

Reyes-Ortiz CA: Diogenes syndrome: The self-neglect elderly. *Comprehensive Therapy* 2001; 27: 117–21.

Reynolds C: Meeting the mental health need of older adults in primary care: How do we get the job done? *Clinical Psychology: Science and Practice* 2003; 10.

Rice DP, Fineman N: Economic implications of increased longevity in the United States. *Annual Review of Public Health* 2004; 25: 457–73.

Richard I, Roudaut C, Saenz A, Pogue R, Grimbergen JE, Anderson LV, Beley C, Cobo AM, de Diego C, Eymard B, Gallano P, Ginjaar HB, Lasa A, Pollitt C, Topaloglu H, Urtizberea JA, de Visser M, van der Kooi A, Bushby K, Bakker E, Lopez de Minain A, Fardeau M, Beckmann JS: Calpainopathy: A survey of mutations and polymorphisms. *American Journal of Human Genetics* 1999; 64: 1524–40.

Ritchie EC, Friedman M, Watson P, Ursano R, Wessely S, Flynn B: Mass violence and early mental health intervention: A proposed application of best practice guidelines to chemical, biological, and radiological attacks. *Military Medicine* 2004; 169: 575–79.

Roach SM: Schizotypal Personality: Neurodevelopmental and psychosocial trajectories. *Annual Review in Clinical Psychology* 2004; 2: 291–326.

Roberto KA, Teaster PB: Sexual abuse of vulnerable young and old women: A comparative analysis of circumstances and outcomes. *Violence against Women* 2005; 11: 473–504.

Roberts LW: Mental illness and informed consent: Seeking an empirically derived understanding of voluntarism. *Current Opinion in Psychiatry* 2003; 16.

Roberts LW, Geppert C, Bailey R: Ethics in Psychiatric Practice: Essential ethics skills, informed consent, the therapeutic relationship, and confidentiality. *Journal of Psychiatric Practice* 2002; 8: 290–305.

Robertsson B, Karlsson I, Styrud E, Gottfries CG: Confusional State Evaluation (CSE): An instrument for measuring severity of delirium in the elderly. *British Journal of Psychiatry* 1997; 170: 565–70.

Robins CJ, Chapman AL: Dialectical Behavior Therapy: Current status, recent developments, and future directions. *Journal of Personality Disorders* 2004; 18: 73–89.

Robins LN, Cottler LB: Making a structured psychiatric diagnostic interview faithful to the nomenclature. *American Journal of Epidemiology* 2004; 160: 808–13.

Robins LN, Helzer JE, Croughan JL, Ratcliff KS: National Institute of Mental Health diagnostic

interview schedule: Its history, characteristics, and validity. *Archives of General Psychiatry* 1981; 38: 381–89.

Robinson DS: The role of dopamine and norepinephrine in depression. *Primary Psychiatry* 2007; 14: 21–23.

Rocca WA, Van Duijn CM, Clayton D, Chandra V, Fratiglioni L, Graves AB, Heyman A, Jorm AF, Kondo K, Mortimer JA, Rocca WA, Shalat SL, Soininen H: Maternal age and Alzheimer's disease: A collaborative re-analysis of case-control studies. EURODEM risk factors research group. *International Journal of Epidermiology* 1991; 20: S21–27.

Rocchi A, Pellegrini S, Siciliano G, Murri L: Causative and susceptibility genes for Alzheimer's disease: A review. *Braun Research Bulletin* 2003; 61: 1–24.

Rockwood K: Causes of delirium. *Psychiatry* 2008; 7: 39–41.

Rockwood K, Mintzer J, Truyen L, Wessel T, Wilkinson D: Effects of a flexible galantamine dose in Alzheimer's disease: A randomized, controlled trial. *Journal of Neurology, Neurosurgery, and Psychiatry* 2001; 71: 589–95.

Rodriguez MA, Wallace SP, Woolf NH, Mangione CM: Mandatory reporting of elder abuse: Between a rock and a hard place. *Annals of Family Medicine* 2006; 4: 403–9.

Roff LL, Burgio LD, Gitlin L, Nichols L, Chaplin W, Hardin JM: Positive aspects of Alzheimer's caregiving: The role of race. *Journals of Gerontology Series B: Psychological Sciences and Social Sciences* 2004; 59: P185–90.

Rogawski MA, Wenk GL: The Neuropharmacological basis for the use of memantine in the treatment of Alzheimer's disease. *CNS Drug Reviews* 2006; 9: 275–308.

Román GC: Vascular dementia revisited: Diagnosis, pathogenesis, treatment, and prevention. *Medical Clinics of North America* 2002; 86: 477–99.

Román GC: Vascular dementia: Distinguishing characteristics, treatment, and prevention. *Journal of the American Geriatrics Association* 2003; 51: S296–304.

Román GC, Tatemichi TK, Erkinjuntti T, Cummings JL, Masdeu JC, Garcia JH, Amaducci L, Orgogozo JM, Brun A, Hofman A: Vascular dementia: Diagnostic criteria for research studies. Report of the NINDS-AIREN International Workshop. *Neurology* 1993; 43: 250–60.

Román GC, Erkinjuntti T, Wallin A, Pantoni L, Chui HC: Subcortical ischaemic vascular dementia. *Lancet Neurology* 2002; 1: 426–36.

Rönnemaa E, Zethelius B, Sundelöf J, Sundström J, Degerman-Gunnarsson M, Berne C, Lannfelt L, Kilander L: Impaired insulin secretion increases the risk of Alzheimer disease. *Neurology* 2008; 71: 1065–71.

Ronninghamstam E: Narcisstic personality disorder: A review. In Maj M, Akiskal H, Mezzich J, Okasha A (eds.), *Personality Disorders*. West Sussex, England: John Wiley, 2005, pp. 277–327.

Roose SP, Sackheim HA, Krishnan KR, Pollock BG, Alexopoulos G, Lavretsky H, Hakkarainen H: Antidepressant pharmacotherapy in the treatment of depression in the very old: A randomized, placebo-controlled trial. *American Journal of Psychiatry* 2004; 161: 2050–59.

Rosack J: FDA orders new warning on atypical antipsychotics. *Psychiatric News* 2005; 40: 1–50.

Rosen WG, Mohs RC, Davis KL: A new rating scale for Alzheimer's disease. *American Journal of Psychiatry* 1984; 141: 1356–64.

Rosenberg PB, Lyketsos CB: Depression in Alzheimer disease. In Charney DS, Evans D (eds.), *The Physician's Guide to Depression and Bipolar Disorder*. New York: McGraw-Hill, 2006.

Rosenblum WI: Structure and location of amyloid beta peptide chains and arrays in Alzheimer's disease: New findings require reevaluation of the amyloid hypothesis and of tests of the hypothesis. *Neurobiology of Aging* 2002; 23: 225–30.

Roth AJ, Massie MJ: Anxiety and its management in advanced cancer. *Current Opinions in Supportive and Palliative Care* 2007; 1: 50–56.

Roth M, Tomlinson BE, Blessed G: The relationship between quantitative measures of dementia and of degenerative changes in the cerebral grey matter of elderly subjects. *Proceedings of the Royal Society of Medicine* 1967; 60: 14–18.

Rowe JW, Kahn RL: Successful aging. *The Gerontologist* 1997; 37: 433–40.

Rowe J, Kahn R: *Successful Aging*. New York: Random House, 1998.

Rubenstein LZ, Abrass IB, Kane RL: Improved care for patients on a new geriatric evaluation unit. *Journal of the American Geriatrics Society* 1981; 29: 531–36.

Rudberg MA, Furner SE, Dunn JE, Cassel CK: The relationship of visual and hearing impairments to disability: An analysis using the Longitudinal Study of Aging. *Journal of Gerontology* 1993; 48: M261–65.

Rudisch B, McDonald WM: Treatment of refractory depression in the elderly: The role of maintenance electroconvulsive therapy. *Current Psychosis and Therapeutics Reports* 2006; 4: 79–83.

Rush AJ, Fava M, Wisniewski SR, Lavori PW, Trivedi MH, Sackeim HA, Niederehe G: Sequenced treatment alternatives to relieve depression (STAR*D): Rationale and design. *Contemporary Clinical Trials* 2004; 25: 119–42.

Rush AJ, Trivedi MH, Wisniewski SR, Nierenberg

AA, Stewart JW, Warden D, Fava M: Acute and longer-term outcomes in depressed outpatients requiring one or several treatment steps: A STAR*D report. *American Journal of Psychiatry* 2006; 163: 1905–17.

Rutter M: Psychosocial resilience and protective mechanisms. *American Journal of Orthopsychiatry* 1987; 57: 316–31.

Rypma B, Prabhakaran V, Desmond JE, Gabrieli JDE: Age differences in prefrontal cortical activity in working memory. *Psychology and Aging* 2001; 16: 371–84.

Sable JA, Jeste DV: Antipsychotic treatment for late-life schizophrenia. *Current Psychiatry Reports* 2002; 4: 299–306.

Sachs GA: *Position Statement: Informed Consent for Research on Human Subjects with Dementia: AGC Ethics Committee*. New York: American Geriatric Society, 2007.

Sachs GA, Shega JW, Cox-Hayley: Barriers to excellent end-of-life care for patients with dementia. *Journal of General Internal Medicine* 2004; 19: 1057–63.

Sackeim HA, Brannan SK, Rush AJ, George MS, Marangell LB, Allen J: Durability of antidepressant response to vagus nerve stimulation (VNSTM). *International Journal of Neuropsychopharmacology* 2007; 10: 817–26.

Safar JG, Geschwind MD, Deering C, Didorenko S, Sattavat M, Sanchez H, Prusiner SB: Diagnosis of human prion disease. *Proceedings of the National Academy of Sciences* 2005; 102: 3501–6.

Sajatovic M: Treatment of bipolar disorder in older adults. *International Journal of Geriatric Psychiatry* 2002; 17: 865–73.

Sajatovic M, Blow F (eds.): *Bipolar Disorder in Late Life*. Baltimore: Johns Hopkins University Press, 2007.

Sajatovic M, Blow FC, Ignacio R, Kales HC: New-onset bipolar disorder in later life. *American Journal of Geriatric Psychiatry* 2005a; 13: 282–89.

Sajatovic M, Madhusoodanan S, Coconcea N: Managing bipolar disorder in the elderly: Defining the role of the newer agents. *Drugs and Aging* 2005b; 22: 39–54.

Sajatovic M, Ramsay E, Nanry K, Thompson T: Lamotrigine therapy in elderly patients with epilepsy, bipolar disorder or dementia. *International Journal of Geriatric Psychiatry* 2007; 22: 945–50.

Sakauye KM, Streim JE, Kennedy GJ, Kirwin PD, Llorente MD, Schultz SK, Srinivasan S: Disaster preparedness for older Americans: Critical issues for the preservation of mental health. AAGP position statement. *American Journal of Geriatric Psychiatry* 2009; 17: 916–24.

Salari S: Patterns of intimate partner homicide suicide in later life: Strategies for prevention. *Journal of Clinical Interventions in Aging* 2007; 2: 441–52.

Salerno JA, Nagy C: Guest editorial: Terrorism and aging. *Journal of Gerontology Series A: Biological Sciences and Medical Sciences* 2002; 57: M552–54.

Salthouse TA: What and when of cognitive aging. *Current Directions in Psychological Science* 2004; 14: 140–44.

Salthouse TA: Relations between cognitive abilities and measures of executive functioning. *Neuropsychology* 2005; 19: 532–45.

Saltzman C (ed.): *Clinical Geriatric Psychopharmacology,* 4th edition. Philadelphia: Wolters Kluwer, 2004.

Salzman C: Late-life anxiety disorders. *Psychopharmacology Bulletin* 2004; 38: 25–30.

Sampson EL, Ritchie CW, Lai R, Raven PW, Blanchard MR: A systematic review of the scientific evidence for the efficacy of a palliative care approach in advanced dementia. *International Psychogeriatrics* 2005; 17: 31–40.

Samuelsson SM, Alfredson BB, Hagberg B, Samuelsson G, Nordbeck B, Brun A, Gustafson L, Risberg J: The Swedish centenarian study: A multidisciplinary study of five consecutive cohorts at the age of 100. *International Journal of Aging and Human Development* 1997; 45: 223–53.

Sanchez FM, Zisselman MH: Treatment of psychiatric symptoms associated with neurosyphilis. *Psychosomatics* 2007; 48: 440–45.

Sánchez R, Alcoverro O, Pagerols J, Rojo JE: Electrophysiological mechanisms of action of electroconvulsive therapy. *Actas espanolas de psiquiatria* 2009; 37: 343–51.

Sanders S, Bowie SL, Bowie YD: Lessons learned on forced relocation of older adults: The impact of Hurricane Andrew on health, mental health, and social support of public housing residents. *Journal of Gerontological Social Work* 2003; 40: 23–35.

Sandlin D: The new joint commission accreditation of health care organizations' requirements for pain assessment and treatment: A pain in the assessment. *Journal of PeriAnesthesia Nursing* 2000; 15: 182–84.

Sansone RA, Levitt JL: *Personality Disorders and Eating Disorders: Exploring the Frontier.* New York: Routledge, 2006.

Santos M, Kovari E, Hof PR, Gold G, Bouras C, Giannakopoulos P: The impact of vascular burden on late-life depression. *Brain Research Reviews* 2009; 62: 19–32.

Sato T, Bottlender R, Schroter A, Moller H-J: Psychopathology of early-onset versus late-onset schizophrenia revisited: An observation of 473 neuroleptic-naive patients before and after first-admission treatments. *Schizophrenia Research* 2004; 67: 175–83.

Sato T, Kienlen-Campard P, Ahmed M, Liu W, Li H, Elliott JI, Aimoto S, Constantinescu SN, Octave SN, Smith SO: Inhibitors of amyloid toxicitybased on β-sheet packing in Aβ40 and Aβ42. *Biochemistry* 2006; 45: 5503–16.

Satter SP, Petty F, Burke WJ: Diagnosis and treatment of alcohol dependence in older alcoholics. *Clinics in Geriatric Medicine* 2003; 19: 743–61.

Satre DD, Mertens JR, Weisner C: Gender differences in treatment outcomes for alcohol dependence among older adults. *Journal of Studies on Alcohol and Drugs* 2004; 65: 638–42.

Saveman BI, Hallberg IR, Norberg A, Eriksson S: Patterns of abuse of the elderly in their own homes as reported by district nurses. *Scandinavian Journal of Primary Health Care* 1993; 11: 111–16.

Savoy J: *Psychotropic Drugs and the Elderly: Fast Facts.* New York: Norton, 2004.

Saxena S, Lawley D: Delirium in the elderly: A clinical review. *Postgraduate Medical Journal* 2009; 85: 405–13.

Saxton J, McGonigle-Gibson KL, Swihart AA, Miller VJ, Boller F: Assessment of the severely impaired patient: Description and validation of a new neuropsychological test battery. *Psychological Assessment* 1990; 2: 298–303.

Sayer NA, Rettmann NA, Carlson KF, Bernardy N, Sigford BJ, Hamblen JL, Friedman MJ: Veterans with history of mild traumatic brain injury and posttraumatic stress disorder: Challenge from provider perspective. *Journal of Rehabilitation Research and Development* 2009; 46: 703–16.

Scalise Jr. RJ: Undue influence and the law of wills: A comparative analysis. *Duke Journal of Comparative and International Law* 2008; 19: 41–10.

Schaie K W: A lifespan developmental perspective of psychological aging. In *The Handbook of Emotional Disorders in Late Life: Assessment and Treatment.* Oxford: Oxford University Press, 2008.

Schneck CH, Mahowald MW: REM sleep behavior disorder: Clinical, developmental, and neuroscience perspectives 16 years after its formal identification in SLEEP. *Sleep* 2002; 25: 120–38.

Schiamberg LB, Gans, D: Elder abuse by adult children: An applied ecological framework for understanding contextual risk factors and the intergenerational character of quality of life. *International Journal of Aging and Human Development* 2000; 50: 329–59.

Schmidt WC, Miller KS, Bell WG, New BE: Public guardianship and the elderly. *Hosp Community Psychiatry* 1982; 33: 491–92.

Schneider AJ, Mataix-Cols D, Marks IM, Bachofen M: Internet-guided self-help with or without exposure therapy for phobic and panic disorders. *Psychotherapy and Psychosomatics* 2005; 74: 154–64.

Schneider LS, DeKosky ST, Farlow MR, Tariot PN, Hoerr R, Kieser M: A randomized, double-blind, placebo-controlled trial of two doses of ginkgo biloba extract in dementia of the Alzheimer's type. *Current Alzheimer Research* 2005; 2: 541–51.

Schneidman E: The Psychological autopsy. *American Psychologist* 1994; 49: 75–76.

Schnurr PP, Lunney CA, Sengupta A, Waelde LC: A descriptive analysis of PTSD chronicity in Vietnam veterans. *Journal of Traumatic Stress* 2003; 16: 545–53.

Schogt B: The suspicious resident. In Conn D, Herrmann N, Kaye A, Rewilak D, Schogt B (eds.), *Practical Psychiatry in the Long Term Care Home.* Cambridge, MA: Hogrefe & Huber, 2007.

Schonfeld L, Dupree LW: Alcohol use and misuse in older adults. *Reviews in Clinical Gerontology* 1999; 9: 151–62.

Schonfeld L, King-Kallimanis BL, Duchene DM, Etheridge RL, Herrera JR, Barry KL, Lynn N: Screening and brief intervention for substance misuse among older adults: The Florida BRITE Project. *American Journal of Public Health* 2010; 100: 108–14.

Schonwetter RS, Han B, Small BJ, Martin B, Tope K, Haley WE: Predictors of six-month survival among patients with dementia: An evaluation of hospice Medicare guidelines. *American Journal of Hospice and Palliative Medicine* 2003; 20: 105–13.

Schuckit MA: Genetics of the risk for alcoholism. *American Journal on Addictions* 2000; 9: 103–12.

Schulberg HC, Bruce ML, Lee PW, Williams JW, Dietrich AJ: Preventing suicide in primary care patients: The primary care physician's role. *General Hospital Psychiatry* 2004; 26: 337–45.

Schultz MAF: Helping patients and families make choices about nutrition and hydration at the end-of-life. *Topics in Advances Practice Nursing eJournal* 2009; 9.

Schultz SK: Depression in the older adult: The challenge of medical comorbidity. *American Journal of Psychiatry* 2007; 164: 847–48.

Schultz SK, Ellingrod VL: Late-life schizophrenia: optimizing treatment. *Current Psychosis and Therapeutics Reports* 2005; 3: 5–8.

Schulz R, Martire LM: Family caregiving of persons with dementia: Prevalence, health effects, and support strategies. *American Journal of Geriatric Psychiatry* 2004; 12: 240–49.

Schulz R, O'Brien A, Czaja S, Ory M, Norris R, Martire LM, Belle SH, Burgio L, Gitlin L, Coon D, Burns R, Gallagher-Thompson D, Stevens, A: Dementia caregiver intervention research: In search

of clinical significance. *The Gerontologist* 2002; 42: 589–602.

Schulz R, Burgio L, Burns R, Eisdorfer C, Gallagher-Thompson D, Gitlin LN, Mahoney DF: Resources for enhancing Alzheimer's caregiver health (REACH): Overview, site-specific outcomes, and future directions. *The Gerontologist* 2003; 43: 514–20.

Schulz R, Martire LM, Klinger JN: Evidence-based caregiver interventions in geriatric psychiatry. *Psychiatric Clinics of North America* 2005; 28: 1007–38.

Schum JL, Lyness J, King DA: Bereavement in late life: Risk factors for complicated bereavement. *Geriatrics* 2005; 60: 18–20, 24.

Scogin F, Welsh D, Hanson A, Stump J, Coates A: Evidence-based psychotherapies for depression in older adults. *Clinical Psychology: Science and Practice* 2005; 12: 222–37.

Seeman MV: Gender differences in the prescribing of antipsychotic drugs. *Focus* 2006; 4: 115–24.

Segal D, Coolige F, Rosowsky E: *Personality Disorders and Older Adults: Diagnosis, Assessment, and Treatment.* Somerset, NJ: John Wiley, 2006.

Seignourel PJ, Kunik ME, Snow L, Wilson N, Stanley M: Anxiety in dementia: A critical review. *Clinical Psychology Review* 2008; 28: 1071–82.

Seitz HK, Stickel F: Alcoholic liver disease in the elderly. *Clinics in Geriatric Medicine* 2007; 23: 905–21.

Selkoe DJ, Schenk D: Alzheimer's disease: Molecular understanding predicts amyloid-based therapeutics. *Annual Review of Pharmacology and Toxicology* 2003; 43: 545–84.

Selwood A, Johnston K, Katona C, Lyketsos C, Livingston G: Systematic review of the effect of psychological interventions on family caregivers of people with dementia. *Journal of Affective Disorders* 2007; 101: 75–89.

Seo HJ, Sohi MS, Patkar AA, Masand PS, Pae CU: Desvenlafaxine succinate: A newer antidepressant for the treatment of depression and somatic symptoms. *Postgraduate Medical Journal* 2010; 122: 125–38.

Seymour J, Benning TB: Depression, cardiac mortality and all-cause mortality. *Advances in Psychiatric Treatment* 2009; 15: 107–13.

Shah A: Are age-related trends in suicide rates associated with life expectancy and socioeconomic factors? *International Journal of Psychiatry in Clinical Practice* 2009; 13: 16–20.

Shanmugham B, Karp J, Drayer R, Reynolds CF, Alexopoulos G: Evidence-based pharmacologic interventions for geriatric depression. *Psychiatric Clinics of North America* 2005; 28: 821–35.

Shaw JA, Egeland JA, Endicott J, Allen CR, Hotstetter AM: A ten-year prospective study of prodromal patterns for bipolar disorder among Amish youth. *Journal of the American Academy of Child and Adolescent Psychiatry* 2005; 44: 1104–11.

Shear K, Frank E, Houck PR, Reynolds III CF: Treatment of complicated grief: A randomized controlled trial. *JAMA* 2005; 293: 2601–8.

Shear MK, Frank E, Foa E, Cherry C, Reynolds III CF, Bilt JV, Masters S: Traumatic grief treatment: A pilot study. *American Journal of Psychiatry* 2001; 158: 1506–8.

Shega J, Emanuel L, Vargish L, Levine SK, Bursch H, Herr K, Karp JF, Weiner DK: Pain in persons with dementia: Complex, common, and challenging. *Journal of Pain* 2007; 8: 373–78.

Shega JW, Levin A, Hougham GW, Cox-Hayley D, Luchins D, Hanrahan P, Stocking C, Sachs GA: Palliative Excellence in Alzheimer's Care Efforts (PEACE): A program description. *Journal of Palliative Medicine* 2004; 6: 315–20.

Sheikh JI, Cassidy EL: Treatment of anxiety disorders in the elderly: Issues and strategies. *Journal of Anxiety Disorders* 2000; 14: 173–90.

Sheikh JI, Swales PJ, Carlson EB, Lindley SE: Aging and panic disorder: Phenomenology, comorbidity, and risk factors. *American Journal of Geriatric Psychiatry* 2004; 12: 102–9.

Shelton A: *Reform Options for Social Security.* Washington, DC: AARP Public Policy Institute, 2008.

Sheng B, Cheng LF, Law CB, Li HL, Yeung KW, and Li KK: Coexisting cerebral infarction in Alzheimer's disease is associated with fast dementia progression: Applying the National Institute for Neurological Disorders and Stroke/Association Internationale pour la Recherche et l'Enseignement en Neurosciences Neuroimaging Criteria in Alzheimer's Disease with Concomitant Cerebral Infarction. *Journal of the American Geriatrics Society* 2007; 55: 918–22.

Sher L: Relation between rates of geriatric suicide and consumption of alcohol beverages in European countries. *Scientific World Journal* 2006; 6: 383–87.

Shinoda-Tagawa T, Leonard R, Pontikas J, McDonough JE, Allen D, Dreyer PI: Resident-to-resident violent incidents in nursing homes. *JAMA* 2004; 291: 591–98.

Shneidman E: The psychological autopsy. *American Psychologist* 1994; 75–76.

Shrestha LB: Life expectancy in the United States. CRS Report for Congress, 2006.

Shuchman M: Approving the vagus-nerve stimulator for depression. *New England Journal of Medicine* 2007; 356: 1604–7.

Shugarman LR, Fries BE, Wolf RS, Morris JN: Identifying older people at risk of abuse during routine screening practices. *Journal of the American Geriatrics Society* 2003; 51: 24–31.

Shulman KI, Cohen CA, Kirsh FC, Hull IM, Champine PR: Assessment of testamentary capacity and vulnerability to undue influence. *American Journal of Psychiatry* 2007; 164: 722–27.

Shulman KI, Peisah C, Jacoby R, Heinik J, Finkel S: Contemporaneous assessment of testamentary capacity. *International Psychogeriatrics* 2009; 21: 433–39.

Shumaker SA, Legault C, Rapp S, Thal LT, Wallace RB, Ockene JK, Hendrix SL, Jones III BN, Assaf AR, Jackson RD, Kotchen JM, Wassertheil-Smoller S, Wactawski-Wende J: Estrogen plus progestin and the incidence of dementia and mild cognitive impairment in postmenopausal women. *JAMA* 2003; 289: 2651–62.

Shumaker SA, Legault C, Kuller L, Rapp SR, Thal L, Lane DS, Fillit H, Stefanick ML, Hendrix SL, Lewis CE, Masaki K, Coker LH: Conjugated equine estrogens and incidence of probably dementia and mild cognitive impairment in postmenopausal women. *JAMA* 2004; 291: 2947–58.

Siddiqi N, House AO, Holmes JD: Occurrence and outcome of delirium in medical in-patients: A systematic literature review. *Age and Ageing* 2006; 35: 350–64.

Sierra F, Hadley E, Suzman R, Hodes R: Prospects for life span extension. *Annual Review of Medicine* 2009; 60: 457–69.

Sigurdsson EM, Knudsen E, Asuni A, Fitzer-Attas G, Sage D, Quartermain D, Frangione B, Wisniewski T: An attenuated immune response is sufficient to enhance cognition in Alzheimer's disease mouse model of immunization with amyloid β-derivatives. *Journal of Neuroscience* 2004; 24: 6277–82.

Silverberg GD, Mayo M, Saul T, Rubenstein E, McGuire D: Alzheimer's disease, normal-pressure hydrocephalus, and senescent changes in CSF circulatory physiology: A hypothesis. *The Lancet* 2003; 2: 506–11.

Silverberg G, Mayo M, Saul T, Carvalho J, McGuire D: Novel ventriculo-peritoneal shunt in Alzheimer's disease cerebrospinal fluid biomarkers. *Expert Review of Neurotherapeutics* 2004; 4: 97–107.

Silverberg GD, Mayo M, Saul T, Fellmann SJ, Carvalho J, McGuire D: Continuous CSF drainage in AD. *Neurology* 2008; 71: 202–9.

Simon GE: Social and economic burden of mood disorders. *Biological Psychiatry* 2003; 54: 208–15.

Simoni-Wastila L, Yang HK: Psychoactive drug abuse in older adults. *American Journal of Geriatric Pharmacotherapy* 2006; 4: 380–94.

Singhal A, Kumar A, Belgamwar RB, Hodgson RE: Assessment of mental capacity: Who can do it? *The Psychiatrist* 2008; 32: 17–20.

Sink KM, Holden KF, Yaffe K: Pharmacological treatment of neuropsychiatric symptoms of dementia. *JAMA* 2005; 293: 596–608.

Siskowski C: Young caregivers: Effect of family health situations on school performance. *Journal of School Nursing* 2006; 22: 163–69.

Skultety KM, Rodriguez RL: Treating geriatric depression in primary care. *Current Psychiatry Reports* 2008; 10: 44–50.

Sleath B, Rubin RH, Campbell W, Gwyther L, Clark T: Physician-patient communication about over-the-counter medications. *Social Science and Medicine* 2001; 53: 357–69.

Sledjeski EM, Speisman B, Dierker L: Does number of lifetime traumas explain the relationship between PTSD and chronic medical conditions? Answers from the National Comorbidity Survey-Replication (NCS-R). *Journal of Behavioral Medicine* 2007; 31: 341–49.

Sleegers K, Lambert J, Bertram L, Cruts M, Amouyel P, Broeckhoven CV: The pursuit of susceptibility genes for Alzheimer's disease: Progress and prospects. Trends in Genetics 2010; 26: 84–93.

Small GW: Pharmacotherapy and other treatments for elderly patients with depression. *Journal of Clinical Psychiatry* 2010; 71: e03.

Smith M, Gerdner LA, Hall GR, Buckwalter KC: History, development, and future of the progressively lowered stress threshold: A conceptual model for dementia care. *Journal of the American Geriatrics Society* 2004; 52: 1755–60.

Smith GS, Gunning-Dixon FM, Lotrich FE, Taylor WD, Evans JD: Translational research in late-life mood disorders: Implications for future intervention and prevention research. *Neuropsychopharmacology* 2007; 32: 1857–75.

Snowden DA: Healthy aging and dementia: Findings from the nun study. *Annals of Internal Medicine* 2003; 139: 450–54.

Snowden D, Kemper S, Mortimer J, Greiner LH, Wekstein DR, Markesbery WR: Linguistic ability in early life and cognitive function and Alzheimer's disease in late life: Findings from the Nun Study. *JAMA* 1996; 27: 528–32.

Snowden J, Arie T: A history of psychogeriatric services. In B Draper (ed.), *Psychogeriatric Service Delivery: An International Perspective.* Oxford: Oxford University Press, 2005, pp. 3–20.

Snowden M, Sato K, Roy-Byrne P: Assessment and treatment of nursing home residents with depression or behavioral symptoms associated with dementia: A review of the literature. *Journal of the American Geriatrics Society* 2003; 51: 1305–17.

Snowdon J, Shah A, Halliday G: Severe domestic squalor: A review. *International Psychogeriatrics* 2007; 19: 37–51.

Snowden M, Steinman L, Frederick J: Treating

depression in older adults: Challenges to implementing the recommendations of an expert panel. *Preventing Chronic Disease* 2008; 5: 1–9.

Soares J, Young A (Eds): *Bipolar Disorder: Brain Mechanisms and Therapeutic Implications.* New York: Informa Healthcare, 2007.

Sokal J, Messias E, Dickerson FB: Comorbidity of medical illnesses among adults with serious mental illness who are receiving community psychiatric services. *Journal of Nervous and Mental Disease* 2004; 192: 421–27.

Solomon PR, Hirschoff A, Kelly B, Relin M, Brush M, DeVeaux RD, Pendlebury WW: A 7-minute neurocognitive screening battery highly sensitive to Alzheimer's disease. *Archives of Neurology* 1998; 55: 349–55.

Somers JM, Goldner EM, Waraich P, Hsu L: Prevalence and incidence studies of anxiety disorders: A systematic review of the literature. *Canadian Journal of Psychiatry* 2006; 51: 100–113.

Sorensen S, Pinquart M, Duberstein P: How effective are interventions with caregivers? An updated meta-analysis. *The Gerontologist* 2002; 42: 356–72.

Spector A, Thorgrimsen L, Woods B, Royan L, Davies S, Butterworth M, Orrell M: Efficacy of an evidence-based cognitive stimulation therapy programme for people with dementia: Randomised controlled trial. *British Journal of Psychiatry* 2003; 183: 248–54.

Spirduso WW, Francis KL, MacRae PG: *Physical Dimensions of Aging.* Champagne, IL: Human Kinetics, 2005.

Spitzer RL, Williams JB, Gibbon M, First MB: The Structured Clinical Interview for DSM-III-R (SCID): I. history, rationale, and description. *Archives of General Psychiatry* 1992; 49: 624–29.

Spungen D: *Homicide: The Hidden Victims: A Guide for Professionals.* Thousand Oaks, CA: Sage Publications, 1998.

Stanley MA, Wilson NL, Novy DM, Rhoades HM, Wagener PD, Greisinger AJ, Cully JA, Kunik ME: Cognitive behavior therapy for generalized anxiety disorder among older adults in primary care: A randomized clinical trial. *JAMA* 2009; 301: 1460–67.

Stanworth R: *Recognizing Spiritual Needs in People Who Are Dying.* New York: Oxford University Press, 2003.

Stathakos D, Pratsinis H, Zachos I, Vlahaki I, Gianakopoulou A, Zianni D, Kletsas D: Greek centenarians: Assessment of functional health status and life-style characteristics. *Experimental Gerontology* 2005; 40: 512–18.

Steffen AM, Gant JR, Gallagher-Thompson D: Reducing psychosocial distress in family caregiver. In Gallagher-Thompson D, Steffen AM, Thompson LW (eds.), *The Handbook of Behavioral and Cognitive Therapies with Older Adults.* New York: Springer, 2008, pp. 102–17.

Steffens DC, Potter GG, McQuoid DR, MacFall JR, Payne ME, Burke JR, Welsh-Bohmer KA: Longitudinal magnetic resonance imaging vascular changes, apolipoprotein E genotype, and development of dementia in the neurocognitive outcomes of depression in the elderly study. *American Journal of Geriatric Psychiatry* 2007; 15: 839–49.

Stein BD, Tanielian TL, Eisenman DP, Keyser DJ, Burnam MA, Pincus HA: Emotional and behavioral consequences of bioterrorism: Planning a public health response. *Milbank Quarterly* 2004; 82: 413–55.

Stein D, Lilenfeld LRR, Wildman PC, Marcus MD: Attempted suicide and self-injury in patients diagnosed with eating disorders. *Comprehensive Psychiatry* 2004; 45: 447–51.

Stein KF, Corte C: Identity impairment and the eating disorders: Content and organization of the self-concept in women with anorexia nervosa and bulimia nervosa. *European Eating Disorders Review* 2007; 15: 58–69.

Steinhausen H-C: The outcome of anorexia nervosa in the 20th century. *American Journal of Psychiatry* 2002; 159: 1284–93.

Stek ML, Wurff van der FFB, Hoogendijk WJG, Beekman ATF: Electroconvulsive therapy for the depressed elderly. *Cochrane Database of Systematic Reviews* 2003; 2.

Stelfox HT, Gandhi TK, Orav EJ, Gustafson ML: The relationship between patient satisfaction and physician communication. *StuderGroup* 2005; 118: 1126–33.

Stern P, Carstenson L (eds.): *Aging Mind: Opportunities for Cognitive Research.* Washington, DC: National Academies Press, 2000.

Stevenson DG, Bramson JS: Hospice care in the nursing home setting: A review of the literature. *Journal of Pain and Symptom Management* 2009; 38: 440–51.

Stevenson JS: Alcohol use, misuse, abuse, and dependence in later adulthood. *Annual Review of Nursing Research* 2005; 23: 245–80.

Stiegel L, Klem E: Information about laws related to elder abuse. American Bar Association Commission on Law and Aging, 2007.

Stocking CB, Hougham GW, Danner DD, Patterson MB, Whitehouse PJ, Sachs GA: Planning for future research participation. *Neurology* 2006; 66: 1361–66.

Stoff DM, Khalsa JH, Monjan A, Portegies P: HIV/AIDS and aging. *AIDS* 2004; 18: 1–2.

Stone M: Borderline and histrionic personality disorders: A review. In M Maj, H Akiskal, J Mezzich, A

Okasha (eds.), *Personality Disorders.* West Sussex, England: John Wiley, 2005, pp. 201-32.

Streeton C, Whelan G: Naltrexone, a relapse prevention maintenance treatment of alcohol dependence: A meta-analysis of randomized control trials. *Alcohol and Alcoholism* 2001; 36: 544–52.

Strober M, Freeman R, Lampert C, Diamond J, Kaye W: Controlled family study of anorexia nervosa and bulimia nervosa: Evidence of shared liability and transmission of partial syndromes. *American Journal of Psychiatry* 2000; 157: 393–401.

Strug DL, Mason SE, Heller FE: An exploratory study of the impact of the year of 9/11 on older Hispanic immigrants in New York City. *Journal of Gerontological Social Work* 2003; 42: 77–99.

Stueve A, O'Donnell LN: Early alcohol initiation and subsequent sexual and alcohol risk behaviors among urban youths. *American Journal of Public Health* 2005; 95: 887–93.

Styron W: *Darkness Visible: A Memoir of Sadness.* New York: Random House, 1990.

Suchowersky O, Gronseth G, Perlmutter J, Reich S, Zesiewicz T, Weiner WJ: Practice Parameter: Neuroprotective strategies and alternative therapies for Parkinson disease (an evidence-based review). *Neurology* 2006; 66: 976–82.

Sudak HS: Predicting suicide rates in the elderly. *American Journal of Psychiatry* 2010; 167: 102.

Sugarman J, Paasche-Orlow M: Confirming comprehension of informed consent as a protection of human subjects. *Journal of General Internal Medicine* 2006; 21: 898–99.

Sunderland T, Linker G, Mirza N, Putnam KT, Friedman DL, Kimmel LH, Bergeson J, Manetti GJ, Zimmerman M, Tang B, Bartko JJ, Cohen RM: Decreased β-amyloid1-42 and increased tau levels in cerebrospinal fluid of patients with Alzheimer disease. *JAMA* 2003; 289: 2094–2103.

Sunderland T, Mirza N, Putname KT, Linker G, Bhupali D, Durham R, Soares H, Kimmel L, Friedman D, Berfeson J, Csako G, Levy JA, Bartko JJ, Cohen RM: Cerbrospinal fluid β-amyloid1-42 and tau in control subjects at risk for Alzheimer's disease: The effect of APOE ε4 allele. *Biological Psychiatry* 2004; 56: 670–76.

Sunderland T, Hampel H, Takeda M, Putnam KT, Cohen RM: Biomarkers in the diagnosis of Alzheimer's disease: Are we ready? *Journal of Geriatric Psychiatry* 2006; 19: 172–79.

Suzuki R, Ye W, Rylander-Rudqvist T, Saji S, Colditz GA, Wolk A: Alcohol and postmenopausal breast cancer risk defined by estrogen and progesterone receptor status: A prospective cohort study. *Journal of the National Cancer Institute* 2005; 97: 1601–8.

Swanberg MM, Cummings JL: Benefit-risk considerations in the treatment of dementia with Lewy bodies. *Drug Safety* 2002; 25: 511–23.

Swegle JM, Logemann C: Management of common opioid-induced adverse effects. *American Family Physician* 2006; 74: 1347–54.

Syme A, Bruce A: Hospice and palliative care: What unites us, what divides us? *Journal of Hospice and Palliative Nursing* 2009; 11: 19–24.

Szapocznik J, Prado G, Burlew AK, Williams RA, Santisteban DA: Drug abuse in African American and Hispanic adolescents: Culture, development, and behavior. *Annual Review of Clinical Psychology* 2007; 3: 77–105.

Szekely CA, Thorne JE, Zandi PP, Ek M, Messias E, Breitner JCS, Goodman SN: Nonsteroidal anti-inflammatory drugs for the prevention of Alzheimer's disease: A systematic review. *Neuroepidemiology* 2004; 23: 159–69.

Tadros G, Salib E: Elderly suicide in primary care. *International Journal of Geriatric Psychiatry* 2007; 22: 750–56.

Talbot K: Motor neuron disease. *Medicine* 2004; 32: 105–7.

Tally RC, Crews JE: Caring for the most vulnerable: Framing the public health of caregiving. *American Journal of Public Health* 2007; 97: 224–28.

Tariot PN, Farlow MR, Grossberg GT, Graham SM, McDonald S, Gergel I: Memantine treatment in patients with moderate to severe Alzheimer disease already receiving donepezil. *JAMA* 2004; 291: 317–24.

Tatara T, Kuzmeskus LB, Duckhorn E, Bivens L, Thomas C, Gertig J, Jay K, Hartley A, Rust K, Croos J: The national elder abuse incidence study. The National Center on Elder Abuse at the American Public Human Services Association in Collaboration with Westat. Newark, DE: University of Delaware, 1998.

Taylor MH, Doody GA: CADASIL: A guide to a comparatively unrecognised condition in psychiatry. Advances in Psychiatric Treatment 2008; 14: 350–57.

Taylor MJ, Freemantle N, Geddes JR, Bhagwager Z: Early onset of selective serotonin reuptake inhibitor antidepressant action: Systematic review and meta-analysis. *Archives of General Psychiatry* 2006; 63: 1217–23.

Taylor WD, Zuchner S, McQuoid DR, Steffens DC, Speer MC, Krishnan KRK: Allelic differences in the brain-derived neurotrophic factor Val66Met polymorphism in late-life depression. *American Journal of Geriatric Psychiatry* 2007; 15: 850–57.

Teaster PB, Roberto KA: Sexual abuse of older adults: APS cases and outcomes. *The Gerontologist* 2004; 44: 788–96.

Teaster PB, Roberto KA, Duke JO, Kim M: Sexual abuse of older adults: Preliminary findings of cases in Virginia. *Journal of Elder Abuse and Neglect* 2000; 12: 1–16.

Teaster PB, Wood EF, Karp N, Lawrence SA, Schmidt WC, Mendiondo MS: Wards of the state: A national study of public guardianship. American Bar Association on Law and Aging, 2005.

Teaster PB, Dugar TA, Mendiondo MS, Abner EL, Cecil KA, Otto JM: *The 2004 Survey of State Adult Protective Services: Abuse of Adults 60 Years of Age and Older.* Washington, DC: National Center on Elder Abuse, 2006.

Teaster PB, Wood EF, Schmidt Jr WC, Lawrence SA: *Public Guardianship after 25 Years: In the Best Interest of Incapacitated People?* American Bar Association, 2007.

Teng E, Ringman JM, Ross LK, Mulnard RA, Dick MB, Bartzokis G, Cummings JL: Diagnosing depression in Alzheimer disease with the National Institute of Mental Health provisional criteria. *American Journal of Geriatric Psychiatry* 2008; 16: 469–77.

Teresi J, Abrams R, Holmes D, Ramirez M, Eimicke J: Prevalence of depression and depression recognition in nursing homes. *Social Psychiatry and Psychiatric Epidemiology* 2001; 36: 613–20.

Teri L, Logsdon RG, McCurry SM: Nonpharmacologic treatment of behavior disturbance in dementia. *Medical Clinics of North America* 2002; 86: 641–56.

Teri L, Logsdon RG, McCurry SM: The Seattle protocols: Advances in behavioral treatment of Alzheimer's disease. In Vellas B, Grundman M, Feldman H, Fitten LJ, Winblad B, Giacobini E (eds.), *Research and Practice in Alzheimer's Disease and Cognitive Decline.* New York: Springer, 2005a, pp. 153–58.

Teri L, McKenzie G, LaFazia. Psychosocial treatment of depression in older adults with dementia. *Clinical Psychology: Science and Practice* 2005b; 12: 303–16.

Teri L, McCurry SM, Logsdon RG, Gibbons LE: Training community consultants to help family members improve dementia care: A randomized controlled trial. *The Gerontologist* 2005c; 45: 802–11.

Teri L, Logsdon RG, McCurry SM: Exercise interventions for dementia and cognitive impairment: The Seattle protocols. *Journal of Nutritional Health and Aging* 2008; 12: 391–94.

Thistlethwaite J: Breaking bad news: Skills and evidence. *InnovAiT* 2009; 2: 605–12.

Thomas VS, Rockwood KJ: Alcohol abuse, cognitive impairment, and mortality among older people. *Journal of the American Geriatrics Society* 2001; 49: 415–20.

Thompson CA, Spilsbury K, Hall J, Birks Y, Barnes C, Adamson J: Systematic review of information and support interventions for caregivers of people with dementia. *BMC Geriatrics* 2007; 7.

Thompson IM, Tangen CM, Goodman PJ, Probstfield JL, Moinpour CM, Coltman CA: Erectile dysfunction and subsequent cardiovascular disease. *JAMA* 2005; 294: 2996–3002.

Thompson L, Coon D, Gallagher-Thompson D, Sommer B, Koin D: Comparison of desipramine and cognitive behavioral therapy in the treatment of elderly outpatients with mild-to-moderate depression. *American Journal of Geriatric Psychiatry* 2001; 9: 225–40.

Thompson S, Herrmann N, Rapoport MJ, Lanctot KL: Efficacy and safety of antidepressants for treatment of depression in Alzheimer's disease: A meta analysis. *Canadian Journal of Psychiatry* 2007; 52: 248–55.

Tibbitts C: The 1961 White House Conference on Aging: Its rationale, objectives, and procedures. *Journal of the American Geriatric Society* 1960; 8: 373–77.

Tielkes CEM, Comijs HC, Verwijk E, Stek ML: The effects of ECT on cognitive functioning in the elderly: A review. *International Journal of Geriatric Psychiatry* 2008; 23: 789–95.

Tiemeier H, van Tuijl HR, Hofman A, Kiliaan AJ, Breteler MMB: Plasma fatty acid composition and depression are associated in the elderly: The Rotterdam Study American. *Journal of Clinical Nutrition* 2003; 78: 40–46.

Timmermans M, Carr J: Neurosyphilis in the modern era. *Journal of Neurology, Neurosurgery, and Psychiatry* 2004; 75: 1727–30.

Toborek M, Lee YW, Flora G, Pu H, Adras IE, Wylegala E, Nath A: Mechanisms of the blood-brain barrier disruption in HIV-1 infection. *Cellular and Molecular Neurobiology* 2005; 25: 181–89.

Tolnay M, Clavaguera F: Argyrophilic grain disease: A late-onset dementia with distinctive features among tauopathies. *Neuropathology* 2004; 24: 269–83.

Toovey S: Influenza-associated central nervous system dysfunction: A literature review. *Travel Medicine and Infectious Disease* 2008; 6: 114–24.

Toseland RW, McCallion P, Gerber T, Banks S: Predictors of health and human services use by persons with dementia and their family caregivers. *Social Science and Medicine* 2002; 55: 1255–66.

Towey J: Five Wishes: Aging with Dignity. A service program developed through a grant from the Robert Wood Johnson Foundation, 1997. Retrieved June 9, 2010, from www.agingwithdignity.org.

Townsend KP, Pratico D: Novel therapeutic opportunities for Alzheimer's disease: Focus on nonsteroidal antiflammatory drugs. *FASEB Journal* 2005; 19: 1592–601.

Travaline JM, Ruchinskas R, D'Alonzo Jr GE: Patient-physician communication: Why and how. *JAMA* 2005; 105: 13–18.

Trzepacz PT, Mittal D, Torres R, Kanary K, Norton J, Jimerson N: Validation of the Delirium Rating Scale-Revised-98: Comparison with the Delirium Rating Scale and the Cognitive Test for Delirium. *Journal of Neuropsychiatry and Clinical Neurosciences* 2001; 13: 229–42.

Tueth MJ: Exposing financial exploitation of impaired elderly persons. *American Journal of Geriatric Psychiatry* 2000; 8: 104–11.

Tulner LR, Frankfort SV, Gijsen GJPT, van Campen JPCM, Koks CHW, Beignen JH: Drug-drug interactions in a geriatric outpatient cohort: Prevalence and relevance. *Drugs and Aging* 2008; 25: 343–55.

Tulving E: Episodic memory: From mind to brain. *Annual Review of Psychology* 2002; 53: 1–25.

Tune LE, Salzman C: Schizophrenia in late life. *Psychiatric Clinics of North America* 2003; 26: 103–13.

Tunzi M: Can the patient decide? Evaluating patient capacity in practice. *American Family Physician* 2001; 15: 299–306.

Turner JA: *Social Security Financing: Automatic Adjustments to Restore Solvency.* Washington, DC: AARP Public Policy Institute, 2009.

Turvey C, Conwell Y, Jones M, Phillips C, Simonsick E, Pearson J, Wallace R: Risk factors for late-life suicide: A prospective, community-based study. *American Journal of Geriatric Psychiatry* 2002; 10: 398–406.

Tuszynski M: Nerve growth factor gene therapy in Alzheimer disease. *Alzheimer Disease and Associated Disorders* 2007; 21: 179–89.

Twamley EW, Padin DS, Bayne KS: Work rehabilitation for middle aged and older people with schizophrenia: A comparison of three approaches. *Journal of Nervous and Mental Disease* 2005; 193: 596–601.

Tyrer P: The anxious cluster of personality disorders: A review. In Maj M, Akiskal H, Mezzich J, Okasha A (eds.), *Personality Disorders.* West Sussex, England: John Wiley, 2005, pp. 349–75.

Uchida H, Suzuki T, Mamo DC, Mulsant BH, Tanabe A, Inagaki A, Masayuki T: Effects of age and age of onset on prescribed antipsychotic dose in schizophrenia spectrum disorders: A survey of 1,418 patients in Japan. *American Journal of Geriatric Psychiatry* 2008; 16: 584–93.

Uchida H, Suzuki T, Mamo DC, Mulsant BH, Kikuchi T, Takeuchi H, Tomita M, Watanabe K, Yagi G, Kashima H: Benzodiazepine and antidepressant use in elderly patients with anxiety disorders: A survey of 796 outpatients in Japan. *Journal of Anxiety Disorders* 2009; 23: 477–81.

Ullman MT: Contributions of memory circuits to language: The declarative/procedural model. *Cognition* 2004; 92: 231–70.

University of Maine Center on Aging: Elder abuse screening protocol for physicians: Lessons learned from the Maine Partners for Elder Protection pilot project. 2007.

Unutzer J, Katon W, Callahan CM, Williams JW, Hunkeler E, Harpole L, Langston C: Collaborative care management of late-life depression in the primary care setting: A randomized controlled trial. *JAMA* 2002; 288: 2836–45.

Unutzer J, Katon W, Callahan CM, Williams Jr JW, Hunkeler E, Harpole L, Oishi S: Depression treatment in a sample of 1,801 depressed older adults in primary care. *Journal of the American Geriatrics Society* 2003; 51: 505–14.

Unutzer J, Schoenbaum M, Druss BG, Katon WJ: Transforming mental health care at the interface with general medicine: Report for the Presidents Commission. *Psychiatric Services* 2006; 57: 37–47.

Unutzer J, Schoenbaum M, Katon WJ, Fan MY, Pincus HA, Hogan D, Taylor J: Healthcare costs associated with depression in medically ill fee-for-service Medicare patients. *Journal of the American Geriatrics Society* 2009; 57: 506–10.

U.S. Department of Health and Human Services, National Institute of Dental and Craniofacial Research: *Oral Health in America: A Report of the Surgeon General.* Rockville, MD: National Institute of Dental and Craniofacial Research, 2000.

U.S. Department of Health and Human Services, Public Health Service, National Institutes of Health, and National Institute on Alcohol Abuse and Alcoholism: *The Physicians' Guide to Helping Patients with Alcohol Problems.* Bethesda, MD: National Institute on Alcohol Abuse and Alcoholism, 1995.

U.S. Department of Health and Human Services, Substance Abuse and Mental Health Services Adminstration, Center for Substance Abuse Treatment: *Substance Abuse among Older Adults.* Treatment Improvement Protocol Series (TIP) 26. DHHS publication no. SMA 98-3179. Rockville, MD: SAMHSA, 1998.

U.S. Department of Health and Human Services, Substance Abuse and Mental Health Services Administration, Center for Mental Health Services: *Mental Health: A Report of the Surgeon General: Executive Summary.* Rockville, MD: SAMHSA, 1999a.

U.S. Department of Health and Human Services, Substance Abuse and Mental Health Services Administration, Center for Substance Abuse Treatment: *Brief Interventions and Brief Therapies for Substance Abuse.* Treatment Improvement Protocol

Series (TIP) 34. DHHS publication no. SMA 99-3353. Rockville, MD: SAMHSA, 1999b.

U.S. Department of Health and Human Services, Substance Abuse and Mental Health Services Administration, Center for Mental Health Services: *Mental Health Response to Mass Violence and Terrorism: A Training Manual.* DHHS Pub. no. SMA 3959. Rockville, MD: SAMHSA, 2004a.

U.S. Department of Health and Human Services, Substance Abuse and Mental Health Services Administration, Center for Substance Abuse Treatment. *Substance Abuse Treatment and Family Therapy.* Treatment Improvement Protocol Series (TIP), no. 39. DHHS Publication no. (SMA) 04-3957. Rockville, MD: SAMHSA, 2004b.

U.S. Department of Health and Human Services, Substance Abuse and Mental Health Services Administration. *Results from the 2003 National Survey on Drug Use and Health: National Findings.* NSDUH Series H-25, DHHS Publication no. SMA 04-3964. Rockville, MD: Office of Applied Studies, 2004c.

U.S. Department of Health and Human Services, Substance Abuse and Mental Health Services Administration, National Institutes of Health: *Report of the Surgeon General on Mental Health,* 1999.

U.S. Department of Health and Human Services, Substance Abuse and Mental Health Services Administration, Office of Applied Studies: *Substance Use by Older Adults: Estimates of Future Impact on the Treatment System.* OAS Analytic Series A-21, DHHS Publication no. SMA 03-3763. Rockville, MD: Substance Abuse and Mental Health Services Administration, 2002.

U.S. Public Health Service: *The Surgeon General's Call to Action to Prevent Suicide.* Washington, DC: Office of the Surgeon General, 1999.

U.S. Public Health Service: *National Strategy for Suicide Prevention: Goals and Objectives for Action.* Rockville, MD: Substance Abuse and Mental Health Services Administration, 2001.

Vaillant G: Aging well. *American Journal of Geriatric Psychiatry* 2007; 15: 181–83.

Vanacore N, Bonifati V, Colosimo C, Fabbrini G, De Michele G, Marconi R, Meco G: Epidemiology of progressive supranuclear palsy. *Neurological Science* 2001; 22: 101–3.

Van Alphen SPJ, Engelen GJJA, Kuin Y, Derksen JJL: The relevance of a geriatric sub-classification of personality disorders in the DSM-V. *International Journal of Geriatric Psychiatry* 2006; 21: 205–9.

Van Citters AD, Bartels SJ: A systematic review of the effectiveness of community-based mental health outreach services for older adults. *Psychiatric Services* 2004; 55: 1237–49.

Vanderplasschen W, Rapp RC, Wolf JR, Broekaert

E: The development and implementation of case management for substance use disorders in North America and Europe. *Psychiatric Services* 2004; 55: 913–22.

VandeWeerd C, Paveza GJ, Fulmer T: Abuse and neglect in older adults with Alzheimer's disease. *Nursing Clinics of North America* 2006; 41: 43–55.

Van Everbroeck B, Dobbeleir I, De Waele M, De Deyn P, Martin J-J, and Cras P: Differential diagnosis of 201 possible Creutzfeldt-Jakob disease patients. *Journal of Neurology* 2004; 251: 298–304.

Van Hilten JJ, Ramaker CC, Stowe R, Ives NJ: Bromocriptine/levodopa combined versus levodopa alone for early Parkinson's disease. *Cochrane Database Systematic Reviews* 2007; 4.

Van Ommeren M, Saxena S, Saraceno B: Mental and social health during and after acute emergencies: Emerging consensus? *Bulletin of the World Health Organization* 2005; 83.

Van Rossum EFC, Binder EB, Majer M, Koper JW, Ising M, Modell S, Holsboer F: Polymorphisms of the glucocorticoid receptor gene and major depression. *Biological Psychiatry* 2006; 59: 681–88.

Van Straaten ECW, Scheltens P, Knol DL, van Buchem MA, van Dijk EJ, Hofman PAM, Barkhof F: Operational definitions for the NINDS-AIREN criteria for vascular dementia: An interobserver study. *Stroke* 2003; DOI: 10.1161/01.STR.0000083050.44441.10.

Vass A, Minardi H, Ward R, Aggarwal N, Garfield C, Cybyk B: Research into communication patterns and consequences for effective care of people with Alzheimer's and their carers. *Dementia* 2003; 2: 21–48.

Venmans A, Nijssen PC, Sluzewski M, van Rooij WJ: Progressive supranuclear palsy. *Journal Belge de Radiologie* 2009; 92: 182–83.

Vergne DE, Nemeroff CB: The interaction of serotonin transporter gene polymorphisms and early adverse life events on vulnerability for major depression. *Current Psychiatry Reports* 2006; 8: 452–57.

Vincent S, Lane R: Rivastigmine in vascular dementia. *International Psychogeriatrics* 2003; 15: 201–5.

Vitali P, Migliaccio R, Agosta F, Rosen HJ, Geschwind MD: Neuroimaging in dementia. *Seminars in Neurology* 2008; 28: 467–83.

Volicer L: *End-of-life Care for People with Dementia in Residential Care Settings.* Chicago: Alzheimer's Association, 2005.

Volicer L, Hurley AC, Blasi ZV: Characteristics of dementia end-of-life care across care settings. *American Journal of Hospice and Palliative Medicine* 2003; 20: 191–200.

Vorm A, Rikkert M: Informed consent in dementia research. *Competence Assessment in Dementia* 2008; 85–91.

Vossen J, Monsieur D, van Os J, Leue C: Serotonin-noradrenalin reuptake inhibitors in the treatment of non-malignant pain syndromes; a systematic review. *Tijdschrift voor Psychiatrie* 2009; 51: 831–40.

Voyer P, McCubbin M, Cohen D, Lauzon S, Collin J, Boivin C: Unconventional indicators of drug dependence among elderly long-term users of benzodiazepines. *Issues in Mental Health Nursing* 2004; 25: 603–28.

Voyer P, McCusker J, Cole MG, St-Jacques S, Khomenko L: Factors associated with delirium severity among older patients. *Journal of Clinical Nursing* 2007; 16: 819–31.

Wade N: Why do we die? Why we live: A new theory of aging. *New York Times,* 2003 www.nytimes.com/2003/07/15/science/15AGIN.html.

Wade LD, Frazier LD: Cultural differences in possible selves during later life. *Journal of Aging Studies* 2003; 17: 251–68.

Wadia PM, Lang AE: The many faces of corticobasal degeneration. *Parkinsonism and Related Disorders* 2007; 13: S336–40.

Wagner B, Maercker A: A 1.5-year follow-up of an Internet-based intervention for complicated grief. *Journal of Traumatic Stress* 2007; 20: 625–29.

Wagner G, Montorsi F, Auerbach S, Collins M: Sildenafil citrate (VIAGRA) improves erectile function in elderly patients with erectile dysfunction: A subgroup analysis. *Journal of Gerontology Series a Biological Sciences and Medical Sciences* 2001; 56: M113–19.

Walaszek A: Clinical ethics in geriatric psychiatry. *Psychiatric Clinics of North America* 2009; 343–59.

Walker MP, Ayre GA, Cummings JL: The clinician assessment of fluctuation and the One Day Fluctuation Assessment Scale: Two methods to assess fluctuating confusion in dementia. *British Journal of Psychiatry* 2000; 177: 252–56.

Wang R, Yan H, Tang X: Progress in studies of huperzine A, a natural cholinesterase inhibitor from Chinese herbal medicine. *Acta Pharmacologica Sinica* 2006; 27: 1–26.

Wang X, Ding H: Alzheimer's disease: Epidemiology, genetics, and beyond. *Neurosci Bulletin* 2008; 24: 105–9.

Washington KT, Bickel-Swenson D, Stephens N: Barriers to hospice use among African Americans: A systematic review. *Health Social Work* 2008; 33: 267–74.

Washington TD: Psychological stress and anxiety in middle to late childhood and early adolescence: Manifestations and management. *Journal of Pediatric Nursing* 2009; 24: 302–13.

Wasteson E, Brenne E, Higginson IJ, Hotopf M, Lloyd-Williams M, Kaasa S, Loge JH: Depression assessment and classification in palliative cancer patients: A systematic literature review. *Palliative Medicine* 2009; 23: 739-53.

Wechsler D: *The Measurement of Adult Intelligence.* Baltimore: Waverly Press, 1944.

Wei LA, Fearing MA, Sternberg EJ, Inouye SK: The Confusion Assessment Method: A systematic review of current usage. *Journal of the American Geriatrics Society* 2008; 56: 823-30.

Weiner HL, Frenkel D: Immunology and immuno-therapy of Alzheimer's disease. *Nature Reviews Immunology* 2006; 6: 404-16.

Weiner MF, Lipton AM (eds.): *The American Psychiatric Publishing Textbook of Alzheimer Disease and Other Dementias.* Arlington, VA: American Psychiatric Publishing, 2009.

Weintraub D, Stern MB: Disorders of mood and affect in Parkinson's disease. *Handbook of Clinical Neurology* 2007; 83: 421-33.

Weiss SJ, Haber J, Horowitz JA, Stuart GW, Wolfe B: The inextricable nature of mental and physical health: Implications for integrative care. *Journal of the American Psychiatric Nurses Association* 2009; 15: 371-82.

Weissman M: A brief history of interpersonal psychotherapy. *Psychiatric Annals* 2006; 36: 553-57.

Weller RO, Nicoll JAR: Cerebral amyloid angiopathy: Pathogenesis and effects on the ageing and Alzheimer brain. *Neurological Research* 2003; 25: 611-16.

Wells J: Health care reform, congress considers first nursing home reforms in two decades. *Public Policy and Aging Report* 2009; 2: 1-5.

Wells JL, Seabrook JA, Stolee P, Borrie MJ, Knoefel F: State of the art in geriatric rehabilitation, part I: Review of frailty and comprehensive geriatric assessment. *Archives of Physical Medicine and Rehabilitation* 2003; 84: 890-97.

Wennberg JE, Fisher ES, Stukel TA, Skinner JS, Sharp SM, Bronner KK: Use of hospitals, physician visits, and hospice care during last six months of life among cohorts loyal to highly respected hospitals in the United States. *British Medical Journal* 2004; 328: 607.

Wetherell JL, Lenze EJ, Stanley MA: Evidence-based treatment of geriatric anxiety disorders. *Psychiatric Clinics of North America* 2005; 28: 871-86.

Wezenberg E, Verkes RJ, Ruigt GS, Hulstijn W, Sabbe BG: Acute effects of the ampakine farampator on memory and information processing in healthy elderly volunteers. *Neuropsychopharmacology* 2007; 32: 1272-83.

Whalley LJ, Dick FD, McNeill G: A life-course approach to the aetiology of late-onset dementias. *The Lancet* 2006; 5: 87-96.

White House Conference on Aging: A Report to the Delegates from the Conference Sections and Special Concerns Sessions. 1971 (Eric ED05851).

White JV, Brewer DE, Stockton MD, Keeble DS, Keenum AJ, Rogers ES, Lennon ES: Nutrition in chronic disease management in the elderly. *Nutrition in Clinical Practice* 2003: 3-11.

Whitehouse P, George D: *The Myth of Alzheimer's.* New York: MacMillan Press, 2008.

Whitton LS: Durable powers as an alternative to guardianship: Lessons we have learned. *Stetson Law Review* 2007-2008; 37: 8-36.

Wieland D, Hirth V: Comprehensive geriatric assessment. *Cancer Control* 2003; 10: 454-62.

Wieland D, Hedrick SH, Rubenstein LZ, Buchner D, Reuben D, Harker J: Inpatient geriatric evaluation and management units: Organization and care patterns in the Department of Veteran Affairs. *Gerontologist* 1994; 34: 652-57.

Wienrich M, Meir D, Ensinger HA, Gaida W, Raschig A, Walland A, Hammer R: Pharacodynamic profile of the M1 agonist talsaclidine in animals and man. *Life Sciences* 2001; 68: 2593-2600.

Wigeratne C, Brodaty H, Hickie I: The neglect of somatoform disorders by old age psychiatry: Some explanations and suggestions for future research. *International Journal of Geriatric Psychiatry* 2003; 18: 812-19.

Wilber K, Reiser T, Harter K: New perspectives on conservatorship: The views of older adults' conservatees and their conservators. *Aging, Neuropsychology, and Cognition* 2001; 8: 225-40.

Wilcox D, Willcox B, Hsuch W, Suzuki M: Genetic determinants of exceptional human longevity: Insights from the Okinawa centenarian study. *AGE* 2006; 28: 313-32.

Wilkinson P: Psychological treatments in the management of severe late-life depression: At least as important as ECT. *International Psychogeriatrics* 2007; 19: 14-18.

Williams BJ, Eriksdotter-Jonhagen M, Granholm A: Nerve growth factor in treatment and pathogenesis of Alzheimer's disease. *Progress in Neurobiology* 2006; 80: 114-28.

Williams JW, Barrett J, Oxman T, Frank E, Katon W, Sullivan M, Cornell J, Sengupta A: Treatment of dysthymia and minor depression in primary care. *JAMA* 2000; 284: 1519-26.

Williams M: *Geriatric Physical Diagnosis: A Guide to Observation and Assessment.* Jefferson (NC): McFarland & Company, 2008.

Williams S, Dale J: The effectiveness of treatment for depression/depressive symptoms in adults with cancer: A systematic review. *British Journal of Cancer* 2006; 94: 372–90.

Williams S, Weinman J, Dale J: Doctor-patient communication and patient satisfaction: A review. *Family Practice* 1998; 15: 480–92.

Williams S, Haskard K, DiMatteo M: The therapeutic effect of the physician-patient relationship: Effective communication with vulnerable older patients. *Clinical Intervention and Aging* 2007; 2: 453–67.

Willis SL, Tennstedt SL, Marsiske M, Ball K, Elias J, Koepke KM, Morris JN, Rebok GW, Unverzagt FW, Stoddard AM, Wright E: Long-term effects of cognitive training on everyday functional outcomes in older adults. *JAMA* 2006; 296: 2805–14.

Wilson R: Advancing age, impending death, and declining cognition. *Neurology* 2008; 71: 874–75.

Wilson RS, Mendez de Leon CF, Barnes LL, Schneider JA, Bienias JL, Evans DA, Bennett DA: Participation in cognitively stimulating activities and risk of incident Alzheimer disease. *JAMA* 2002; 287: 742–48.

Wimo A, Winblad B, Stoffler A, Wirth Y, Mobius H: Resource utilization and the cost analysis of memantine in patients with moderate to severe Alzheimer's disease. *Pharmacoeconomics* 2003; 21: 1–14.

Wislowski A, Cuellar N: Voting rights for older Americans with dementia: Implications for health care providers. *Nursing Outlook* 2006; 54: 68–73.

Wisniewski SR, Belle SH, Coon DW, Marcus SM, Ory MG, Burgio LD, Burns R, Schulz R: The Resources for Enhancing Alzheimer's Caregiver Health (REACH): Project design and baseline characteristics. *Psychology and Aging* 2003; 18: 375–84.

Wissow LS: Communication and malpractice claims: Where are we now? *Patient Education and Counseling* 2004; 52: 3–5.

Wolf R: Elder abuse and neglect: An update. *Reviews in Clinical Gerontology* 1997; 7: 177–82.

Wolinski FD, Mahncke HW, Kosinski M, Unverzagt FW, Smith DM, Jones RN, Stoddard A, Tennstedt SL: The ACTIVE cognitive training trial and predicted medical expenditures. *BMC Health Services Research* 2009; 9: 109.

Wolkove N, Elkholy O, Baltzan M, Palayew M: Sleep and aging: Sleep disorders commonly found in older people. *Canadian Medical Association Journal* 2007; 176: 1299–304.

Wong MS, Chan SW: The experience of Chinese family members of terminally ill patients: A qualitative study. *Journal of Clinical Nursing* 2007; 16: 2357–64.

Worden JW: *Grief Counseling and Grief Therapy: A Handbook for the Mental Health Practitioner,* 4th edition. New York: Springer Publishing Co., 2008.

World Health Organization: *Cancer Pain Relief and Palliative Care: Report of a WHO Expert Committee.* Geneva, World Health Organization, 1990.

World Health Organization: The World Health Report, 2001: *Mental Health: New Understanding, New Hope.* Geneva: World Health Organization, 2001.

World Health Organization: Abuse of the elderly. In Krug E, Dahlberg LL, Mercy JA, Zwi AB, Lozano R (eds.), *World Report on Violence and Health.* Geneva: WHO Press, 2002.

World Health Organization: *International Statistical Classification of Diseases and Related Health Problems.* Geneva: WHO Press, 2007.

Wragg R, Jeste D: Overview of depression and psychosis in Alzheimer's disease. *American Journal of Psychiatry* 1989; 146: 577–87.

Wright RM, Warpula RW: Safer prescribing for the elderly patient. *Journal of the American Podiatric Medical Association* 2004; 94: 90–97.

Wutzler U: Differential diagnosis of somatoform disorders in elderly patients. *MMW Fortschritte der Medizin* 2007; 149: 90–92.

Wyllie MG: The underlying pathophysiology and causes of erectile dysfunction. *Clinical Cornerstone* 2005; 7: 19–26.

Xiong GL, Daubert GP: Wernicke-Korsakoff syndrome. Retrieved from eMedicine from WebMD 2009 http://emedicine.medscape.com/article/288379-overview.

Yager J, Devlin MJ, Halmi KA, Herzog DB, Mitchell JE, Powers P, Zerbe KJ: *Practice Guidelines for the Treatment of Patients with Eating Disorders,* 3rd edition. Washington, DC: American Psychiatric Association, 2006.

Yamashita TE, Phair JP, Muñoz A, Margolick JB, Detels R, O'Brien SJ, Jacobson LP: Immunologic and virologic response to highly active antiretroviral therapy in the Multicenter AIDS Cohort Study. *AIDS* 2001; 15: 735–46.

Yan E, Tang CSK, Yueng D: No safe haven: A review on elder abuse in Chinese families. *Trauma, Violence and Abuse* 2002; 3: 167–80.

Yank V, Rennie D: Reporting of informed consent and ethics committee approval in clinical trials. *JAMA* 2002; 287: 2835–38.

Yao G, Gallagher-Thompson D (eds.): *Ethnicity and the Dementias.* Washington, DC, Taylor & Francis, 2006, pp. 187–203.

Yates WR (2009 October 26). Anxiety disorders. Retrieved February 22, 2010, from EMedicine WebMD website: http://emedicine.medscape.com/article/286227-overview.

Yates, WR (2010, March 2). Somatoform disorders: Treatment and medication. Retrieved from eMedicine. http://emedicine.medscape.com/article/294908-treatment.

Yatham LN, Kennedy SH, O'Donovan C, Parikh S, MacQueen G, McIntyre R, Gorman CP: Canadian Network for Mood and Anxiety Treatments (CANMAT) guidelines for the management of patients with bipolar disorder: Consensus and controversies. *Bipolar Disorders* 2005; 7: 5–69.

Yee JL, Schulz R: Gender differences in psychiatric morbidity among family caregivers: A review and analysis. *The Gerontologist* 2000; 40: 147–64.

Yesavage JA, Brink TL, Rose TL, Lum O, Huang V, Adey M, Leirer VO: Development and validation of a geriatric depression screening scale: A preliminary report. *Journal of Psychiatric Research* 1983; 17: 37–49.

Yeung WJ, Chan Y: The positive effects of religiousness on mental health in physically vulnerable populations: A review on recent empirical studies and related theories. *International Journal of Psychosocial Rehabilitation* 2007; 11: 37–52.

Yohannes AM: Depression and anxiety in elderly patients with chronic obstructive pulmonary disease. *Age and Ageing* 2006; 35: 457–59.

Young EA, Garfinkel SN, Liberzon I: Stress and anxiety disorders. In AP Arnold, AM Etgen, SE Fahrbach, RT Rubin, and DW Pfaff (eds.), *Hormones, Brain, and Behavior,* 2nd edition. Boston: Elsevier, 2009; pp. 2875–97.

Young J, Inouye SK: Delirium in older people. *British Medical Journal* 2007; 334: 842–46.

Young RC: Evidence-based pharmacological treatment of geriatric bipolar disorder. *Psychiatric Clinics of North America* 2005; 28: 837–69.

Young RC, Gyulai L, Mulsant BH, Flint AMB, Beyer JL, Shulman KI, Reynolds CF: Pharmacotherapy of bipolar disorder in old age: Review and recommendations. *American Journal of Geriatric Psychiatry* 2004; 12: 342–57.

Ystad MA, Lundervold AJ, Wehling E, Espeseth T, Rootwelt H, Westlye LT, Andersson M, Adolfsdottir S, Geitung JT, Fjell AM, Reinvang I, Lundervold A: Hippocampal volumes are important predictors for memory function in elderly women. BMC Medical Imaging 2009; 9: 1–15.

Yum SY, Caracci G, Hwang MY: Schizophrenia and eating disorders. *Psychiatry Clinics of North America* 2009; 32: 809–19.

Zarate Jr CA, Manji HK: The role of AMPA receptor modulation in the treatment of neuropsychiatric diseases. *Experimental Neurology* 2008; 211: 7–10.

Zerr I, Kallenberg K, Summers D, Romero C, Taratuto A, Helnemann U, Breithaupt M, Varges D, Meissner B, Ladogana A, Schurr M, Haik S, Collins S, Jansen G, Stokin G, Pimental J, Hewer E, Collie D, Smith P, Roberts H, Brandel J, van Duijin C, Pocchairi M, Begue C, Cras P, Will R, Sanchez-Juan P: Updated clinical diagnostic criteria for sporadic Creutzfeldt-Jakob disease. *Brain* 2009; 132: 2659–68.

Zhang BH, El-Jawahri A, Prigerson HG: Update on bereavement research: Evidence-based guidelines for the diagnosis and treatment of complicated bereavement. *Journal of Palliative Medicine* 2006; 9: 1188–1203.

Zhang M, Katzman R, Salmon D, Jin H, Cai G, Wang Z, Liu WT: The prevalence of dementia and Alzheimer's disease in Shanghai, China: Impact of age, gender, and education. *Annals of Neurology* 2004; 27: 428–37.

Zhang X, Grabowski DC: Nursing home staffing and quality under the Nursing Home Reform Act. *Gerontologist* 2004; 44: 13–23.

Zisserson RN, Oslin DW: Alcoholism and at-risk drinking in the older population. *Geriatric Times* 2003; 4.

Zubenko GS, Zubenko WN, McPherson S, Spoor E, Marin DB, Farlow MR, Sunderland T: A collaborative study of the emergence and clinical features of the major depressive syndrome of Alzheimer's disease. *American Journal of Psychiatry* 2003; 160: 857–66.

Zwakhalen SMG, Hamers JPH, Abu-Saad HH, Berger MPF: Pain in elderly people with severe dementia: A systematic review of behavioural pain assessment tools. *BMC Geriatrics* 2006; 6 (www.biomedcentral.com/1471-2318/6/3).

Zweig RA, Agronin ME: Personality disorders. In ME Agronin, GJ Maletta (eds.), *Principles and Practice of Geriatric Psychiatry.* Philadelphia: Lippincott Williams & Wilkins, 2006, pp. 449–70.

INDEX

About the Authors

Donna Cohen received her B.S. from Duke University and her Ph.D. from the University of Southern California. She has been a faculty member in the Department of Psychiatry and Behavioral Sciences at the University of Washington (1976–1981), professor and head of the Division of Geriatric Psychiatry at Albert Einstein College of Medicine/Montefiore Medical Center (1981–1986), and professor, College of Public Health, and deputy director, University Center on Aging, University of Illinois at Chicago (1986–1992).

In 1992 Dr. Cohen joined the faculty of the University of South Florida in Tampa, Florida. She is professor and head of the Violence and Injury Prevention Center in the Department of Aging and Mental Health Disparities, Louis de la Parte Florida Mental Health Institute, College of Behavioral and Community Sciences. She was previously chair of the department (1992–1998) and founding director of the university's Institute on Aging (1993–1996).

Dr. Cohen specializes in the areas of aging, mental health, Alzheimer disease, family caregiving, long-term care, and violence. She has published six books (two with Carl Eisdorfer) and more than 190 articles. Dr. Cohen's contributions have established guidelines and standards of health care practices in geriatric mental health, and she is a well-known advocate for policy reform at the national and state levels. From 1988 to 1992 Dr. Cohen headed a national effort to develop a plan for a 1991 White House Conference on Aging, which was finally held in 1995.

Dr. Cohen has testified in Congress on health care, long-term care, Alzheimer disease, depression and suicide and homicide-suicide, abuse and family violence, age discrimination, and veterans' affairs. She has served on many national scientific and technical advisory groups, including several NIA study sections, the American Association of Suicidology, and the National Committee for the prevention of Elder Abuse.

Carl Eisdorfer received his Ph.D. in ╷ from New York University, his M.D. ╷ graduate training in psychiatry at D╷ sity, and a Certificate in Health Syst ╷ ment from Harvard University. He v ╷ of Behavioral Sciences at the Duke ╷ ity Medical Center (1967–1972) and ╷ its Center on Aging and Human De╵ (1970–1972).

He then became chairman of the ╷ of Psychiatry and Behavioral Science ╷ versity of Washington in Seattle (19 ╷ where he founded and directed the ╵ Institute on Aging. He left Seattle t╷ fessor of neuroscience and of psychi╷ Albert Einstein Medical School and ╷ president and CEO of Montefiore M ╷ (1981–1986).

In 1986, Dr. Eisdorfer came to th╷ of Miami as professor and chair of t ╷ ment of Psychiatry and Behavioral ╵ professor of psychology and of famil ╷ munity medicine. He founded and d ╷ university's Center on Aging as well ╷ ioral Health Program.

Dr. Eisdorfer has written or edite╷ 330 scientific and professional publi ╷ behavioral sciences, mental health, c ╷ derly people, and health policy. His ╷ *Caring for the Elderly* and *Loss of Sel╵* wrote with Donna Cohen). He has s ╷ president of the Gerontological Soci╷ ica, the American Society on Aging, ╷ American Federation for Aging Rese ╷ been honored by many organization╵ the American Psychiatric Associatio╷ can Psychological Association, and t ╷ tional Psychogeriatrics Association. ╷ only recipient of both the Kent Awa╷ service and the Kleemeir Award for ╷ the Gerontological Society of Ameri╷ he received a Lifetime Achievement ╷ the American Association for Geriat